"Challenging one-dimensional readings of Freud's *Beyond the Pleasure Principle*, this book builds on the finding that the text was composed in two stages (1919–1920), each articulating distinct theoretical constructions around its central concepts—the life drives and the death drives—as they relate to trauma. With clarity and originality, the book traces the elaboration of these theories and their complex interplay across biophysics, biology, and evolutionary thought. The result is a nuanced and illuminating study that deepens our understanding of the conceptual architecture of psychoanalytic theory."

– **Ulrike Kistner**, *Emiritus Professor of Philosophy, University of Pretoria, South Africa*

"*Reading Freud's* Beyond the Pleasure Principle is a sweeping endeavour. Taking up the original argument developed in his coauthored *Seduction, Drive and Repetition* (2025) concerning the persistence of trauma—including seduction—in Freud's conception of transference neuroses, Westerink turns here to the two strikingly different versions of Freud's *Beyond the Pleasure Principle* (1919 and 1920). Covering works from Freud's 1895-1896 "Project" through his late group psychology, he follows the evolution of the drives in Freud and traces the genealogy of the pleasure and reality principles down to Freud's ultimate theory of life versus death drives. Following the model of trauma inaugurated by the clinic of hysteria, Freud's analytic work gradually turns to a "pathoanalysis of human existence." Striving to adapt German Darwinism (Haeckel's recapitulation theory), what begins as a study of the evolutionary stages of sexuality moves toward a much broader, philogenetically inherited scheme, whose ambition is to make psychoanalysis an authentic, genetic, anthropology. Throughout his arguments, Westerink shows how Freud integrated materialist mechanism (Helmholtz), Darwinism and its variants, biology, and physics into a conception of the history and fundamental interrelatedness of organic substances—in short, of life itself. In the process, the meaning of consciousness is reconceived and the cellular theory of his time reframed in such a way that the famous hiatus between the physical and the psychic emerges as a metabiology and a reconceived dualism. This book is thus vastly more than a study of *Beyond the Pleasure Principle.* It is a crucial odyssey through the history of decisive sciences in the late nineteenth century and beyond. Avoiding the traps of organicism and vitalism, it is a map of a new philosophy of life. Westerink proceeds from long years of psychoanalytic study, and collaboration. His work with Philippe Van Haute on sexuality and trauma make Westerink a foremost authority both in critical Freudian studies and henceforth in the history of science."

– **Bettina Bergo**, *Professor of Philosophy, University of Montreal, Canada*

"This book creates a fresh and polysemic space for re-encountering Freud's *Beyond the Pleasure Principle.* Herman Westerink subtly and compellingly recalibrates the Freudian text to contemporary debates, while rigorously unpacking the plural field of Freud's influences and affinities. Avoiding any attempt to harmonise this event-text, Herman Westerink inhabits its contradictions with striking precision but also with excitement for Freud's speculative thinking. Ultimately, this book takes psychoanalysis seriously in its clinical anthropology dimension and it shows, through Freud's text, the unique potential that psychoanalysis has in rethinking biology. Herman Westerink offers brilliant insights into Freud's curiosity about the traumatic character of the origin of life. Freud emerges as a thinker of catastrophes, while *Beyond the Pleasure Principle* emerges as the site of not one, but several drive theories. This volume will produce an important mark in both psychoanalytic and philosophical debates."

– **Raluca Soreanu**, *Psychoanalyst & Professor of Psychoanalytic Studies, University of Essex, UK*

Reading Freud's *Beyond the Pleasure Principle*

Reading Freud's Beyond the Pleasure Principle presents a new reading of this foundational text, based on the hypothesis that the work was written in two phases. Herman Westerink explores the idea that Freud put the first version of 1919 aside because he found the conclusions he drew from his line of reasoning difficult, if not impossible, to accept. The book considers which clinical and theoretical problems Freud wanted to address in the first version of the text, what arguments he developed, and in what way these explorations and arguments resulted in implications he considered problematic. Returning to the text in 1920, Westerink asserts that Freud introduced theories of the life and death drives as a response and possible solution to the problems and implications of his 1919 inquiries.`

This book will be a significant reference for academics and scholars of Freud, psychoanalytic studies, trauma, critical theory, philosophy and the history of science. It will be of great interest to psychoanalysts in practice and in training.

Herman Westerink is Associate and Endowed Professor at the Center for Contemporary European Philosophy, Radboud University Nijmegen, the Netherlands. He has published many books and articles on Freudian psychoanalysis, sexuality and religion.

History of Psychoanalysis

Series Editor
Peter L. Rudnytsky

This series seeks to present outstanding new books that illuminate any aspect of the history of psychoanalysis from its earliest days to the present, and to reintroduce classic texts to contemporary readers.

Other titles in the series:

The Vicissitudes of Psychoanalysis in Soviet Russia, 1930–1980
Lizaveta van Munsteren

Freud's British Family
Reclaiming Lost Lives in Manchester and London
Roger Willoughby

Sigmund Freud's Inner Divisions
Personal and Theoretical
Ken Fuchsman

Sigmund Freud on the Way to Paris, 1873–1885
Foundations of Psychoanalysis
Giosuè Ghisalberti

Reading Freud's Beyond the Pleasure Principle
Trauma and Life
Herman Westerink

Between Genius and Tragedy
A Psychoanalytic Portrait of Viktor Tausk
Francisco Balbuena Rivera

For further information about this series please visit https://www.routledge.com/The-History-of-Psychoanalysis-Series/book-series/KARNHIPSY

Reading Freud's *Beyond the Pleasure Principle*

Trauma and life

Herman Westerink

Routledge
Taylor & Francis Group
LONDON AND NEW YORK

Designed cover image: Getty Images

First published 2026
by Routledge
4 Park Square, Milton Park, Abingdon, Oxon OX14 4RN

and by Routledge
605 Third Avenue, New York, NY 10158

Routledge is an imprint of the Taylor & Francis Group, an informa business

British Library Cataloguing-in-Publication Data
A catalogue record for this book is available from the British Library

Library of Congress Cataloging-in-Publication Data
A catalog record has been requested for this book

ISBN: 978-1-041-15623-9 (hbk)
ISBN: 978-1-041-15622-2 (pbk)
ISBN: 978-1-003-68041-3 (ebk)

DOI: 10.4324/9781003680413

Typeset in Times New Roman
by Taylor & Francis Books

In memory of Philippe

Contents

Acknowledgements

The idea to jointly write a monograph on Freud's *Jenseits des Lustprinzips* arose during the time Philippe Van Haute and I were in the final stages of completing our monograph *Seduction, Drive and Repetition: Freud's Metaphysics of Trauma* in late 2021. In that book, there is a chapter devoted to this metapsychological text and, in particular, the way Freud explores several fundamental aspects of his trauma theory. The fact that his text has been widely received in contemporary continental philosophy and psychoanalytic theorizing, and has given rise to a broad variety of interpretations, was sufficient reason to systematically further study the text from the starting point that it was written in two stages, in which very different clinical reflections and theoretical constructs are explored. After we had made an initial rough sketch of the contents, the collaboration was cut short by Philippe's death in November 2022. That this monograph came about is unthinkable without my colleague and close friend with whom I had the pleasure of working for many years and with whom I read and discussed this text on many occasions.

In the past few years, the collaboration with Jenny Willner in the project of a text edition and commentaries of *Beyond the Pleasure Principle* has had a substantial impact on the development of my reading of this text. I am deeply indebted to her ground-breaking study of Freudian and Ferenczian bioanalysis. I would like to thank her for her many inspiring comments and suggestions. Also, the other authors in the volume *Towards the Limits of Freudian Thinking: Critical Edition and Readings of Beyond the Pleasure Principle* – Ulrike May, Ulrike Kistner and Jakob Staberg – provided valuable insights into the complexity of Freud's text.

In recent years, I have been fortunate to have had the opportunity to read and discuss *Beyond the Pleasure Principle* with numerous colleagues and students in reading groups, lectures and at conferences and symposia. I would like to thank the members of the *Freud Research Group* of the *International Society for Psychoanalysis and Philosophy* – Ulrike May, Daniela Finzi, Britta Günther, Ruud Welten, Elisabeth Schäfer, Beatriz Santos, Ednei Soares, Marlen Bidwell-Steiner, Céline Surprenant, Isabelle Alfandary, Sam Adriaenssens, Esther Hutfless, Dominik Drexel, Wolfgang Müller-Funk and Marcus Coelen. From this group, I would like to warmly thank Ulrike

Kistner in particular for her critical reading of the book manuscript and her thought-provoking suggestions to the text. I am grateful to the *Nijmegen Freud Reading Group* – Philip Eijndhoven, Ingrid van de Ven, Jackie Scharroo and Maarten Lange – and to the philosophy students in the course "Great texts in continental philosophy". My thanks also go to Raluca Soreanu for her valuable questions and suggestions on every occasion we met. I would like to thank Richard Simanke and Bettina Bergo for making available their work on Freud's metapsychology and for discussing his work. I am grateful to my fellow colleagues of the *Center for Contemporary European Philosophy* of the Radboud University Nijmegen for the thought-provoking conversations on psychoanalysis and philosophy – Rachel Aumiller, Ype de Boer, Annabelle Dufourcq, Katrine Smiet, Gert-Jan van der Heiden, Marjolein Oele, Tim Miechels, Robin Riemersma, and Rafael Gargano. In particular, I would like to thank Arjen Kleinherenbrink for his helpful corrections, suggestions and comments to the book manuscript, and Manja Kisner and Anna Vinkelman for valuable insights I gained from their research on the concept of *Trieb* in German Idealism.

Finally, I would like to thank Susan Dunsmore for copy-editing the text, and Saloni Singhania and Daniela Amodeo for guiding me through the publication process.

Introduction

In July 1920, Freud finished writing the manuscript of *Jenseits des Lustprinzips* (*Beyond the Pleasure Principle*). Since its publication, this text has been recognized as a key text in Freud's metapsychology. It is a text in which he critically discusses several of the most fundamental concepts and principles in his psychoanalytic theories. Above all, it is the text in which he famously introduces the concepts of death drives and life drives. This new drive theory has no doubt been central to a broad variety of psychoanalytic and philosophical readings and diverging interpretations of the text. This fact should not surprise us. According to Ernest Jones, Freud wrote the text "in the hope of clarifying some problems that had long puzzled him", but the result was a text with "occasional gaps in the reasoning" and "trains of thought by no means easy to follow" (Jones 1957: 266, 276–278). Indeed, in the text we do not find a coherent and consistent line of reasoning and a stable conceptuality. The text is more characterized by an unwieldy tangle of intertwined theoretical problems and questions, clinical observations and everyday phenomena, and references to very diverse and sometimes contradictory sources. The text as we know it from the *Gesammelte Werke* and the *Standard Edition* seems to mirror the processes of assimilation and dissimilation Freud regards as characteristics of the life and death drives: an agglomeration of haphazard pieces; a crystallization, as it were, but without the cleavages and fragments being made invisible (compare Freud 1933a: 59).

To a large extent, the lack of inner consistency can be explained when we consider that *Beyond the Pleasure Principle* was written in two phases. Since Ilse Grubrich-Simitis discovered two manuscript versions in the Freud Archive in the Library of Congress, we know that the first published edition of *Beyond the Pleasure Principle* is in fact a composition of two versions written in two different periods (Grubrich-Simitis 1993: 182ff; May 2024). Freud completed a first draft of the manuscript in April 1919. He then decided not to publish the text, and for more than a year he let it rest. His attention meanwhile turned to writing other texts such as "The Uncanny" and "The Psychogenesis of a Case of Homosexuality in a Woman". During the same period between April 1919 and May 1920, Freud was studying contemporary publications in biology that would be incorporated into the second version of *Beyond the Pleasure Principle* and the fourth edition of *Three Essays*. An initial "simple-minded idea" in the Spring of 1919 (Freud & Ferenczi 1996a: 354) would form the starting point for *Group Psychology and the Analysis of the Ego* – a text that would eventually be completed in March 1921. From correspondence, we know that Freud was working on "group psychology and death drives" in the Winter of 1919–1920 (Freud & Eitingon 2004: 194). This is, in fact, the first mention of the term "death drives". What is certain is that in May of that year Freud was working on *Beyond the Pleasure Principle*, adding substantial new theoretical material. In July, he announced that the work had been completed (Freud & Ferenczi 1996b: 32; Freud & Eitingon 2004: 213). This second version of *Beyond the Pleasure Principle* is an extension of the first. It contains *grosso modo* the first five chapters that, bar a few added – and significant – passages, remained unaltered in the second version. The entire sixth chapter was inserted between the fifth and the final chapter. In this way, the original sixth chapter became the seventh in the second version. This seventh chapter is a thoroughly revised version of the original final chapter. In the years following its publication in 1920, Freud would add short comments and passages scattered throughout the text – mostly in footnotes – in the 1921, 1923 and 1925 editions.

Comparing the 1919 and 1920 versions of *Beyond the Pleasure Principle*, one can hardly avoid the conclusion that they articulate different theoretical trains of thought that cannot easily be harmonized. This is particularly evident when we compare Chapters 5 and 6 where Freud elaborates the concept of the drives. Since we know that he first introduced the theory of the death drives and life drives only in the 1920 version, we can assume that he did not have the intention of writing a metapsychological paper introducing this new drive theory in 1919. This begs the question, how are the first and second version of the text related?

The reading of *Beyond the Pleasure Principle* presented in this book explores the hypothesis that Freud put the first version of the text aside because he found the conclusions he drew from his line of reasoning difficult, if not impossible, to accept. I argue that the two versions are at least partly contradictory and irreconcilable. The added sections from the 1920 version do not simply continue the argument of the first five chapters but respond to and correct the insights gained from the discussion of the drives, the pleasure principle and the compulsion to repeat. We therefore need to ask which clinical and theoretical problems Freud wants to explore in the first version of the text, what arguments he develops, and in what way these explorations and arguments resulted in implications he considered problematic. Next, we need to inquire in which way the new drive theory and associated issues introduced in the sixth chapter are a response to the problems and implications of his inquiries in the first version of the text.

There are clear indications that Freud, in the process of reflecting on the arguments put forward in the first version of the text, was well aware of creating new theoretical inconsistencies when introducing the new drive theory in the second version. For example, in a 1925 footnote to his ideas on the conservative character of all drives (Chapter 5), he writes that "the reader should not overlook the fact that what follows is the development of an extreme line of thought". And he adds, "later on, when account is taken of the sexual drives, it will be found that the necessary limitations and corrections are applied to it" (Freud 2024: 57).[1] Having said this, a number of passages formulated in 1920 and in the later editions can be seen as attempts to nuance or cover up tensions and contradictions in the text. This is particularly the case in the transition from the fifth to the sixth chapter. For example, after having argued in Chapter 5 that all drives are conservative, Freud adds the phrase "apart from the sexual drives" in 1920 (Freud 2024: 60).[2] This insertion is meant to announce the new drive theory developed in Chapter 6.

This tendency to nuance or cover up possible inconsistencies is continued in Freud's discussions of the drive theory in the years following the first publication of the text. In several texts from the period 1920–1925, he repeatedly argues that various trains of thought on the concept of the drives, and notably the concept of the death drive(s) in *Beyond the Pleasure Principle*, highlight aspects of what he presents – and defends – as a consistent theory. In "Two Encyclopedia Articles", for example, Freud writes that the death drives (in the plural) correspond with the process of "dissolution in the organism"; they follow the aim of "leading the living creature to death", and "manifest themselves as destructive and aggressive impulses" (Freud 1923a: 258).[3] In passages such as these and others, he presents his theory of the drives, and notably his concept of the death drive(s), as coherent and as an important and innovative theoretical step. The new drive conceptuality and theory are presented as "new solution to the problem of the drives" (Freud 1925d: 57). Freud's attempts to present *Beyond the Pleasure Principle* as a text in which eventually a new coherent theory of the drives is introduced undoubtedly contributed to the fact that most readings of *Beyond the Pleasure Principle* treat this text as indeed an inquiry into various aspects of one drive theory. This theory then either allows for a systematic reconstruction or for a rejection of (parts of) this drive theory because of theoretical inconsistencies and/or the lack of clinical evidence and relevance (for example, Lear 2000: 84–90; 2005: 160–162; Van Haute & Geyskens 2007).

It should come as no surprise, then, that in philosophical and psychoanalytical reflections on *Beyond the Pleasure Principle*, it is precisely the concept of the death drive(s) – and to a far lesser extent the life drives – that dominates most readings of the text. After all, when one is unaware of or ignores the fact that there are two versions of the text, the reader is confronted with different lines of thought that pose a challenge to any attempt at reconstructing a consistent drive theory. Readers tend to highlight specific passages as particularly significant for Freud's overall view of the drives. Thus, the death drives are (or the death drive is) defined in terms of auto-destruction, allo-aggression and violence, of organic elasticity and inertia, of brute repetition and the compulsion to repeat, of unbinding of and withdrawal from libidinally invested object relations, of mastery that manifests itself in the creation of protective shields, of fragmentation and annihilation as a result of trauma, or of the production of new forms and identities through psychic destruction. However, these different interpretations gain plausibility only to the extent that they disregard passages in the text that threaten to undermine or contradict a certain reading.

In this study, no attempt is made to harmonize Freud's various trains of thoughts and speculations. Instead, this study aims at systematically exploring the different clinical and theoretical problems that Freud discusses, his premises and arguments, and the implications and potentials of the various lines of thought. In order to provide such a reading of *Beyond the Pleasure Principle*, this book offers a historical contextualization of the text and explores the central concepts and composition of ideas relative to Freud's relevant earlier writings and to an existing body of scientific literature and debates, notably in the domains of biophysics, biology and evolutionary theory.

In Chapter 1, the focus is on the concept of the pleasure principle as Freud thematizes it particularly in the first and last chapters of *Beyond the Pleasure Principle*. It is notably in these two chapters that Freud inserts and adds extensive passages in 1920, respectively. This is an important fact, and it is the first significant indication that Freud needs to adjust and correct his theoretical assumptions and the implications of his speculations about drives in the 1919 version of the text, and in the light of the new drive theory he introduces in 1920. More specifically, in the first version, Freud associates the pleasure principle with the tendency towards the elimination of tension and excitation. He regards this principle to be the psychic manifestation of the conservative nature of all drives and their insistence on elimination of tension through a return to the inanimate. This changes with the introduction of the new drive theory. The pleasure principle will now be associated with Fechner's principle of constancy and tendency towards stability. The pleasure principle primarily describes the psychic tendency to establish a homeostatic optimum between decreasing and increasing tension and excitation.

In Chapter 2, the clinical observations and phenomena that led Freud to question his theoretical premises and assumptions are discussed. This specifically involves the study of traumatic neuroses. In his pre-psychoanalytic years, Freud had already dealt with the aetiology of these neuroses, but in the process of psychologizing and sexualizing trauma, Freud's attention had shifted to the psychoneuroses (especially hysteria). With the vast increase in numbers of traumatized soldiers (war neuroses) at the end of the First World War, the question of psychoanalytic interpretation and treatment of traumatic-neurotic patients becomes topical. The study of these neuroses forces Freud to rethink the aetiology of the psychoneuroses and the part played by sexuality. The study of traumatic neuroses not only incites him to conceptualize trauma beyond the sexual and thus beyond neurotic conflict, but also beyond our common understanding of perception, experience and memory.

In Chapter 3, we delve into Freud's much-discussed references to biology and evolutionary theory. These references have often been regarded as reflecting Freud's biologism and positivist reductionism, i.e., the expression of the conviction that psychoanalysis should be founded on firm scientific facts and that psychic life can be explained in physicalist and biological terms. The argument presented in this chapter is to the contrary. These references can be seen as an integral part of Freud's contribution to the bioanalytical project that he and Sandor Ferenczi started in the preceding years. The aim of this project was to transfer psychoanalytic concepts to organic processes and to identify the psychic principles and mechanisms manifest in phylogeny and ontogeny. As such, it can be seen as the most radical consequence of the pathoanalytical perspective Freud had developed in earlier writings: the human constitution and psychic life can best be studied from the perspective of the various psychopathologies. In addition, in this chapter we will also explore the very different perspectives on phylogeny and ontogeny developed in the 1919 and 1920 versions of the text. This includes a discussion of the sometimes contradictory sources and positions Freud at crucial moments in the text relies on in his arguments.

In Chapter 4, Freud's drive theories will be discussed. I will elaborate in detail the central hypothesis of this book: Freud introduces the theory of life drives and death drives in the 1920 version of *Beyond the Pleasure Principle* in response to the highly problematic implications of his 1919 speculations on trauma, repetition and drives. In the 1919 version of *Beyond the Pleasure Principle* Freud's analyses of the traumatic neuroses and the compulsion to repeat culminate in a theory of the drives as urges to restore a previous situation and to eliminate tension and excitation. The initial thoughts on this conservative character of all drives have implications Freud cannot accept. They tend towards drive monism and provide no answer to the question of which principles are at work "beyond" the pleasure principle. Instead of working towards a new articulation of inner psychic conflict, his train of thoughts leads to the conclusion that all motive forces and principles in psychic life resist enforced modifications from external sources. It is only a year later that Freud introduces a theory of life drives and death drives in order to restore a dualistic approach and rethink the "beyond" of the pleasure principle, more concretely, the inner sources of tension and excitation the pleasure principle will seek to eliminate. This leads to the conclusion that the life drives are "beyond" the pleasure principle, whereas the death drives maintain the conservative character Freud previously assigned to all drives. In this chapter, I will argue, the introduction of the concept of life drives depends on the application of the libido theory to the relationship between cells. The concept of the life drives derives not only from the biological literature, but notably also from the analyses of binding processes between individuals in groups. Also, in this chapter the relation between the various drive theories in *Beyond the Pleasure Principle* and the references to biological and evolutionary theories will be continued. Whereas in the 1919 theory of the drives, the enforced "traumatic" modifications in the processes of adaptation and acquisition of characteristics are highlighted, the new drive theory focuses attention on the life drives producing change and development. These life drives are creative forces. Freud appears to introduce a vitalist principle that brings him unexpectedly close to his contemporary Henri Bergson. A short comparison with Bergson's *Creative Evolution* provides the opportunity to rethink the life and death drives in terms of plastic-proliferating forces and an internal tendency towards adhesiveness and viscosity. In the final part of this book, I will thus propose a theory of the life and death drives "beyond" dualism.

Throughout the various chapters I will regularly critically discuss various significant philosophical readings of *Beyond the Pleasure Principle* in order to show the implicit and explicit choices that have been made in the interpretation of this text. I will confront these readings with the reading presented in this book based on the two versions of the text and the hypothesis of Freud responding to the first version in the second version. At the very least, the two versions of *Beyond the Pleasure Principle* constitute two divergent trains of thought in which key concepts such as life, drives, pleasure and trauma are articulated in different ways and lead to different metapsychological constructions. This book is an attempt to reconstruct Freud's trains of thought and arguments in this text and to think through their philosophical premises and implications.

Notes

1 In the published 1920 version, this footnote was formulated differently: "A correction of this extreme view of the self-preservative instincts follows" (Freud 1920g: 39).
2 In the 1921 edition of the text, Freud italicizes this insertion in order to underscore its significance (Freud 1920g: 41).
3 In *The Ego and the Id*, we find similar views with regards to the death drive (now in the singular) (Freud 1923b: 40). And in *An Autobiographical Study*, he writes that the "*instinct of death* or *destruction*" can be regarded as an "impulsion towards the restoration of a situation which once existed but was brought to an end by some external disturbance" (Freud 1925d: 57; Freud's italics).

Chapter 1

The pleasure principle

The economic perspective

The starting point for our reading of the 1919 version and the 1920 edition of *Beyond the Pleasure Principle* is the one Freud himself articulates in the opening paragraphs of the first chapter: the concept of the pleasure principle (*Lustprinzip*). In the first sentence of *Beyond the Pleasure Principle*, Freud states that he had thus far always assumed and taken for granted that the course taken by psychic events is automatically regulated by the pleasure principle:

> we believe, that the course of these events is invariably set in motion by an unpleasurable tension [*Spannung*], and that it takes a direction such that its final outcome coincides with a lowering of that tension – that is, with an avoidance of unpleasure or a production of pleasure.
>
> (Freud 1920g: 7)

A few lines further down, Freud writes that "unpleasure corresponds to an *increase* in the quantity of excitation [*Erregung*] and pleasure to a *diminution*" (Freud 1920g: 8; Freud's italics). He adds that the determining factor in the increase or decrease of feelings of unpleasure and pleasure is not the quantity of excitation as such, but "increase or diminution in the quantity of excitation *in a given period of time*" (Freud 1920g: 8; Freud's italics).[1] Unpleasure is particularly felt when there is strong and sudden decrease or increase of tension and excitation in a relatively short period of time. A few sentences later, Freud continues arguing that, indeed, clinical practice had caused him to believe "that the mental apparatus endeavours to keep the quantity of excitation present in it as low as possible [*möglichst niedrig*] or at least to keep it constant". This latter hypothesis would only be "another way of stating the pleasure principle" (Freud 1920g: 9).

Freud further remarks that "strictly speaking", it is incorrect to assume that psychic life is indeed automatically regulated by the pleasure principle. What can be said, Freud writes, is that there is a "strong *tendency* [*Tendenz*]

DOI: 10.4324/9781003680413-1

towards the pleasure principle" (Freud 1920g: 9; Freud's italics). After all, the endeavour to keep excitation as low as possible or constant is disrupted, again and again, by internal and external forces (drives and stimuli). This implies, first of all, that there is no assured psychic stability or rest. But, as we will see in the course of our reading of *Beyond the Pleasure Principle*, Freud questions the assumption of automatic regulation of psychical events; and this is what leads him to inquire into the very conditions and origins of psychic functions and regulative principles. The pleasure principle cannot be assumed *a priori*, but should be regarded as part of a psychic response to modifying forces. In other words, it needs to be established as part of a totality of pacifying responses to problems posed to human beings in particular and to living beings in general. In the final chapter of the text, Freud returns to this "tendency" which aims to "free the psychic apparatus entirely from excitation or to keep the amount of excitation in it constant or to keep it as low as possible" (Freud 1920g: 62). He adds that he cannot "yet decide with certainty in favour of any of these ways of putting it". His indecision here concerns the question as to whether the psychic apparatus aims at a zero amount of excitation or at a constant quantity.

As several authors have shown, Freud's indecision on the question as to whether the elimination of excitation or constancy of excitation is the aim of the pleasure principle's regulation of psychic processes, results in a contradiction (Sulloway 1979; Laplanche 1985; Fletcher 2013). Is the pleasure principle a tendency towards discharge of excitation to zero? Or is it a tendency towards (static or dynamic) equilibrium? Fechner's principle of tendency towards stability, to which Freud refers in the first chapter, would be at odds with the pleasure principle, according to which the aim would be to eliminate any quantity of excitation in the psychic system.

One of the references to Fechner is embedded in Freud's statement that "the pleasure principle follows from the principle of constancy". Sulloway, Laplanche and others have argued that if Freud gives "priority to zero over constancy" (Laplanche 1985: 113), it seems impossible to maintain that the pleasure principle follows from the principle of constancy. After all, if priority were given to the principle of constancy, it is contradictory to argue that a tendency towards reduction of excitation to zero can be the aim of psychic life. After all, the constancy principle points towards a psychic apparatus as a homeostatic system in which a certain optimum range of excitation is maintained. Diversions in both directions – excess of excitation or lack of excitation – would be felt as unpleasure which the psychic apparatus would seek to avoid. If the aim is to maintain excitation at a certain level, both discharges and recharges (influx) of excitation can produce pleasure; both accumulation or depletion of tension or excitation can produce unpleasure.

So far, we have said that Freud in the first chapter of *Beyond the Pleasure Principle* poses the problem in terms of drives that produce tension and excitation versus a pleasure principle that aims to regulate and pacify this tension and excitation. In the course of the text, however, the relation between drives and the pleasure principle is defined in a very different way. The main argument for Laplanche's conclusion that Freud gives "priority [to] zero over constancy" does not so much derive from his "undecided" formulations of the pleasure principle in the first and last chapters of the text, but from the conceptualization of the drives in Chapter 5 of *Beyond the Pleasure Principle*. There Freud defines all drives as "conservative" and ultimately as urges to return to the initial state of things, i.e., the state of inertia and absence of tension, the inanimate that precedes life (Freud 1920g: 36, 38). In Chapter 7, Freud reflects on the relation between these drives and the pleasure principle. He repeats that all drives "would be concerned with the most universal endeavour [*Streben*] of all living substance – namely to return to the quiescence of the inorganic world" (Freud 1920g: 62). The pleasure principle as "tendency" (*Tendenz*), Freud writes, can therefore be said to be operating in the service (*im Dienste steht*) of the "function" (*Funktion*) of the drives, that is, of the endeavour to lead the living substance back to the quiescence of the inorganic world. The pleasure principle is the psychic equivalent of a more fundamental endeavour. Hence, Freud's conclusion in the last chapter is that the "tendency" of the pleasure principle operates in the service of the drives and their aim to return to the quiescence of the inorganic world provides the decisive argument for the priority of zero over constancy. And, indeed, in arguing that the pleasure principle stands in the service of drives that seek the elimination of tension, Freud cannot but prioritize zero over constancy. On this point we can agree with Laplanche.

Seen from this perspective, Freud's statement that "the pleasure principle follows from the principle of constancy" and that this principle "which we thus attribute to the mental apparatus is subsumed as a special case under Fechner's principle of the *tendency towards stability*" (Freud 1920g: 8) does not seem to make sense. In other words, the references to Fechner in the first chapter of *Beyond the Pleasure Principle* appear to undermine the pleasure principle as function in the service of all drives. However, the references to Fechner in the first chapter of *Beyond the Pleasure Principle* are not part of the 1919 version of the text. In fact, in the trains of thought that dominate the first version of the text, the notions of constancy or stability of levels of excitation are hardly relevant. The references to Fechner, along with notions of constancy and stability of levels of excitation, were inserted a year later in the 1920 version of the text. The question then arises why Freud inserted references in a text that had thus far led to the conclusion that the pleasure principle and the conservative drives seek the elimination of all excitation. What prompted Freud to rethink the pleasure principle in other terms?

From unpleasure to the pleasure principle

The combination of contradictory definitions of (the aim of) the pleasure principle is not new; it can be traced back to Freud's earliest psychoanalytic texts, letters and drafts from the mid-1890s. In "Project for a Scientific Psychology", Freud argues that the "basic principle of neuronal activity" is the "principle of inertia" (Freud 1950c: 296) which provides the motive for any reflex movement, namely, to fend off and keep itself free from any external stimulus (*Reiz*) that produces excitation. The principle of inertia describes the organism's spontaneous reactions to external stimuli aimed at fleeing from the stimulus (*Reizflucht*) and returning to a situation of absence of excitation. Such absence and return to inertia are felt as pleasure. Yet, Freud adds that, in advanced organisms – more complex than unicellular organisms – this principle of inertia had to be abandoned, since such organisms not only have to respond to external stimuli that trigger the irritable external surface, but also to internal stimuli originating in cells and organs from which the organism cannot withdraw. Every complex organism is subjected to the continuous influx of internal stimuli. This results in a modification of the inertia principle into "an endeavour at least to keep the $Q\dot{\eta}$ [quantity of energy in the nervous system, HW] as low as possible and to guard against any increase of it – that is, to keep it constant" (Freud 1950c: 297).[2] Here Freud already mentions what in *Beyond the Pleasure Principle* will be termed the "tendency towards the pleasure principle" (Freud 1920g: 9).

The evolutionary perspective in early writings such as "Project for a Scientific Psychology" provides Freud with an argument for upholding the two definitions of the aim of the pleasure principle. The inertia principle in reality only applies to the most primitive organic life forms: the unicellular protists. Due to external influences, organic life gradually acquires characteristics that increase the complexity of organisms. This growing complexity of organisms implies the production of internal stimuli in one part of the organism, creating excitation and workload in other parts or systems. The adaptation to the *Not des Lebens*, the external influences that force organisms to change and develop, leads to the modification of the inertia principle into a principle of constancy (Freud 1950c: 297).

In "Project for a Scientific Psychology", Freud mentions the principle of inertia, but he does not yet refer to a (un)pleasure principle. This step is taken in *The Interpretation of Dreams* where Freud introduces the concept of the "unpleasure principle" (Freud 1900a: 600). The formulations in this text are quite similar to those which are taken up later in *Beyond the Pleasure Principle.* Thus, he states: "We are … driven to conclude that these releases of pleasure and unpleasure automatically regulate the course of cathectic processes" (Freud 1900a: 574). And somewhat later in the text he writes that "the accumulation of excitation … is felt as unpleasure" which "sets the apparatus in action with a view to repeating the experience of satisfaction, which involved a diminution of excitation and was felt as pleasure" (Freud 1900a: 598).

The apparatus to which Freud is here referring is the "primitive psychical apparatus"; it is constructed like a "reflex apparatus" which aims to immediately discharge along a motor path any sensory excitation impinging on it (Freud

1900a: 538, 565, 598). An example would be the experience of fright, that is, the sudden and unexpected influx of stimulus from the outside that causes a painful excitation. One can think here of the fright experienced in a life-threatening situation, such as the perception of an armed person approaching, or an object on the course of collision. The appropriate motor reaction would then be to "withdraw the apparatus from the perception", or more concrete, to actually flee the scene in which a concrete danger appears "till the perception has disappeared" (Freud 1900a: 600). The flight reaction is the typical response to the sudden increase of external stimuli.

This view is continued throughout Freud's writings. In "Instincts and Their Vicissitudes", his starting point for a discussion of the concept of the drive is the "physiological" perspective – i.e., the perspective from physics – which starts from the notion of an external stimulus (*Reiz*) and a subsequent reflex reaction, "according to which a stimulus applied to living tissue (nervous substance) *from* the outside is discharged by action *to* the outside, that is, by withdrawal from the influence of the stimulus" (Freud 1915c: 118). In an advanced organism, such as a human being, this simple scheme becomes more complicated. After all, there are also inner forces – the drive is defined "as a constant force" (*wie eine konstante Kraft*) – that do not have a momentary character but continuously act upon the nervous and psychic systems causing unpleasure.[3] In this case, there is no possibility of flight. The most efficient way of discharge of the excitation (and hence unpleasure) caused by the drives is either an alteration of the inner sources of the stimulation – for example, satisfying hunger through food intake – or alterations of external circumstances that allow for such satisfaction, or both.

In "Formulations on the Two Principles of Mental Functioning", Freud had explored these alterations of external circumstances. He argues that these are possible through the development of the psychic functions of attention, memory, judgement, and (strategic) thought (Freud 1911b: 220–221), which allow human beings to protect themselves against the forces of nature and gain some mastery over the circumstances in which they live, for example, by distributing available goods. The pleasure principle is here (again) articulated in relation to phylogenetic and ontogenetic developments. In the most primitive psychic apparatus, the tendency towards pleasure only consists of drawing back "from any event that might arouse unpleasure" (Freud 1911b: 219). Strictly speaking, this is what describes the unpleasure principle. The fact that Freud will speak of the pleasure principle from now onwards is related to the modifications and adaptations effected by higher organisms such as human beings in the course of their development. They will increasingly direct their sense-organs towards the external world, and pro-actively engage with a world in which they no longer only await (dis-)appearances of objects that may or may not provide unpleasure and pleasure. The primitive reflex processes of discharge of excitation are now "converted into *action*" (Freud 1911b: 221; Freud's italics) in order to alter the external world in such a way that it will provide and assure pleasure at a later moment in time.

From these texts we can conclude that what Freud had first named the unpleasure principle was primarily derived from the idea of a reflex apparatus's response to the momentary influx of external stimuli. This implied the tendency to withdraw from incoming stimuli, to maintain or return to a situation without excitation, to reduce unpleasure to a minimum, and – in the course of evolution – to produce protective and strategic capacities against the impact of external stimuli. In "Instincts and Their Vicissitudes", Freud argues that the drives are a constant source of excitation in all organic life forms. The drive is essentially an amount of force (*Summe von Kraft*) exercising pressure (*Drang*) on the psychic apparatus. In this situation, the psychic apparatus is obliged "to renounce its ideal intention of keeping off stimuli", and to develop various capacities to receive (*auffangen*), master (*bewältigen*), inhibit (*hemmen*) and regulate (*regulieren*). It gets involved in increasingly complex activities (*verwickelten, ineinandergreifenden Tätigkeiten*) in order to manage the invincibility of the unavoidable afflux of drive stimuli (Freud 1915c: 119–123). For this reason, the drives can be said to be the "motive force" for further evolutionary developments and the production of the psychic capacities human beings (and other living beings) have in altering circumstances so that pleasure can be assured. Compared to primitive organisms, advanced organisms – notably human beings – have more complex ways of endeavouring to master unpleasurable excitations. For Freud, evolution and development (*Entwicklung*) equal complexifying (*verwickeln*) psychic life. But unlike in the case of external stimuli, Freud does not refer to this process as "purposive" or "expedient" (*zweckmäßig*) in overcoming the initial helplessness of the organism vis-à-vis the pressure of drive stimuli. On the contrary, the drives are those forces from which "one cannot withdraw". The living being paradoxically cannot but seek the reduction of tension "to the lowest possible level" (Freud 1915c: 120) through psychic capacities of receiving and inhibiting – hence accepting and maintaining – pressure and the demand for psychic work. In this context, the terms *das Seelische* (Freud 1915c: 122) or *das seelische/psychische Apparat* denote an intermediate network of processes designed to protect the individual from the irregular and life-threatening immediacy of influx and discharge.

The tendency towards the pleasure principle

In the first chapter of *Beyond the Pleasure Principle*, Freud argues that both the economic perspective on psychic functioning and clinical facts "caused us to believe in the dominance of the pleasure principle in mental life" (Freud 1920g: 9). This is a general reference to his studies of the various psychoneuroses and the conflicts between the ego and the sexual drives that are typical of these neuroses (Freud 1911b: 219). Freud notes that while the ego passes through its development into more complex organizations, sexual drives can turn out to be incompatible with the aims and demands of the ego drives. These sexual drives will then be repressed, but also continue to seek immediate or substitutive satisfaction, that is, discharge of excitation. If these drives succeed in this aim, this satisfaction is "felt by the ego as unpleasure" (Freud 1920g: 11). Freud refers to such situation as a "breach" in the pleasure principle, a temporary interruption in the dominance of the pleasure principle due to sexual drives endeavouring to obtain satisfaction.[4] The dominance of the pleasure principle is always contested and never fully assured.

There are more reasons to question the dominance of the pleasure principle. For example, the perceptual unpleasure we have already discussed does not contradict the pleasure principle, Freud argues, since the external perception of stimuli generating unpleasure will and can normally be dealt with through appropriate motor reactions, such as flight (Freud 1920g: 11). But it does show that the psychic apparatus is repeatedly challenged to discharge unpleasure. Since it is impossible not to have perceptions, it is also impossible to maintain a psychic state in which pleasure is assured. The fact that pleasure (and satisfaction) cannot always be realized immediately or at least within a very limited amount of time, and that one may find "the temporary toleration of unpleasure as a step on the long indirect road to pleasure" (Freud 1920g: 10), does not contradict the pleasure principle. Concerning the necessary postponement of pleasure and the toleration of unpleasure in circumstances in which immediate satisfaction is impossible, Freud had already argued in "Formulations on the Two Principles of Mental Functioning" that the substitution of the pleasure principle by the reality principle does not imply the abandonment of the intention to seek pleasure. On the contrary, it implies not deposing but merely safeguarding the pleasure principle, since a possible momentary and immediate pleasure is only given up in order to attain an assured pleasure at a later moment (Freud 1911b: 223). The reality principle thus illustrates the tendency towards the pleasure principle, even in a situation of felt unpleasure.

Excitation and/as pleasure

The clinical observations that lead Freud to assume the tendency towards or dominance of the pleasure principle raise the fundamental question whether pleasure should only be defined in terms of the absence of unpleasure. Is pleasure merely the feeling accompanying the elimination of excitation? In *The Interpretation of Dreams*, Freud had answered this question in the positive. The psychic apparatus aims to decrease unpleasure through discharge of the influx of stimuli. This would then result in an experience of satisfaction (pleasure), and the production of a "memory-trace" (*Erinnerungsspur*) of both the excitation produced by a stimulus (such as the need for nourishment) and the perception of satisfaction (the actual food intake). So, the next time such stimulus arises, the psychic apparatus will seek to "re-establish the situation of the original satisfaction". In other words, the psychic apparatus will wish to repeat (*Wiederholung*) the satisfaction and the way it was attained (Freud 1900a: 566). We repeat because certain past experiences provided pleasure.

In *Three Essays of the Theory of Sexuality*, Freud returns to this issue of the repetition of pleasurable experiences in the context of his discussion of infantile sexuality. He argues that the first sexual pleasure is associated with food intake, that is to say, with the satisfaction of the need for nutrition. Such satisfaction could be described in terms we are familiar with: hunger is felt as increase of excitation – food intake produces decrease of excitation. But this is not the case for sexual pleasure, Freud writes. During nourishment (breast-feeding) the little child discovers a kind of pleasure other than that of the satisfaction of hunger through nutrition. It discovers that the rhythmic sucking and the warm flow of milk that touches the lips and the sensitive inside of the mouth produce a kind of excitation that is pleasurable (Freud 1905d: 180). In this situation the lips and mouth are discovered as erogenous zones, that is, as sensitive body parts and organs capable of receiving stimuli from the outside or inside, and of experiencing a sexual excitation that in itself is satisfactory (Freud 1905d: 168 n.). Freud argues that "the need for repeating the sexual satisfaction now becomes detached from the need for taking nourishment" and the child will engage in autoerotic sexual activities such a sensual sucking that reproduce the original pleasurable sensations (Freud 1905d: 182). For Freud, infantile sexuality consists of nothing but physically pleasurable and satisfactory activities originating from the excitability of erogenous zones.[5] From now on, these first pleasurable activities will be the original experiences that a child will seek to re-experience. From this perspective, the pleasure principle, when applied to infantile sexuality, could be defined in terms of the repetition of experiences of pleasurable excitations through autoerotic activities.[6]

The inquiries into infantile sexuality lead to the conclusion that sexual pleasure corresponds to (increase of) excitation. Freud is well aware that this conclusion is at odds with what he had named the unpleasure principle. In the third essay of *Three Essays on the Theory of Sexuality* (on the transformations of sexuality in puberty), he explicitly states that the "tension of sexual excitement", which from an economic perspective would have to be considered unpleasurable, "is undoubtedly felt as pleasure". If so, "how, then, are this unpleasurable tension and this feeling of pleasure to be reconciled?" (Freud 1905d: 209). Freud finds part of an answer to this question during his inquiries into the transformations of sexuality in puberty. This period of puberty is one in which the erotogenic zones become subordinated to the primacy of the genital zone, sexuality becomes object-oriented, and the sexual aim is no longer autoerotic pleasure but "the discharge of the sexual products" in the service of the reproductive function (Freud 1905d: 207). This transformation of infantile sexuality into pubertal and adult sexuality provides Freud with the argument that the sexual excitations provide a certain amount of pleasure that "leads to an increase of tension which in its turn is responsible for producing the necessary motor energy for the conclusion of the sexual act" (Freud 1905d: 210). In other words, in order to experience pleasure at the discharge of sexual products, a person first needs to be aroused and stimulated. One can only experience pleasure at discharge of tension when enough tension produced. Pleasure at excitation is no longer an aim but a means to an end. The concepts of "fore-pleasure" (*Vorlust*) and "end-pleasure" (*Endlust*) are introduced by Freud to conceptualize both forms of pleasure and situate these pleasures in a double chronology: the development from infantile sexual activities into pubertal sexuality; the adult sexual activities as composed of foreplay and ejaculation. Freud refers to this train of thought in the final chapter of *Beyond the Pleasure Principle* when he writes the following:

> We have all experienced how the greatest pleasure attainable by us, that of the sexual act, is associated with a momentary extinction of a highly intensified excitation. The binding [*Bindung*] of a drive impulse would be a preliminary function designed to prepare the excitation for its final elimination in the pleasure of discharge.
>
> (Freud 1920g: 62)

Fore-pleasure is not explicitly mentioned here but could be conceptualized in this context as the preliminary process of the binding of the sexual drives and excitation to concrete representations in order to make possible the final discharge of excitation.

In the 1919 version of *Beyond the Pleasure Principle*, the idea of sexual excitation as pleasurable is strikingly absent. The reason for this absence of references to rhythmic repetitions of pleasurable feelings of excitation is determined by the theoretical and clinical problems Freud wants to address. The most pressing clinical issue concerns the traumatic neuroses and repetitions of frightful "states" which were in no way associated with sexual pleasure (Freud 1920g: 12ff., 31ff). In *The Interpretation of Dreams*, Freud had already argued that fright was in fact a case of the "antithesis" of a primary experience of satisfaction. In fright, we find a sudden and momentary increase of unpleasurable excitation, and a subsequent reaction of flight. An impressive experience produces a memory trace such that the first experience and initial reaction will be the model for all later reactions to frightful experiences. Once the perception of something frightening reappears, the reaction will be repeated until the perception disappears. The psychic apparatus will seek to avoid such perception of the original fright and, which amounts to the same thing, avoid the memory of the perception of fright. This avoidance is, according to Freud, nothing but "the repetition of the previous flight from the perception" (Freud 1900a: 600). In *Beyond the Pleasure Principle*, this antithesis is the starting point: fright is what characterizes traumatic neuroses, and this fright can be defined in terms of an unanticipated confrontation with danger (Freud 1920g: 12), that is, with an external source of huge quantities of excitation. In the context of the discussion of the impact of momentary and sudden changes in quantities of excitation, the idea that excitations can be pleasurable when moderate and rhythmically repeated is not relevant.

Towards the priority of constancy

What reasons did Freud have in 1920 to include references to Fechner's *Einige Ideen zur Schöpfungs- und Entwicklungsgeschichte der Organismen* (1873) in his elaborations on the pleasure principle in the first chapter of *Beyond the Pleasure Principle*? Why would Freud introduce references to Fechner's principle of the tendency towards stability and declare that the pleasure principle follows from the principle of constancy (Freud 1920g: 9)? We have to understand these references as part of the trains of thought developed in the second version of the text from 1920. In Chapter 6, Freud only mentions the pleasure principle once, namely in the following passage:

> The dominating tendency of psychic life is the effort to reduce, to keep constant or to remove internal tension due to stimuli (the 'Nirvana principle', to borrow a term from an English author Barbara Low) – a tendency which finds expression in the pleasure principle; and our recognition of that fact is one of our strongest reasons for believing in the existence of death drives.
>
> (Freud 1920g: 55–56)

Here we once again find the indecision regarding the pleasure principle – reduction of tension (excitation), removal of tension, or constancy. It is not without significance that the word order is reversed here, in comparison with formulations we have encountered thus far: reduction and constancy come first. This is understandable in light of the sentences which precede this passage and in which Freud addresses the two tendencies that characterize life. On the one hand, there is a tendency towards "abolition of chemical tensions, that is to say, to death". On the other hand, Freud argues, the "union with the living substance of a different individual increases those tensions, introducing what may be described as fresh 'vital differences' which must then be lived off". And he adds: "as regards this dissimilarity there must of course be one or more optima" (Freud 1920g: 55). He suggests here that the theory of the life drives and death drives introduced in the 1920 version of the text can be articulated in terms of an interplay between increasing and decreasing quantities of excitation. Contrary to what Freud had argued in the first edition of the text, not all functions and tendencies aim at the reduction of tension. The life drives are in fact "breakers of the peace" (Freud 1920g: 63), continuously producing new forms and hence increasing tensions.

This train of thought has implications for the concepts of pleasure and unpleasure. In the final paragraphs of the 1920 version of the text, Freud states that the life drives produce tensions that can be felt as "either pleasurable or unpleasurable" (Freud 1920g: 63). What he has in mind here are tensions and excitations produced in the interaction between cells, organs and body parts. Such excitations can be pleasurable in the way Freud had described in *Three*

Essays, that is, as rhythmically repeated sensations that only become unpleasurable when disturbed by sudden increases and surplus of excitation (see Freud 1920g: 33). If excitations produced by the life drives can be pleasurable, it is difficult to uphold the idea that all drives and the pleasure principle seek to reduce tension to zero by returning to the quiescence of the inorganic. In order to underscore the possibility of pleasurable tension, Freud introduces the references to Fechner's tendency towards approximate stability in the first chapter. The mention of "one or more optima" in the interaction between life drives and death drives can find support, he reasons, in the principle of constancy (of a certain level of energy, tension, excitation) and the principle of the tendency towards stability. Hence, whereas, in the first version of *Beyond the Pleasure Principle*, zero does indeed have priority of constancy, the introduction of the concept of the life drives in the second version of the text results in prioritizing constancy over zero.

Why would Freud mention Fechner so explicitly? What he finds in Fechner's *Einige Ideen* is the formulation of a theory on a tendency towards stability that appears to be congruent with the first law of thermodynamics (the conservation of energy) and the main theories from evolutionary biology Freud calls upon in *Beyond the Pleasure Principle*, notably Haeckel's recapitulation theory (Fechner 1873: iv–v; Seeck 2021). Fechner tries to harmonize physiological and biological perspectives on the fundamental forces and principles at work in inorganic matter and organic life.[7] The starting point of his argument is that the principle of the conservation of energy sets limits to the possibilities of stability. There can never be absolute stability – absence of energy, movement and change – in a system in which a certain amount of energy is present. Yet, whereas the quantity of energy is constant, the quality of energy is not. To be more precise, the "form" or organization in which energy is contained can change (Fechner 1873: 35). According to Fechner, processes in the organization of both inorganic matter and organic life gradually tend towards more stability in terms of stable movements (such as planetary systems) or periodic, circular and rhythmic repetitions (such as blood circulation, the recapitulation of phylogeny in ontogeny, or the life cycle of birth and death). Fechner adds that in organic life, this tendency towards stability will be continuously disturbed by external influences demanding new expedient adaptations. Moreover, the tendency towards stability will repeatedly be disrupted through internal chemical and metabolic processes in molecules and cells producing displacements (*Diffusionen*), defusions (*Auflösungen*) and fusions (*Verschmelzungen, Verbindungen*) within the organism, and through the incorporation of particles from the outside (for example, food intake) (Fechner 1873: 4–12).[8] Even though life tends towards more stability, it is characterized by numerous internal and external disturbances and disruptions. According to Fechner, these dynamics also apply to psychic life. In this context, he refers to sensations of pleasure and unpleasure relative to diversions from psychophysical stability in the circulation of energy and changing levels of excitation (Fechner 1873: 94–95; Freud 1920g: 8).

And there is more. In Fechner, Freud also finds confirmation of a perspective on evolution in which the development from the most primitive to the most advanced – and even from the inorganic to the organic – was thought not only in terms of differences in molecular, metabolic or chemical processes, but also in terms of the complexity of organization. This intuition can already be found in Freud's earliest zoological article on the morphological continuity between primitive fish (such as the lamprey) and the higher, more advanced fishes (Wilson 2004: 2). In writings such as "Project for a Scientific Psychology", *The Interpretation of Dreams, Three Essays* and notably also *Beyond the Pleasure Principle*, this intuition continues to be upheld. The fundamental characteristics of nervous and psychic systems one finds in advanced organisms such as human beings can also be found in the earliest forms of organic life (Freud 1920g: 26). The difference between the two is merely a matter of degree of complexity in the organization of basically the same principles, processes and functions.

However, when it comes to the conservative nature of living substance and the death drives, we should not overlook some difficulties. Fechner's principle of the tendency towards stability is a progressive tendency in organic life, that is, a progression towards more stability which includes a tendency in the organic towards the inorganic, a tendency within life towards death. After all, death is a more stable situation than life.[9] Life progresses towards future death. In Freud's copy of Fechner's *Einige Ideen*, notably in the passages where Fechner mentions the transition from organic to inorganic states, we find markings and underscoring by Freud (Fechner 1873: 36, 91; Davies & Fichtner 2006; Seeck 2021: 147–148). This may not be surprising, given the fact that the problematics of life and death play such a prominent part in *Beyond the Pleasure Principle*. Yet for Freud, contrary to Fechner, the tendency of the organic towards the inorganic is not progressive, but regressive. Life seeks to return to death. Having said this, Freud's peculiar reading of *Einige Ideen* does help us to understand the references to Fechner in the second version of *Beyond the Pleasure Principle*. What Freud takes from Fechner is a theory in which the "principle of constancy" can be interpreted in terms of a continuous "descent towards death". At the same time, the principle of constancy expresses the idea of the continuous generation of new tension and excitations. Concerning the pleasure principle, this means that Freud is convinced that he can actually maintain two formulations. In line with the tendency towards stability, he argues that the pleasure principle expresses the tendency to eliminate excitation and to return to an inorganic state (Freud 1920g: 63). In line with the new drive theory, he will at the same time claim that for as long as the life drives produce new excitations, an organism will seek "one or more optima" of tension and excitation. Hence, with the introduction of the life drives and death drives in the 1920 version of the text, the pleasure principle comes to describe the tendency towards approximate homeostasis between the poles of rising and falling quantities of excitation.

The references to Fechner also shed some light on Freud's relation to nineteenth-century natural sciences, notably physics and physiology. Several authors have pointed out that Freud's metapsychological theories and his fundamental conceptuality are deeply rooted in these sciences.[10] The references to concepts such as force, pressure, energy, tension, inertia and constancy indicate that Freud adopts the conceptuality from nineteenth-century physics, which at the time provides the paradigms for all sciences, including physiology and psychology.[11] For example, Freud's definition of the drive in "Instincts and Their Vicissitudes" as "constant force" follows from an "angle of physiology" that adopts laws and principles from physics. Drives are forces or amounts of energy that cause movement in matter and bodies. For Freud, these forces cause excitations in the various organs and sensitive organic tissues and surfaces (such as mucous membranes) and in the nervous and psychic systems. In other words, these systems never act out of themselves. They are first of all reactive systems – they are reflex apparatuses. They move, change and work only in reaction to a force or energy that operates from their outside. Force and energy pressure bodies, systems or apparatuses; they are what Helmholtz in his famous *Über die Erhaltung der Kraft* had named *Bewegungskräfte* (Helmholtz 1847: 3–7) – quantities of force or energy that produce movement, i.e., modifications in (physical) matter and (psychic) systems. As such, they pose problems to which the reflex apparatuses respond by slowing down the incoming amounts of force/energy, and by converting these amounts to be used for specific and effective actions and movements. Any excess or surplus of force/energy will have to be discharged in order to continue the efficient functioning of a system. For Freud, as for many of his predecessors and contemporaries, force and energy are fundamental – metaphysical – concepts explaining the movements, dynamics and development of complexity in the body and the psychic apparatus. When Freud introduces Fechner in the first chapter of the second version of *Beyond the Pleasure Principle*, he does so to give credit to the man who had systematically introduced the law of energy conservation into psychology; it was Fechner who put forward the idea that all organic life and psychic systems are subjected to this law – an idea that had been of crucial importance for the development of psycho-physics.[12]

We don't know when exactly Freud read *Einige Ideen*, but fact is that he was already familiar with some of Fechner's writings in the 1890s (see Freud 1950c: 315) and probably earlier, having been taught by Theodor Meynert.[13] We also know that it is through teachers and predecessors such as Ernst von Brücke and his successor Sigmund Exner, Ernst Mach and Ewald Hering that Freud must have been introduced to the Helmholtzian school of biophysics and psychophysics, and its applications in neurophysiology and psychology, at an early stage in his career. Important associates in the 1890s, such as Wilhelm Fliess and Joseph Breuer, were also scholars strongly influenced by this school. We also know that Freud was strongly influenced by scholarship in psycho-physics more generally.[14] From the Viennese physicist Ernst Mach – Freud held several books of his books in his library, including *Beiträge zur Analyse der Empfindungen* from 1886 – for example, Freud was able to glean some of the general assumptions guiding his 1895 "Project" and *Beyond the Pleasure Principle.* [15] Mach had criticized both mechanistic and vitalist approaches while focussing his research on the body as sensitive (*empfindliche*) – or what Freud will call irritable (*reizbare*) or excitable (*erregbare*) – matter. This sensitivity implies that organic substances have the ability to respond to and interact with whatever forces and objects impinge on them from outside, producing sensations (including sensations of pleasure and unpleasure). From this starting point, Mach will argue that what is generally considered as ego and consciousness can best be considered the result of gradual psychic structuring and organization of sensations such that the organism can survive in its environment and maintain an inner homeostatic equilibrium (Fechner's stability). The crucial aspects of this structuring of sensations are perception of stimuli (through stimulation of the sense organs), awareness of one's position in space and time, and memory of perceived and experienced sensations (Mach 1886; also Assoun 1981: 73–89; Schloegel & Schmidgen 2002; Bergo 2025). The latter aspect is of crucial importance for understanding the evolution of species as process of further adaptation and increasing psychic complexity, based on the memories and experiences of previous generations. Without this first psychic structuring through a distinction between transitory perceptions, on the one hand, and memories produced by impressive and/or repeated experiences, on the other, life would be characterized by mere immediate and inefficient – hence destabilizing and even life-threatening – reflexes to continuous and chaotic sensations.

Observations and speculations

What characterizes *Beyond the Pleasure Principle* is not a simple adherence to the theories of his predecessors. Freud's use of principles and concepts from (psycho-)physics and other scientific disciplines (notably biology) shows a creative use of concepts in his metapsychology. *Beyond the Pleasure Principle* testifies to this. The two main versions of the text present different references to both principles from physics and biology that – as we will also see in the next chapters – are difficult to reconcile. This could be seen as merely a failure on Freud's part to produce a coherent and consistent theory, but it also and more importantly illustrates his active engagement in discussions and debates on fundamental concepts and paradigms in the natural and life sciences that, according to Freud, do not have a "rigid" and dogmatic character, but are in fact "constantly being altered in their content" (Freud 1915c: 117). It is hence the fundamental undecidedness of the natural sciences with regards to the definition of their conceptuality that provides Freud with an argument for the use of concepts and theories in an idiosyncratic way in his "speculations" that are informed by clinical and theoretical problems and questions.[16]

But this is not all there is to say about Freud's "speculative" references to physics and biology in what he calls his metapsychology. The regular appearance of the term "speculation" in *Beyond the Pleasure Principle* indicates that Freud is well aware of the limits of psychoanalysis and the distinction between empirical observations, on the one hand, and "auxiliary postulates" and "speculative assumptions", on the other (Freud 1915c: 124; 1920g: 7). For Freud, psychoanalysis is first and foremost a clinical practice of empirical observations that calls for metapsychological reflection in which concepts from other scientific fields are introduced and applied in order to establish principles, mechanisms and relations and interdependencies between observed phenomena. Freud adds that these concepts allow ideas to be pursued that seem far-fetched but may nevertheless provide insight into clinical phenomena (Freud 1920g: 59). Concepts such as forces or drives are "outside the scope of psychology", beyond the realm of the empirical (Freud 1915c: 123; 1940a: 158–159). They are theoretical "fictions" (Freud 1900a: 603) that are part of the "speculative superstructure of psychoanalysis, any portion of which can be abandoned or changed without loss or regret the moment its inadequacy has been proven" (Freud 1925d: 32–33). Concepts such as drive or apparatus are merely working hypotheses "to be retained only so long as it proves useful, and it will make little difference to the results of our work of description and classification" if they are replaced by other concepts (Freud 1915c: 124). Metapsychology is speculative in that it makes use of abstract ideas that as such have no empirical content and are not observable except through their effects. The drives, Freud writes, are only known through their aims, that is, through their manifestation in concrete satisfaction (Freud 1915c: 123). In other words, like his predecessors and contemporaries, Freud is aware of a problem that Kant had already clearly formulated: in the search for causes of observable facts in nature or life, one inevitably realizes that such causes can only be considered as concepts elaborated by reason. They are theoretical constructions that explain and organize facts. Seen from this perspective, Freud's "hypotheses", "speculations" and "fictions" are "beyond" the empirical observations. In this way, Freud is profoundly Kantian (Fulgencio 2005; Alfandary 2021).[17]

This Kantian character of Freud's view of the relation between the empirical and the metapsychological helps us to understand his references to the "dynamic" perspective of psychic life. In his *Metaphysische Anfangsgründe der Naturwissenschaft*, Kant (2004 [1786]) had started from the distinction between empirical knowledge, on the one hand, and systematizing conceptual "constructions" and "transcendental principles", on the other .[18] From here he proceeded to argue that, from a metaphysical point of view, the natural sciences are sciences that study movement (since "matter is that what is movable in space"). This includes inquiries not only into the quantities and qualities of matter, but also into the "moving forces". Here Kant distinguishes between "mechanics" (including chemical reactions) as movement caused by interactions between portions of matter, and "dynamics" as movement caused by "basic movement forces" of attraction and repulsion (as evidenced, for example, in gravity, elasticity or inertia) (Kant 2004). It is in the Kantian sense of the word that Freud applies the "dynamic point of view" to the systematic (speculative) reflection on psychic phenomena as effects of interacting – conflicting and cooperating – forces, tendencies and principles (see, for example, Freud 1900a: 610–611; 1916–1917a: 67, 374).

Pleasure principle and mastery

In a footnote in "Formulations on the Two Principles of Mental Functioning", Freud argues that in earliest infancy the primitive psychic apparatus is the "slave of the pleasure principle", seeking immediate satisfaction of needs (Freud 1911b: 220). The child reveals its felt unpleasure at an increase of excitation by ineffective screaming and beating. The child is dominated by the pleasure principle without being able to actively pursue and find satisfaction (pleasure). Later, when the older child can take cognizance of the reality of the external world, "it learns to employ these manifestations of discharge intentionally as methods of expressing its feelings". As a result, the reality principle (see below) is being set up, allowing the child to actively and intentionally engage with its environment (Freud 1911b: 219). In other words, in the course of life, the inefficient pleasure principle becomes an effective tendency.

In Chapter 2 of *Beyond the Pleasure Principle*, this train of thought is brought to the fore again; here Freud presents a detailed analysis of play observed in his own one-and-a-half-year-old grandson Ernst. The little child would repeatedly throw away a small wooden reel with a piece of string tied around it over the edge of his curtained cot and pull the reel by the string back into the cot again. These activities of throwing and pulling were accompanied by uttering o-o-o-o (*fort*) and *da*. Freud interprets this play as the repeated theatrical staging of an unpleasurable experience – the departure of the mother as the person who satisfies the child's needs. But this apparent meaning of the child's play does not lead Freud to affirm a mere oedipal interpretation in which the play signifies object relations and loss of an original unity with mother. On the contrary, the actual psychic work of the child consists in managing a surplus of excitation felt as unpleasure by binding these excitations to representations. The repetitions therefore cannot be reduced to oedipal schemata reproduced in substitute object relations, but must be seen as exhibiting a pulsional character while serving the pleasure principle.

In this play, the child seeks to "bind" the unpleasurable situation of increased excitation to representations of absent and present objects by repeatedly throwing and pulling back the reel attached to the string (Freud 1920g: 14–17). According to Freud, the great "cultural achievement" of this little child consists in its renunciation of immediate drive satisfaction (*Triebverzicht*) in a situation in which it was "overpowered" by momentary influxes of excitation felt as unpleasure, possibly even pain. In this situation, it sought to discharge the excitation through inadequate motor reflexes such as screaming and beating. Through the repetitive activities in the play, the little boy could work over the unpleasurable sensations, such that they could be psychically processed and yield pleasure as their final outcome. In this way, unpleasurable situations can become a subject to be "remembered" (*Gegenstand der Erinnerung machen*). That is to say, these experiences can eventually be recognized as experiences belonging to the past.[19]

The child's play marks a transition towards more efficient attempts at assuring pleasure by taking an active position motivated by a drive for mastery (*Bemächtigungstrieb*).[20] According to Freud, this drive for mastery at first "makes itself independent" (*sich unabhängig macht*) from sensations of pleasure and unpleasure. In order to be able to pursue its aim (satisfaction), this drive pressures the child to repeatedly stage an unpleasurable experience. The way in which play can lead to active mastery is by repeatedly allowing the unpleasurable and painful experience (*Erlebnis*) to be re-staged and to associate the experience with the representation of the coming and going of the mother. Repetition in play strengthens mastery over both the inner and outer world, and thus prepares for more assured pleasure (Freud 1920g: 35). In other words, the drive for mastery is the motor force in the production of pleasure at the expense of former inefficient attempts to eliminate unpleasure.[21] Seen in his way, play reveals the transition from inadequate attempts to immediately discharge excitation to zero, towards the situation in which unpleasure is tolerated as long as assured pleasure can be attained – in this case, repeatedly attained. Having said this, the very activity of throwing and pulling is also pleasurable, if we consider that muscular movements of contractions and relaxations produce pleasurable sensations (*Lustcharakter der Bewegungsempfindungen* – Freud 1905d: 202). Muscular activity – which is inherent in the form and function of the muscles – is pleasurable in itself and the drive for mastery seeks to repeat (re-experience or continue) this pleasure in relation to objects.

According to Freud, there are more reasons why the repetitions we find in the child's play are not "beyond" and "independent" of the pleasure principle. He notes that there may be a satisfaction of aggressive impulses involved (Freud 1920g: 16). He mentions impulses of revenge and hostility manifesting themselves in the child's activities. To be more precise, Freud hints at discharge of excitation in anger and annoyance: he observes his grandson angrily throwing toys on the floor. The mention of revenge and hostility in relation to anger and annoyance is telling for Freud's views on aggression: the lack of proper distinction between different forms of aggression, and the tendency, in his writings from *Three Essays*onwards, to reduce all aggressive impulses to a sadistic component of the sexual drives.[22] The references to hostility and revenge could easily be taken to suggest an oedipal interpretation of the child's anger: the objects thrown away would be replacements of actual significant persons. However, it is far from self-evident that rage and anger would be mere manifestations of sexualized drive impulses, and as such would aim at exercising power over an object (the mother) or doing away with a hated rival (father).[23] On the contrary: one could argue that rage and anger are first of all characterized by outbursts of excitation inadequately and senselessly directed at random objects in the way Breuer had described in the theoretical part of *Studies on Hysteria.* [24] Anger and rage illustrate the immediate motor discharge of increased excitation that "cannot be levelled out by associative activity" (Breuer & Freud 1895d: 201). Outbursts of anger or rage are not informed and guided by adequate ideas and representations; this is what explains their manifestation in inexpedient screaming and beating. A person is overwhelmed by a sudden influx of amounts of excitation, and the immediate automatic reaction is that of discharge. Such outbursts thus only "serve the tendency 'to keep the [intra-]cerebral excitation constant'" (Breuer & Freud 1895d: 202).[25] Rage produces immediate relief, which is felt as pleasure. Freud suggests that this pleasure at immediate discharge of excitation is a motive for repeating the unpleasurable situation associated with the absence of the mother. The pleasure at the discharge of excitation in anger thus contributes to the process of mastering unpleasurable sensations. Consequently, the repetitive activities will allow the child to develop more efficient anger management when it can actively direct aggressive impulses from random objects to more specific – oedipal – objects. Again, play is an oedipal staging of what essentially comes down to drive management.

The transition from immediate and inadequate discharge of excitation towards more efficient anger management is an aspect of the child's play in which several achievements are attained. First, there is toleration of unpleasure in a situation in which the inefficient pleasure principle dominates psychic life. Second, there is the binding of excitation to representations in the psychic apparatus. Third, there is the first displacement of anger towards objects instead of being overwhelmed by excitation resulting in inexpedient screaming and beating.[26] Fourth, the child's play shows a certain mastery over external circumstances and – more importantly – over internal excitations in such a way that pleasure can be produced. And, fifth, through play, the child transforms an actual unpleasurable experience into a memory of past events.

The child's play illustrates the primal function of the psychic apparatus – namely that of mastering stimuli (*Reizbewältigung*) that threaten to overpower and distress the helpless and defenceless child (compare Freud 1914c: 85; 1915c: 120). The drive for mastery is the motive force not only for actively gaining control over objects in the child's environment, but also, and more so, for mastering the drive stimuli that threaten to overwhelm the psychic apparatus from the inside. In this context, *bemächtigen* and *bewältigen* indicate two analogous active processes through which the child is able to produce pleasure at and through its own activities of binding drive energy to representations of presence and absence of significant objects, and learning to distinguish between present and past.

Freely mobile and bound processes

It has been argued (Laplanche & Pontalis 1973: 218–219; Fong 2016: 24ff.) that the child's attempts to actively engage with reality point to first attempts at gaining control over objects and circumstances. Moreover, this active engagement can be associated with what Freud calls "binding" (*Bindung*) (Freud 1920g: 31–33). Through play, the child can inhibit and master amounts of excitation overpowering the psychic apparatus by binding them to concrete and more stable representations in space and time – concrete, the present and absent mother and father. Freud confirms this suggestion in more general statements in the opening passages of Chapter 5 of *Beyond the Pleasure Principle*:

> Since all drive impulses [*Triebregungen*] have the unconscious systems as their point of impact, it is hardly an innovation to say that they obey the primary process. Again, it is easy to identify the primary psychical process with Breuer's freely mobile cathexis [*frei bewegliche Besetzung*] and the secondary process with changes in his bound or tonic cathexis [*gebundene oder tonische Besetzung*]. If so, it would be the task of the higher strata of the mental apparatus to bind [*binden*] the drive excitation reaching the primary process. A failure to effect this binding [*Bindung*] would provoke a disturbance analogous to a traumatic neurosis; and only after the binding has been accomplished would it be possible for the dominance of the pleasure principle (and of its modification, the reality principle) to proceed unhindered. Till then the other task of the mental apparatus, the task of mastering or binding excitations [*die Erregung zu bewältigen oder zu binden*], would have precedence – not, indeed, in opposition to the pleasure principle, but independently of it and to some extent in disregard of it.
>
> (Freud 1920g: 34–35)

The notion of the binding of free mobile cathexis into bound cathexis is not new in Freud's work. We already find this idea in the 1895 "Project for a Scientific Psychology" in the context of his discussions of the conditions for the "introduction of the ego" and the "secondary process". Starting points are, first, "the conception of neuronal excitation as quantity [of energy, HW] in a state of flow", which Freud also refers to as "*Q*" (Freud 1950c: 296), and, second, the neuronal reception and discharge of this quantity.[27] From this starting point – and guided by an existing psycho-physicist literature – he sets out to inquire into the conditions for psychic organization. According to Freud, the very fact of irritability and excitability of "surfaces" and tissues poses problems for living beings, and sets in motion processes of response with the aim of resolving the problem of destabilizing and modifying life-threatening stimuli. The psychic organization results from repeated (*wiederholte*) responses to the problem of irritability.[28] In this context, Freud points to the role of the ego as "inhibiting" and slowing down the quantities of inflowing energy with the aim of efficient discharge. For Freud, this ego is nothing but "the totality of the ψ cathexes". That is to say, it constitutes the totality or "complex"[29] of stable contact barriers (*Kontaktschranken*), permanent traces (*dauernde Spuren*), side cathexes (*Seitenbesetzungen*), neural pathways (*Wege*) and facilitations (*Bahnungen*), which the excitations will follow before being discharged. The term ego describes a certain organization and management of excitations and tensions (produced by stimuli) such that these can be received and arranged before being converted or discharged (Freud 1950c: 296ff, 323, 369).

How is this ego able to organize and stabilize cathexes? According to Freud, transient perception does not have lasting effects on psychic organization; in fact, if the psychic apparatus were to merely consist of the function of perception, it would remain nothing but an *ad hoc* reflex apparatus. The capacity to organize and stabilize incoming excitations depends on the ego's ability to expect and anticipate an influx of stimuli. The ego's "attention" (*Aufmerksamkeit*), defined as a "state of expectation" (*Erwartungszustand*), allows the ego to anticipate incoming amounts of excitation. Such attention and anticipation, Freud argues, are based on the fact that the psychic apparatus – more specifically, impermeable neurons loaded with resistance that do not easily allow energy to pass through – can store enduring and lasting impressions such that the apparatus becomes permanently modified. This capacity to store impressions is assigned to memory (*Gedächtnis*). Memory is to be understood as the storage of information about past situations and experiences, which enables humans to learn what to expect and anticipate. Whether impressions are stored as memories is based mainly on the "magnitude" of the impression (*Größe des Eindruckes*) and the "frequency" with which the same impression is "repeated" (*Häufigkeit der Wiederholung*). Memorizing equals a process of learning. Anticipation and expectation are seen as a capacity that the ego will "biologically acquire" through "education" (*Erziehung*) and "development" – notably through repeated confrontations with sources of unpleasure (Freud 1950c: 300, 324, 360–361, 369–370). Here, Freud appears to be profoundly Humean when assuming that impressions are not organized according to *a priori* categories (Kant) but only lead to knowledge of causal relations through repetition (or "constant conjunction") of a series of identical observations (Hume 1777: 1.3.6).

In "Project for a Scientific Psychology", this process of transforming free mobile cathexes into more stable organized cathexes is referred to as a process of "binding" (Freud 1950c: 395); its opposite is "unbinding" (*Entbindung*), that is, the sudden "release" of energy insisting on discharge (Laplanche & Pontalis 1973: 51). Freud describes this process in physicist and biological terms, while at the same arguing that it is linked to modes of attention, expectation, thought and judgement (Freud 1950c: 368–369). Through these psychic activities and the repetitive involvement in processes of binding, a person becomes increasingly adept at organizing incoming amounts of excitation in stable networks of "ideas", and increasingly efficient in discharging excitation at the proper moment in time and occasion (Freud 1950c: 325).[30]

In the fourth chapter of *Beyond the Pleasure Principle*, Freud elaborates on the psychic processes involved in managing external and internal stimuli (excitations). He argues that notably in more advanced organisms, such as human beings, there is no effective protective shield against, and hence no automatic regulation of, amounts of internal excitation that "extend into the higher system directly and in undiminished amount" (Freud 1920g: 29), thus giving rise to feelings of unpleasure. In this context, Freud introduces the distinction between "quiescent" ("bound") and "mobile" ("free") energy (Freud 1920g: 26, 34), which Breuer had pioneered in the theoretical part which he had contributed to *Studies on Hysteria* (Breuer & Freud 1895d: 194 n.),[31] and which Freud used in his seventh metapsychological chapter of his *Interpretation of Dreams* (Freud 1900a: 599ff). Freud identifies this "mobile energy" (*frei bewegliche Besetzung*) with the primary process that dominates unconscious processes – as he had already done in "Project". In the unconscious, energy can freely pass from one representation to another, thus creating associations that appear senseless in waking life. This is what becomes manifest in dreams (and hallucinations). Dreams show that in the unconscious systems, "cathexes can easily be completely transferred, displaced and condensed" (Freud 1920g: 34). Any representation can pass its cathectic energy to one or more other representations, or different representations can concentrate their cathectic energy in a single representation. These unconscious processes do not in any way consider the reality and the prevailing order such as, for example, the time sequence or spatial structure. This primary process aims only at achieving satisfaction at any cost, as quickly and directly as possible and eventually in a hallucinatory way (Freud 1920g: 32).

Freud distinguishes the primary process from the secondary process that characterizes (pre-)consciousness. In the secondary process, the mobile flow of energy is "bound" and mediated in a more stable network of representations that take into account the realities of time and space.[32] This latter aspect Freud had already explored in "Formulations on the Two Principles of Mental Functioning": "the conversion of freely displaceable cathexes into 'bound' cathexes" is a necessary step in the restraint upon motor discharge and the development of psychic capacities (judging, remembering, thinking), taking into account the significance of external reality (Freud 1911b: 220–221). According to Freud, this binding of energy to representations within stable spatial and temporal coordinates can be seen as condition for the "dominance of the pleasure principle (and its modification, the reality principle)" (Freud 1920g: 35).[33] The child's play is Freud's example of such process of binding. Repetition in play presents an effective way of processing the influx of drive stimuli that threaten to overwhelm and paralyze the higher psychic functions. Play illustrates the psychical activity of binding drive stimuli to representations of appearing and disappearing objects.

It is a striking fact that several of the initial ideas in "Project" are carried over into *Beyond the Pleasure Principle*. We know that Freud abandoned his neurological "Project" and decided against its publication, so it is puzzling why so many theoretical elements from that text return in *Beyond the Pleasure Principle* – notably the inquiries into the conditions of psychic life and its elementary structures and principles. How can we understand this return of concepts and ideas first systematically addressed in "Project"? The reasons for the abandonment of the "Project" have been discussed at length by Sulloway (1979: 118–131) and others,[34] and provide clues for an answer. If the "Project" can be seen as an attempt to provide insight into the constitutional (here, neurophysiological) factors through which clinical phenomena could be explained or understood, it failed to provide answers to the most pressing problems Freud would be concerned with in the years to come: a theory of (organic) repression, the question of the choice of neuroses, and the importance and characteristics of sexuality. *Three Essays* and its inquiries in the physiological processes defining sexuality is the first major result of this line of research in which questions concerning the conditions of psychic life (secondary processes, consciousness, ego-functions) are hardly considered. It is only in *Beyond the Pleasure Principle* and the discussion of clinical phenomena, such as the compulsion to repeat (in traumatic neuroses), that Freud is once again confronted with questions and problems that demand fundamental reflection on the conditions of psychic life. It is in this context that he returns to clinical and theoretical insights that pre-date his attempts to develop the sexual aetiology of the psychopathologies. The question of the "beyond" of the pleasure principle takes him back to ideas developed "before" the theory of sexuality and the related first drive theory of 1905.

The pleasure principle and the reality principle

The idea that the dominance of the pleasure principle is related to the secondary process may come as a surprise, considering that, in the opening chapter of *Beyond the Pleasure Principle*, Freud had made the following remarks:

> We know that the pleasure principle is proper to a *primary* method of working on the part of the mental apparatus, but that, from the point of view of the self-preservation of the organism among the difficulties of the external world, it is from the very outset inefficient and even highly dangerous.
>
> (Freud 1920g: 10; Freud's italics)

This reference to the primary process is in line with what we have said so far. Freud starts from the assumption that the psychic apparatus is automatically regulated by the pleasure principle. It seeks the discharge of tension. This would be the case for both primary and secondary processes (compare Freud 1900a: 597ff.). But the analyses of the dreams of traumatic neurotic patients repeating highly unpleasurable situations (see Chapter 2) lead Freud to question this assumption. It would appear that there first has to be some psychic activity that creates the possibility for the regulation of psychic life by the pleasure principle. This leads Freud to associate the "dominance" of the pleasure principle with its effectiveness. In other words, Freud starts to make a distinction between a primary process characterized by the psychic apparatus being passively overwhelmed by the influx of amounts of drive energy and excitation, on the one hand, and a secondary process regulated by the active and efficient discharge of excitation, on the other. The "dominance" of the pleasure principle now results from the process of binding that distinguishes between the two processes.

This raises the question as to whether and how the (dominance of the) pleasure principle can and must be distinguished from the reality principle. In order to answer this question, we would need to briefly return to the text in which Freud had introduced the concept of the reality principle. We have already seen that Freud (in "Formulations on the Two Principles of Mental Functioning") takes up an evolutionary perspective that can also be detected in earlier writings, such as "Project". In the most primitive psychic apparatus, the pleasure principle merely aims at withdrawing from any external stimulus that arouses unpleasure. The introduction of the concept of the pleasure principle in "Formulations on the Two Principles of Mental Functioning" resulted from thinking through the kind of modifications (adaptations) one finds in higher organisms such as human beings. Higher organisms develop through an increasingly pro-active engagement with their environment. The primitive processes of discharge of excitation are converted into actions aimed at influencing and controlling the external world in such a way that it will provide an assured pleasure. In "Formulations", Freud does not further elaborate on the distinction between a primitive unpleasure principle and a more advanced pleasure principle in order to describe the two tendencies; instead, he introduces a new distinction: pleasure principle and reality principle. For Freud, this reality principle does not depose the pleasure principle but safeguards it (Freud 1911c: 223).

In *Beyond the Pleasure Principle*, this train of thought is confirmed. The main motive for the replacement of the pleasure principle by the reality principle is given with the former's inefficiency and the difficulties faced by human beings in interaction with the external world. Freud explains:

> This reality principle does not abandon [*aufzugeben*] the intention of ultimately obtaining pleasure, but it nevertheless demands and carries

> into effect the postponement [*Aufschub*] of satisfaction, the abandonment of a number of possibilities of gaining satisfaction and the temporary toleration of unpleasure as a step on the long indirect road [*auf den langen Umwege*] to pleasure.
>
> (Freud 1920g: 10)

The reality principle, in which the pleasure principle is safeguarded, describes the more efficient way to pursue and assure pleasure while taking account of the material and cultural environment. In the opening passages of Chapter 5, Freud is now telling us that it is only after the binding of drive energy to representations is accomplished that efficient regulation of psychic life by the pleasure principle is possible. But does binding not imply the consideration of external reality? The binding of energy to representations in space and time – and the example of the child's play – suggest as much. In other words, Freud implicitly tends to equate the (dominance of the) pleasure principle with the reality principle. The dominance of the pleasure principle indicates the efficacy of the ego in defending itself against drive impulses and using drive energy for "cultural achievements" (compare Freud 1920g: 15).

Beyond the pleasure principle?

These trains of thought are also relevant in view of the question of the "beyond" of the pleasure principle. If the dominance of the pleasure principle and the reality principle are associated with the secondary process, it appears that the question of the "beyond" can be answered with reference to the primary process and unbound drive energy. Beyond the pleasure principle we would find unbound drive energy and the process of its binding. Is this indeed the conclusion from the 1919 edition of *Beyond the Pleasure Principle*? As we will see in our discussion of the drive theory (see Chapter 4), the fact that Freud defines all drives as "conservative" and as urges seeking to "return to the quiescence of the inorganic" leads him to conclude that the relation between the drive impulses and the pleasure principle – or between primary and secondary processes – is not a matter of opposing systems or inner conflict (Freud 1920g: 62). On the contrary, it seems that the two processes are characterized by two variations of the same principle of the reduction of tension: As tendency, the pleasure principle stands in the service of the "function" of all drives. Freud refers to this endeavour towards the elimination of tension by coining a new concept – that of "pleasure drive" (*Lusttrieb*) (Freud 2013: 91; 2024: 78). There is continuity between the function of the pleasure drive (drive for pleasure) and the tendency of the pleasure principle.[35] This notion of the "pleasure drive", introduced in the 1919 version of the text but deleted from the 1920 published edition, is the radical consequence drawn from the idea that "the aim of all life is death" and thus at zero tension (Freud 1920g: 38).

According to Freud, "this raises the question of whether feelings of pleasure and unpleasure can be produced equally from bound and from unbound excitatory processes" (Freud 1920g: 63). His answer to this question is that feelings of pleasure and unpleasure do not depend on the process of binding and the regulation of psychic life by the pleasure principle. These feelings do not exclusively correspond to the pleasure principle's regulations in the secondary process. Feelings of pleasure and unpleasure are also produced in the primary process. Here, they are "far more intense" and "direct". While the pleasure drive seeks the elimination of tension (excitation), the primary process is further characterized by unanticipated "frequent interruptions" (*häufige Durchbrüche*) of fresh amounts of stimuli that enter the psychic apparatus and produce feelings of unpleasure. In the primary process, all tension and excitation has an interruptive and uninhibited character, so the "feeling of tension" (*Spannungsempfindung*) is always more intense. It is only in the secondary process that tension and unpleasure are anticipated and mastered. In the 1919 version of the text, Freud concludes:

> Perhaps the so-called feelings of tension that our consciousness mediates internally, along with feelings of pleasure and unpleasure, should actually be attributed to the bound processes, whereas the direct feelings of pleasure and unpleasure should be attributed to the unbound processes and the processes of discharge. Perhaps the occurrence of pleasurable and unpleasurable tension will be rendered more comprehensible to us by means of this distinction. I consider it superfluous to try to excuse either the timidity or the uncertainty of these speculations. Whoever wishes to isolate the actuality behind them should turn his attention to the phenomenon of the compulsion to repeat.
>
> (Freud 2024: 79)[36]

In the 1920 version of the text, this passage is deleted and replaced by a passage that phrases similar speculations in the form of questions.[37] Also, the two references to the "pleasure drive" are deleted and – in the second reference – replaced by "struggle for pleasure" (*Luststreben* – striving for pleasure). In both the 1919 and 1920 passage on the feelings of tension and the feelings of unpleasure and pleasure, Freud suggests that it is only in the secondary process that tension is tamed (*gebändigt*), actively processed, and mastered such that pleasure is assured (reality principle).

The "speculations" on the pleasure drive in relation to the pleasure principle reveal a fundamental problem Freud is facing in the final chapter of the 1919 version of *Beyond the Pleasure Principle.* The prioritization of the "economic point of view", from the first paragraphs of the text onwards, leads Freud to conceptualize the "dynamic" factor – the forces that produce movement – in economic terms. But if it is true that the "pleasure drive" governs the primary process, can one still maintain that the drives are forces producing internal unpleasurable tensions that need to be discharged? Freud suggest something to this effect when he writes: "The pleasure drive, which governs all psychical life, is in this respect no different from the other organic drives, which somatic excitation conveys to the psychical" (Freud 2024: 78). The reference to "other organic drives" (*andere organische Triebe*) suggests that Freud seeks to maintain the idea that there must be drives that produce fresh tension and excitation felt as (intense) unpleasure. But what are these organic drives if, as Freud argues in the previous chapter of the 1919 edition of the text, all drives are conservative and aim at the elimination of tension? This question remains unanswered in the 1919 version of the text.

And there is another complicating problem. We recall that in the 1919 version of the text, tension in the primary process is felt as unpleasure; discharge is felt as pleasure. This seems to leave no room for the possibility of drives producing pleasurable tension. And yet, in *Three Essays* and elsewhere, Freud had argued that the sexual drives can find satisfaction at pleasurable tension – notably in rhythmically repeated autoerotic activities and fore-pleasure. Doesn't Freud disregard the fact that drives can produce pleasurable tensions?[38]

Final remarks

From "Project for a Scientific Psychology" onwards, Freud emphasizes that the main task of the psychic apparatus is to manage the influx of drive impulses and stimuli because of the associated feelings of unpleasure. The problem is not the quantities of impulses and stimuli as such, but the unpleasurable feelings generated by the excessiveness and suddenness of "interruptions". The psychic apparatus seeks pleasure. But what exactly is pleasure? Is it the absence of all tension and excitation? Is it a specific tension or excitation produced by sexual processes (Freud 1905d: 209)? If so, what then is the difference between sexual and non-sexual tension or excitation? In the two main versions of *Beyond the Pleasure Principles* Freud's reflections on these questions can be clearly distinguished. His focus on the traumatic neuroses in the 1919 version of text lead him to consider only increases of highly unpleasurable amounts of drive energy that have no apparent relation to pleasurable sexual excitation. Pleasure at excitation is irrelevant in Freud's discussion of these neuroses. The traumatic neuroses are "beyond" the sexual. But things change in the second version of the text when he introduces the life drives and with it the possibility of pleasurable sexual tension and excitation. It is in this context that Freud will explicitly address the question whether the traumatic neuroses originate from an unexpected strong increase of sexual excitation, such that this excitation is no longer felt as pleasurable. We will further discuss this in Chapter 2.

Notes

1 The italics in this quotation are in *The Standard Edition of the Complete Psychological Works* of Sigmund Freud but not in the German text. I use the *Studienausgabe* (Fischer Verlag, Frankfurt) of Freud's works for the references to the original texts in German (Freud 1969–1975).

2 We note here that in 1893 Freud writes – very much in line with Joseph Breuer's views, among others – that "the nervous system endeavours to keep constant something in its functional relations that we may describe as the 'sum of excitations'" (Freud 1940d: 153). In other texts from the 1890s, such as "Draft D" and "Draft K", we also find references to fundamental tendencies in psychic life such as "the law of constancy" (Freud 1985c: 187, 221). In other words, even in these early writings, we see Freud formulating and applying different principles: constancy and inertia.

3 In "On the Grounds for Detaching a Particular Syndrome from Neurasthenia under the Description 'Anxiety Neurosis'" (1895), that is, before the introduction of the concept of drive in his theories, Freud had already defined endogenous excitation (*endogene Erregung*) as "constant force" (Freud 1895b: 112).

4 This seems to undermine the economic perspective on the pleasure principle, as this statement appears to imply that the neurotic unpleasure results from repressed drives seeking satisfaction, that is to say, the diminution of excitation. But why exactly would such drive satisfaction be contrary to the pleasure principle? Freud admits that he is confronted here with the puzzling and as yet unanswered question as to how repression turns "a possibility of pleasure into a source of unpleasure" (see also Fletcher 2013: 287–288).

5 Compare Freud's definition of the "drive" in the first edition of *Three Essays*:

> In addition to a 'drive', which is not itself sexual and which has its source in motor impulses, we can discern in the partial drives a contribution from an organ receiving stimuli (e.g., the skin, the mucous membrane, or a sense organ). An organ of this kind will be described in this connection as an 'erogenous zone' – as being the organ whose excitation lends the drive a sexual character.
>
> (Freud 1905d: 168; 2016: 29)

Note that in this first definition of the concept of "drive", the drive can only be said to have a sexual character through the excitation of an erogenous zone. It is only through such excitation that a "force" can be said to be "sexual".

6 For a more detailed and thorough reading of *Three Essays*, see Van Haute & Westerink (2021).

7 Even in earlier key texts we find Freud bringing together perspectives from physiology (physics) and biology (e.g., Freud 1905d; 1915c; 1950c). On this issue in relation to *Beyond the Pleasure Principle*, see also May (2024).

8 The consummation of energy through food intake in particular stands in the service of the conservation of energy in an organism that uses and discharges energy in activities.

9 In this context, Fechner argues that his principle of the tendency towards stability is a reformulation of Helmholtz's first law of thermodynamics (principle of energy conservation). In fact, he presents his ideas as a supplement to this law which he conceives as expressing the tendency towards more stable forms in which energy is conserved (Fechner 1873: 34–35). That is why this tendency towards stability cannot be interpreted as a reformulation of the second law of thermodynamics, i.e., the law of entropy. After all, this law specifies that within a closed system all energy will dissipate.

10 See, among others, Sulloway (1979), Gödde (1999), Simanke (2020), Tran The et al. (2020) and Seeck (2021).

11 Strictly speaking, the concept of inertia can be traced as least as far back as Newtonian physics and the law of inertia stating that an object remains at rest or in motion at a constant speed unless impressed by an external force. We should note here that the Freudian notion of "psychical inertia" is at odds with the Newtonian concept: in Freud's view, inertia indicates the tendency towards zero tension (Macdonald 2024).

12 Freud's references to Fechner include one in which he credits the man who had first coined the concept of *Lustprinzip*. Fechner introduced this concept in an 1846 text, *Über das höchste Gut* (Willner 2024a: 237).

13 In "*An Autobiographical Study*", Freud states that he had always been open to Fechner's ideas and "followed that thinker upon many important points" (Freud 1925d: 59).

14 Despite there being no copy in Freud's personal library, Sigmund Exner's (1894) *Entwurf zu einer physiologischen Erklärung von psychischen Erscheinungen* should be mentioned here to underscore the importance of psycho-physicist studies in the Viennese context. In his *Entwurf*, Exner attempts to show that all psychic phenomena, including the higher functions such as consciousness, can be explained by the continuous state of irritability (*Erregungszustände*) of the nervous system (Exner 1894: 3). This aim shows remarkable parallels with Freud's "Project".

15 Another scholar in this field referenced by Freud is Theodor Lipps. Freud's copies of his *Grundtatsachen des Seelenlebens* (1883) and *Komik und Humor* (1898) include many marginal markings and underscores, notably in the chapters on fundamental psychological principles such as psychic force and psychic energy, excitation, pleasure and unpleasure, and psychic associations and representations (Lipps 1883; 1898; Freud 1985c: 324–325; Davies & Fichtner 2006).

16 An example: at first sight, it may seem that Freud's theory of the drives as urges aiming at an inanimate state (Freud 1920g: 38) is congruent with Fechner's principle of stability (see, e.g., Sulloway 1979: 406). Yet, Fechner does not define stability in terms of a "return" to an original state. He explicitly rejects such a possibility when arguing that any theory asserting that organic life originates from inorganic matter is contrary to the law of energy conservation (Fechner 1873: 41). In fact, in his "cosmorganic" universe, there is no such thing as inanimate matter. Inherent to all matter are movement, the tendency to self-preservation and "processes of consciousness" (Fechner 1873: 96, 99; also Willner 2024a: 238–239).

17 When Freud argues that psychoanalysis is an "empirical science" and should be sharply distinguished from philosophies as "systems" that seek to grasp the universe as a whole from a few basic concepts (Freud 1923a: 253–254), he does not dismiss Kant and hence does not align himself with Hume's scepticism. What Freud criticizes in philosophy is what he refers to as "completed" theories that leave no room for correction or modification. What characterizes Freud's work is the fact that the variety of clinical observations (related to the variety of psychopathologies and individual cases) give rise to a variety of "speculations" and hypotheses that question or undermine previous ones.

18 In his famous lectures, *Über die Grenzen des Naturerkennens: Die sieben Welträtsel* from 1872 and 1880, Émil du Bois-Reymond – one of Freud's admired teachers – takes his starting point in Kant's text on the natural sciences in order to argue against an unrestricted epistemological optimism in the natural sciences. When it comes to questions, such as the essence of or relation between matter and force, mind and body, or the source and cause of movement and sensations, the scientist is confronted with the limits of his empirical observations and knowledge (du Bois-Reymond 1891).

19 I will return to this issue of remembering as assigning experiences to the past in Chapter 2.

20 This concept of the drive for mastery had first been introduced in *Three Essays on the Theory of Sexuality* where it is presented as an original non-sexual drive that

manifests itself in muscular activity and violent behaviour towards objects (animals, playmates) (Freud 1905d: 188, 193; Van Haute & Westerink 2021: 52, 66). In *Beyond the Pleasure Principle* these aspects of the drive for mastery are mentioned again: the muscular activities of throwing and pulling; the hostility towards and revenge at the absent mother. For Freud, there is no doubt that both, the muscular activities and the expression of hostility, are pleasurable sensations. In later texts, he regards the drive for mastery as a manifestation of the death drives turned towards external objects, finding satisfaction in their destruction (Freud 1924c: 163).

21 On this issue, compare also Fong (2016: 18–19, 24–26).

22 Notably in the case study of the Rat Man, Freud argues that his patient's outbursts of anger must be interpreted in terms of hatred of the father, and that this hatred can be traced back to the sadistic component of the sexual drives. For Freud, all aggression is sexual aggression, and all aggression is bound to representations and aimed at objects. On Freud's views of aggression, see Van Haute and Geyskens (2013) and Westerink (2015).

23 If indeed the child discharges excitation in rage, the mastery we find in the child's play cannot self-evidently be interpreted as attempts at violently dominating objects or as expression of sadistic cruelty. Such an interpretation – based on Laplanche and Pontalis' association of *Bemächtigung* and *Bewältigung* – has been put forward by Derrida in *The Post Card.* Derrida interprets the latter in terms of the first, which leads him to conclude that both concepts indicate the violent exercise of power within a network of objects. Hence, there would be a "drive for power" that is always already aimed to dominate objects (Derrida 1987: 404–405; Fong 2016: 148 n.). According to Derrida, the idea of a desire for power as that which propels the drives forward would bring Freud very close to Nietzsche's concept of the "will to power". We should note, however, that this will to power as a will "to master something" through struggle does not have a libidinal character and is not aimed at pleasure (Nietzsche 1901: 342).

24 The reason for introducing Breuer here is that Freud himself refers to Breuer's distinction between "quiescent (or bound) and mobile cathectic energy in the elements of the psychical systems", that is, between a "freely flowing cathexis that presses on towards discharge and a quiescent cathexis" (Freud 1920g: 26–27, 31). Breuer's elaborations of anger and rage are to be understood in the context of his theoretical formulations of the psychic apparatus' attempts at managing the influx of excitations.

25 From Breuer's elaborations on the topic of anger, we can deduce another motive for Freud paying attention to the relative efficient mastery of excitation that one finds in the child's play. Breuer opposes the idea of anger management through "deeds and words" that may level out the increase of excitation and establish psychical equilibrium with the vicissitudes of fright. Fright is characterized by the paralyzing of both movements (motor reflexes) and associations (representations). In fright, excitation increases without it being employed in associative or motor activities. If the excitations are not gradually levelled out, traumatic neurosis may result (Breuer & Freud 1895d: 202–203).

26 That such can be seen as "cultural achievement" is something Freud had already explored in his study on Michelangelo's Moses statue. In that text Freud argues that the statue captures the moment of Moses' contained anger. It thus shows that Moses is able to control his anger, avoiding the direct outburst of rage against his people (Freud 1914b).

27 Similar ideas can be found in the 1895 text, "On the Grounds for Detaching a Particular Syndrome from Neurasthenia under the Description 'Anxiety Neurosis'" (Freud 1895b: 93). On the notion of "binding" and "unbinding" (release of pleasure/unpleasure), see Laplanche and Pontalis (1973: 50–51).

28 The idea that irritability and excitability (*Erregbarheit*), i.e., the capacities to receive and respond to stimuli, are fundamental characteristics of organic life can be traced back to early Romantic medicine and the critique of mechanical explanations of change and movement. Excitability is an inner capacity for activity and development (that nevertheless requires stimulation from the outside).

29 The term "complex" seems to be borrowed from Ernst Mach who frequently mentions "complexes of elements" (*Complex von Elementen*), indicating a complex of sensations, perceptions, and memories that produce further psychic responses and developments (Mach 1886).

30 It is beyond the scope of my reading of *Beyond the Pleasure Principle* to provide a detailed analysis of all theoretical aspects of this text that find their first articulations in "Project". Such study would no doubt reveal many similarities, notably with regards to the processing of excitations, the pleasure principle, the primary and secondary processes, the binding of excitations to representations and the development of ego-functions through repetition. Since, however, "Project" was never published during Freud's lifetime, there are obviously no explicit references to this text in *Beyond the Pleasure Principle.*

31 In fact, Breuer does not make a distinction between unbound and bound energy. Breuer argues that the nerve cells are in a constant state of excitation/tension (equilibrium) that can also be described in terms of "free" or "tonic" energy which "lies quiescent in the chemical substance of the cell". When disturbed, this produces a "form of kinetic energy" – a term borrowed from Helmholtz – which will be discharged in motor activities. Freud replaces Breuer's quiescent tonic energy with "freely mobile" energy and thus reverses the relation between quiescent and mobile energy. This reversal shows that Freud reasons from the assumption of a certain amount of energy that needs to be discharged, whereas Breuer starts from the idea that the nervous apparatus always seeks to maintain constancy. On this issue, see Holt (1962).

32 In this context, Freud refers to Immanuel Kant's a priori "forms of thought" (categories) that organize incoming perceptions. Freud links these forms of thought, including those of space and time, with the structuring and binding of unconscious representations in the (pre-)conscious system. According to Freud, these a priori forms of thought are suspended, as it were, in the unconscious (Freud 1920g: 28).

33 From binding as a condition for the pleasure principle, Deleuze draws the conclusion that Eros merges as the foundation of the pleasure principle (Deleuze 1991: 113). This reading is not self-evident when we consider the fact of two versions of *Beyond the Pleasure Principle.* In the 1919 version, Freud writes about the binding of drives to representations, whereas, in the 1920 version, he mentions the libidinal binding between cells, organs, etc., which includes the production of excitation (contrary to the aims of the pleasure principle).

34 See also, more recently, Bergo (2025).

35 To my knowledge, this is the only mention of the "pleasure drive" in Freud's writings.

36 Freud was not satisfied with this "speculation"; he penned a hand-written and unfinished formulation which was crossed out in turn and was not integrated into the 1920 edition:

> There is a competing view, however, which would aim to correlate feelings of tension with the absolute quantity and level of cathected energy, while correlating pleasure and unpleasure with changes in quantity over time. The two possibilities are not compatible with each other and…
>
> (Freud 2024: 79–80)

37 According to Freud:

> Our consciousness communicates to us feelings from within not only of pleasure and unpleasure but also of a peculiar tension which in its turn can be either pleasurable or unpleasurable. Should the difference between these feelings enable us to distinguish between bound and unbound processes of energy? or is the feeling of tension to be related to the absolute magnitude, or perhaps to the level, of the cathexis, while the pleasure and unpleasure series indicates a change in the magnitude of the cathexis within a given unit of time?
>
> (Freud 1920g: 63)

38 In "The Economic Problem of Masochism", Freud explicitly admits that he had overlooked the fact that "there are pleasurable tensions and unpleasurable relaxations of tension" and that sexual excitation is the most striking example of "a pleasurable increase of stimulus". Hence, it was not enough to refer to an increase or a decrease of quantities of excitation as the criteria for the definitions of pleasure and unpleasure. A qualitative factor would also have to be taken into account, more specifically "the rhythm, the temporal sequence of changes, rises and falls in the quantity of stimulus" (Freud 1924c: 160). According to Freud, this might lead to the conclusion that the principle of discharge of tension and excitation which eventually culminated in the notion that "the aim of all life is death" would have to be complemented with a revised theory of the pleasure principle. Such a theory would have to take into account the fact that drives can find satisfaction in pleasurable rhythmically repeated excitations.

Chapter 2

Traumatic neuroses and repetition

Kriegsneurosen as traumatic neuroses

The second chapter of *Beyond the Pleasure Principle* starts with a clinical phenomenon that seems to falsify the premise of the "automatic regulation" of psychic life through the pleasure principle. The First World War had confronted Freud and his followers with "puzzling disorders" that posed a challenge for psychoanalysis – both clinically and theoretically: the war neuroses (Freud 1919d: 207). Patients suffering from severe war neuroses compulsively repeat their traumatic experiences "which include no possibility of pleasure" (Freud 1920g: 20). In these war neuroses, one finds patients returning to highly disturbing, frightening traumatic situations (Freud 1920g: 13). But how to explain such compulsion to repeat (*Wiederholungszwang*) highly unpleasurable situations if the psychic apparatus is supposed to automatically seek pleasure? Are there other principles or forces at work "beyond" the pleasure principle? If so, what would be the consequences for psychoanalytic theory?

In an introductory lecture on fixation to traumas, Freud had already briefly referred to these war neuroses. It appears self-evident for him that "the illnesses which are being produced with special frequency precisely at the present time by the war" can be seen as "traumatic neuroses" (Freud 1916–1917a: 274). This is the starting point for further explorations in the following years (Freud 1919d: 209; 1920g: 12). For Freud, these neuroses are similar to the phenomena that the German neurologist Hermann Oppenheim had first identified in the 1880s in terms of a pathology arising from "railway collisions and other alarming accidents involving fatal risks" (Freud 1916–1917a: 274). According to Freud, these traumatic neuroses are "in essence" not the same as the psychoneuroses psychoanalysis had studied and theorized. He expresses his hope that psychoanalysis will, in the near future, succeed in bringing the traumatic neuroses "into harmony with our views". He expects psychoanalysis to provide a full understanding of these traumatic neuroses from the perspective of the aetiology of the psychoneuroses. For now, Freud argues, it is enough to realize a few aspects common to the two types of neuroses, namely the hysteriform symptoms that admit of analysis, and the significance of fixation to the

DOI: 10.4324/9781003680413-2

moment of the traumatic accident. That traumatic-neurotic patients repeat the traumatic situation (Freud 1916–1917a: 274–275) appears to be analogous to the way in which psychoneurotic patients are fixated "to a particular portion of their past, as though they could not manage to free themselves from it" (Freud 1916–1917a: 273). What we would thus, at first sight, find in the psychoneuroses and the traumatic neuroses are fixations to a traumatic scene "which within a short period of time presents the mind with an increase of stimulus too powerful to be dealt with or worked off in the normal way" through effective motor reactions or psychical activities, such as verbalization. In other words, both types of neuroses point towards traumata that can be defined in purely economic terms. Trauma is the sudden increase of stimulus resulting in permanent disturbances, since the ego is unable to perform its "task" of effectively discharging the surplus of energy.

By interpreting the war neuroses as traumatic neuroses without further argument, Freud finds himself on familiar ground in so far as his own psychoanalytic theorizing in the early 1890s can be said to originate from discussions on traumatic neurosis and traumatic hysteria.[1] In *Beyond the Pleasure Principle*, he states that "the symptomatic picture presented in traumatic neurosis approaches that of hysteria", and that the cause of the war neuroses cannot be found in "organic lesions of the nervous system" (Freud 1920g: 12). These remarks echo his position in studies on hysteria and trauma from that earliest period of his psychoanalytic work, and his discussions of his predecessors' theories. Oppenheim's treatise, *Die traumatischen Neurosen* (1899), would have it that traumatic neuroses are caused by a grave mechanical shock such as a railway accident[2] directly or indirectly damaging the nervous tissues. This would result in so-called functional disturbances for which no identifiable and perceptible organic lesion could be found. In addition, Oppenheim mentioned a psychological factor, namely fright. The fact that a person was unprepared and caught by surprise was a factor that contributed to the production of somatic symptoms. However, the question as to how a psychic reaction of fright could influence organic structure or explain the specificities of symptom formations, remained unresolved. For Charcot, the traumatic neuroses identified by Oppenheim were not a separate diagnostic category, but a subcategory of hysteria (*traumato-hystérie*). The similarities with hysterical symptom formation led him to conclude that these neuroses were not caused by the traumatic impact of a mechanical shock and the subsequent fright reaction. Such shock was only an *agent provocateur* which would give way to the development of hysteria in individuals with an inherited neuropathic predisposition (Breuer & Freud 1895d: 6; Westerink & Van Haute 2025: 24ff). The cause of traumatic hysteria, according to Charcot, is not the actual traumatic impression (shock) but the underlying neuropathic disposition resulting from a series of inherited acquired characteristics (degeneracy). The same goes for fright – it can trigger the development of hysterical symptoms, based on a neuropathic disposition.

In his early writings, Freud had followed Charcot in the assumption that traumatic neuroses are a form of hysteria. However, he draws groundbreaking conclusions from problems inherent in the theories of his predecessors. First, if hysteria is a functional disorder that has an organic, and in Charcot's understanding, hereditary cause that cannot be anatomically localized, there are two options. Either one assumes that a functional lesion is indeed a true organic lesion that respects the anatomy of the nervous system, or one asserts the contrary –"that the lesion in hysterical paralyses must be completely independent of the anatomy of the nervous system" (Freud 1893c: 169). The latter position implies that the hysterical symptoms must be explained by factors other than organic lesions or neuropathic dispositions. Second, if fright and possibly other affects can produce hysterical symptoms, one could conclude that hysteria is not a neurological but a psychological problem (Freud 1893c: 170–171). The text we are referring to here – "Some Points for a Comparative Study of Organic and Hysterical Motor Paralyses" – continues with a decisive step. Every impression or experience, Freud writes, is provided with a "certain quota of affect" (e.g., fright, shame), of which the ego needs to rid itself via a motor reaction (e.g., weeping, raging) or psychical acts (e.g., verbal utterances). If the surplus of affect is not discharged, the psychical system cannot maintain its optimum of tension. In that case, "the memory of the impression attains the importance of a trauma" and becomes the cause of hysterical symptoms (Freud 1893c: 172). Trauma is neither the result of an external shock and its immediate after-effects, nor is it an *agent provocateur* activating a neuropathic disposition. What defines trauma is the fact that a certain impression is remembered. "*Hysterics*", Freud concludes, "*suffer mainly from reminiscences*" (Breuer & Freud 1895d: 7; Freud's italics) or, which amounts to the same thing, hysterics suffer from psychic trauma (Freud 1985c: 250).

In the process of the psychologization (sexualization and internalization) of trauma, Oppenheim's traumatic neuroses soon disappear from Freud's considerations only to reappear in the years shortly before writing *Beyond the Pleasure Principle*. In his 1915 *Der Krieg und die traumatischen Neurosen*, Oppenheim had restated his earlier theories, arguing that one would have to assume mechanical shocks damaging "the delicate organization of the nervous tissue directly or indirectly" in such a way that it left no perceptible anatomical traces (Oppenheim 1915: 4–5). These views, articulated in the context of the First World War and the rapidly increasing numbers of shell-shocked patients, were rebuked at a special meeting of German neurologists and psychiatrists in Munich in September 1916, which focused on the war neuroses as a problem of supreme national interest. The participants in this conference largely opposed Oppenheim, reasoning that patients suffering from what they called "terror neurosis" were actually *Kriegshysteriker* "fleeing into illness" as an attempt to escape the horrors – fear, tension, grief, life-threatening situations – of war (Fischer-Homberger 1975: 86ff; Lerner 2010). They rejected the references to mechanical shocks and organic lesions as the single or main cause for war neuroses. Instead, some psychiatrists preferred Charcot's views on the terrors of war as *agent provocateurs* of a neuropathic (hysterical) disposition, while others placed emphasis on "wish complexes" or a "will to illness" as motive causes in patients merely pursuing accident insurance compensations and war pensions.[3]

This debate in Munich on the war neuroses or *Kriegshysterie* was highly consequential for the discussion of this phenomenon among psychoanalysts in the following years. From the proceedings of the Fifth Psychoanalytic Congress, held in Budapest in September 1918, and devoted to the topic of the war neuroses, we can clearly see the main contributors – Sándor Ferenczi, Karl Abraham, Ernst Simmel and Ernest Jones – each in their own way arguing that psychoanalysis could make an important contribution to these debates in psychiatry and neurology. After all, psychoanalysis does not focus solely on mechanical shocks and subsequent organic lesions or on self-suggestions, nor does it identify a neuropathic disposition as the decisive aetiological factor. Instead, Ferenczi and Jones, in particular, claim that psychoanalysis offers a theory that takes account of both accidental and constitutional factors, and their interactions (Ferenczi 1919a: 20; Jones 1919: 75).[4] Since the medical (psychiatric, neurological) studies of the war neuroses had, up to that point, focused on the significance of actual factors (shock, fright), Ferenczi claims, psychoanalysis would be able to contribute to the investigation of constitutional and dispositional factors. In this context, he mentions two pertinent issues. First, there is the definition of "constitution" in terms of a sexual constitution in *Three Essays*. In this context, Freud had highlighted the inherently conflictual character of sexuality – the polymorphous perverse tendencies versus the spontaneous first organic repressions. The question then arises as to whether and how the sexual constitution and the inherent conflicts play a role in the aetiology of the war neuroses. Second, there is the question of the relation between ontogeny and phylogeny. If neurotic symptoms always indicate "regression to earlier and already conquered developmental stages in onto- and phylogeny" (Ferenczi 1919a: 23), the question should be raised: to what developmental stage(s) do the symptoms of the war neuroses regress?

The disappearance of traumatic neurosis and the sexualization of trauma

In the 1893 text on the organic and hysterical paralyses, the notion of trauma remains rather unspecific and basically refers to any undischarged surplus of affect. This changes in the following years, culminating in what is generally known as the seduction theory. Freud formulates this theory in several texts from 1896, among others, in "The Aaetiology of Hysteria". In this text, he argues that if, for example, a hysterical symptom such as vomiting can first be traced to the fright experienced in a railway accident, this accident inevitably must have triggered a memory of an impression that is better able to explain the characteristics of this specific symptom, for example, the disgust felt at the sight of a cadaver or rotten fruit. Freud distinguishes between the "suitability as a determinant" of a trauma and the "traumatic force" that emanates from it (Freud 1896c: 193). The fright experienced during a railway accident is likely to be impressive enough to be traumatizing, but it cannot explain the specific symptom of hysterical vomiting. The fright is a suitable determinant but cannot explain the traumatic force producing the vomiting. The disgust felt at the sight of a rotting cadaver can. In other words, the symptom cannot be explained from one traumatic impression but needs to be understood as the effect of an associated series of impressions that have all produced surplus unpleasure. The actual traumatic impression – in this example, the fright in the railway accident – is merely the last in a series of associated impressions. In other words, pathogenesis cannot be understood from one singular cause, but only from a temporal sequence of associated traumatic scenes. From here Freud continues, arguing that a reconstruction of the chain of interconnected memories eventually and inevitably will lead to "the field of sexual experience" (Freud 1896c: 199) and more specifically to sexual experiences in the earliest childhood as the period before the development of sexual life (Freud 1896c: 202).

In this line of reasoning, we can witness the disappearance of traumatic neurosis as a determining factor. The fright experienced at a mechanical shock in the example just mentioned is merely the most recent impression in a sequence of traumatic scenes. The accident cannot be the single external cause of the specificities of hysterical symptoms – it is only the awakening of earlier sexual experiences that explain these symptoms. The paradigmatic example of this particular kind of causal reasoning is the case of Emma Eckstein in the 1895 "Project for a Scientific Psychology" (Freud 1950c: 353–355). At the age of 8, Emma was abused by a drugstore assistant who had touched her genitals through her clothes. Initially, this event had seemingly no pathogenic effect. She was apparently unharmed and the experience did not prevent her from revisiting the same shop shortly after. But this changes four years later at the start of puberty. Emma enters a clothing store and sees two men, one of whom she finds sexually attractive, laughing at her clothes. The men's smile reminds her of the grin on the shopkeeper's face. This memory now surfaces at the edge of her consciousness, and Emma, who is now an adolescent, understands the sexual meaning of what happened a few years before, and runs away in a state of fright. It is thus in retrospect (*nachträglich*) that the first scene in the drugstore is understood and becomes traumatic.[5] This case presents a striking illustration of the temporality of trauma in Freudian theory. The first experience takes place at a premature age and, since Emma does not yet have knowledge of sexual difference and the function of the genital organs, she does not yet understand what is happening to her. In fact, Emma was not in any way conscious of the significance of the event; the abuse was not experienced as such as it occurred (Caruth 1996: 18). It is only in the second scene that the first experience obtains sexual meaning. The affect of fright in this case is no longer related to a mechanical shock. In fact, the reaction of fright is not caused by the experience of the laughing men, but by the memory this scene awakens – the scene at the age of 8 in the drugstore. The fright can be seen as an immediate first reaction to a memory that is about to enter consciousness.[6]

What exactly was it that caused Emma's experiences to have a traumatic effect? At the heart of the psychological theory of the aetiology of the neuroses – the seduction theory – one finds the notion of inner psychic conflict. Freud argues that every psychical impression is provided with a certain quota of affect of which the ego divests itself either by means of a reaction or activity of discharge, or by means of repression when the ego is unable or unwilling to get rid of the surplus of affect (Freud 1893c: 171–172). In short, the ego is in conflict with an affect-laden representation. Hysteric patients do not simply suffer from memories of unpleasurable events – they also suffer from an inner conflict between the ego and the affects associated with the memories. This can be illustrated through the Emma case. The first scene seemingly did not produce a conflict between the ego and a number of impressions. It was only after having understood the significance of the first scene that the unconscious memory produces an inner conflict between her ego and representations that only now produce the surplus of affect (anxiety). It is in this second moment that these affect-laden impressions will be repressed and cause hysterical symptom formations. The memories from which hysterics suffer are always memories that afterwards (*nachträglich*) produce a conflict between the ego and affect-laden representations.

At the heart of this seduction theory lies the assumption that the first sexual experiences in childhood – when the child is still an asexual being – will only afterwards, that is, from puberty onwards, produce traumatic effects and thus become meaningful (Van Haute & Geyskens 2004: 10ff).[7] It is the child's asexuality that explains why early confrontations with adult sexuality remain without immediate impact. But Freud soon realizes that this assumption is not sustainable. Both the infantile sexual activities aiming at sexual satisfaction of the later obsessional neurotics, and the sexual perversions that appear to be fixations and repetitions of infantile pleasurable sexual activities,[8] undermine the idea of the child's asexuality and point towards an infantile sexual life that cannot be explained from encounters with adult sexuality or cultural representations. In order to map the components of infantile sexuality, Freud avers, one needs to inquire into the constitutional elements, i.e., the physiological processes that define this infantile sexuality (Freud 1985c: 268ff; Van Haute & Geyskens 2004: 23ff). Freud's efforts eventually culminate in the first edition of his *Three Essays on the Theory of Sexuality*, which was published in 1905. This text introduces a radical theory of infantile sexuality in terms of polymorphous-perverse physiological processes and activities that are constitutive for human psychic life in general and the aetiology of the psychoneuroses in particular (Van Haute & Westerink 2021). It is also the text in which

Freud systematically introduces the concept of drives. The inner psychic conflicts between the ego and sexual representations will from now on be interpreted as the expression of the two fundamental drives: the self-preservative (or ego-) drives and the sexual drives. While focusing attention on the force of the sexual drives, repression and the return of the repressed, the immediate and overwhelming experiences of terror and fright moved into the background.

From this disappearance of the traumatic neuroses in the context of a psychologization, sexualization and internalization of trauma, we can begin to understand why the war neuroses as traumatic neuroses posed an intriguing problem for Freud and his followers. In the above-mentioned introductory lectures on fixation and trauma, Freud writes that despite apparent analogies between the psychoneuroses and the traumatic neuroses, there are fundamental differences in the pathogenesis. Whereas in the traumatic neuroses, one finds a single impact from the outside producing an increase of stimulus within a short period of time, the study of the psychoneuroses resulted in the model represented by the Emma case. Here one encounters "a greater wealth of determinants for the onset of the illness" (Freud 1916–1917a: 276). In this model, apparent traumatic experiences can be traced back to one or several reinterpreted past experiences and fixations that at that point in time passed off without doing any damage. This is contrary to the traumatic neuroses and war neuroses in which "the attack corresponds to a complete transplanting of the patient into the traumatic situation" (Freud 1916–1917a: 274–275). No wonder Freud in another introductory lecture from the same series writes that psychoanalysis is "even today far from understanding" the traumatic neuroses (Freud 1916–1917a: 381).

Traumatic neuroses and narcissistic conflicts

The challenges posed by the war neuroses were inventoried and discussed at the Fifth Psychoanalytical Congress held in Budapest in September 1918 (Schröter 2023: 257–272). In his introduction to the proceedings of this conference, Freud writes that these neurotic disturbances provide psychoanalysis with the opportunity of firmly establishing itself as an esteemed practice in the domain of psychiatry, if it can be convincingly shown that some of the aspects characterizing these neuroses have already been recognized and described in psychoanalytic practice and theory. These concern the psychogenetic origins of symptoms, that is, the unconscious conflicts between ego and sexual drives as motor forces for the production of these symptoms, and the so-called "flight into illness" as a form of self-protection against the life-threatening effects of inner conflicts (Freud 1919d: 207–208). If indeed it could be shown that the war neuroses – and the familiar traumatic neuroses – have their origin in a conflict between the ego and the sexual drives, these neuroses could be fully integrated into a theory of the aetiology of the psychoneuroses.

However, Freud realizes that the theory of the sexual aetiology of the neuroses was originally put forward "only in relation" to the transference neuroses such as hysteria. The application of this theory to what he had grouped under the term "narcissistic neuroses" – notably paranoia and melancholia – had met with difficulties. In the Schreber case, Freud had raised the fundamental question whether Schreber's *Weltuntergangskastastrophe* could be explained from "a general detachment of the libido from the external world", or whether one had to assume that such detachment included "a corresponding disturbance in the ego-cathexes" (Freud 1911c: 73–74). After all, from a theory of sexual drives and ego-drives one might want to assume that disturbances in the distribution of libido would not have an effect on the ego's adaptive relation to the external world. However, the case of the paranoiac Schreber also seemed to point towards disturbances in the adaptive functions. This called into question the fundamental distinction between ego-drives and sexual drives. This was precisely what Carl Gustav Jung in his 1912 *Wandlungen und Symbole der Libido* would conclude. In severe cases of paranoia and psychoses – and notably in stuporose and catatonic automats – there is not only libidinal detachment from the external world, but also a failure to maintain self-preservative adaptation to and orientation in this world (Jung 1912: 135).[9]

In the case of Schreber's paranoia, Freud had salvaged the drive theory by arguing that the amount of sexual energy detached and withdrawn from external reality is invested in the ego and used for its aggrandisement. This amounted to a return to a stage of narcissism in which the own ego is the sexual object. In the study of melancholia, Freud found a similar process: the withdrawal of libido from a specific loved object resulted in displacement of the libido onto the ego. Here, this libido was not used for the ego's aggrandisement but, on the contrary, to establish identification with the lost and reproached object. Through identification, the reproaches towards this object were internalized and continued, resulting in severe self-reproaches on the part of the ego. Paranoia and melancholia could thus be interpreted from a theory that not only relied on the distinction between ego-drives and sexual drives but also took into account the libidinal investment in objects. The studies of these neuroses showed that the theory of the sexual aetiology of the transference neuroses could thus be extended to the domain of these narcissistic neuroses.[10]

In the 1919 text on the war neuroses, the question is whether the traumatic neuroses and war neuroses can also be understood from a theory of sexual aetiology. Clearly, Freud writes, these neuroses evolve around a conflict in the ego: "the ego is defending itself from a danger which threatens it from without or which is embodied in a shape assumed by the ego itself" (Freud 1919d: 210). According to Freud, the war neuroses can be described in terms of "conflicts in the ego" between the old "peaceful ego" and its newly formed parasitic "warlike ego" – an ego that is produced in the situation of a war that demands aggression, heroism, sacrifice and the inevitable confrontation with life-threatening danger (Freud 1919d: 208–209). What is feared is an internal enemy capable of over-riding self-preservation. The question can then be raised whether this enemy is an internalized external danger or in fact represents the sexual drive. If the latter is the case, the war neuroses could be seen as narcissistic neuroses. The ego's defence against the warlike ego could then be interpreted in terms of the projection of the internal danger onto the outside world, giving the war neuroses the appearance of traumatic neuroses. The war-neurotic patient could be said to "flee into" a traumatic neurosis in order to fend off the internal danger (Freud 1919d: 209). According to Freud, this is indeed the case: the internal danger can be traced back to the components of any neurotic conflict – ego-drives versus sexual drives (Freud & Ferenczi 1996a: 305).

In this train of thought, it seems as if Freud introduces a distinction between the traumatic neuroses and the war neuroses in order to be able to integrate the latter into a theory of the sexual aetiology of the psychoneuroses. As a consequence, the classical traumatic neuroses (resulting from a mechanical shock) would be situated – again – "beyond" a psychoanalytic theory and practice. Yet, Freud is not satisfied with such a conclusion. He writes: "The traumatic neuroses of peace will also fit into the scheme as soon as a successful outcome has been reached of our investigations into the relations which undoubtedly exist between fright, anxiety and narcissistic libido" (Freud 1919d: 210). What the study of the traumatic neuroses and war neuroses should therefore be focusing on, according to Freud, is first of all the aspect of fright. After all, this is the defining aspect of any traumatic neurosis, and inquiries into fright and anxiety will answer the question of the relation to other neuroses.[11] In a letter to Jones from February 1919, Freud writes on this issue the following:

> [The traumatic neurosis of peace] is a narcissistic affection … Angst is a protection against shock (Schreck). Now the condition of the tr. N. seems to be that the soul had no time to recur to this protection and is [overrun] taken by the trauma unprepared. Its 'Reizschutz' is overrun, the principal and primary function of keeping off excessive quantities of 'Reiz' frustrated. Then narc. Lib. is given out in shape of the signs of 'Angst'. This is the mechanism of every case of primary repression, a traumatic neurosis thus to be found at the bottom of every case of Übertraggs-neurose.
>
> (Freud & Jones 1993: 334)

In this passage, we already find elements that will be further elaborated in *Beyond the Pleasure Principle* – fright and unpreparedness, the breaching of the protective shield against stimuli, and the preparedness for anxiety (*Angstbereitschaft*).[12] Also, in this letter to Jones, Freud suggests that the traumatic neuroses may shed light on the most elementary and fundamental functions in psychic life and as such may provide new insights into the aetiology of other neuroses.

The inquiries into fright in the traumatic neuroses are at the heart of the first edition of *Beyond the Pleasure Principle.* It is striking that Freud in this text does not continue the line of argumentation from his "Introduction" on the war neuroses. He does not expand on the idea that the war neuroses can be considered narcissistic neuroses manifesting a conflict within the ego. On the contrary, in the only relevant reference to this text, Freud writes that the war neuroses "may very well be traumatic neuroses which have been *facilitated* by a conflict in the ego" (Freud 1920g: 33; my italics). The word "facilitated" may here not fully suffice as the translation of the German *erleichtert* – relieved, eased. The war neuroses in which we find a conflict in the ego are in fact "eased" traumatic neuroses. What does Freud mean by this? In the sections preceding the reference to the ego conflict, he argues that the traumatic neuroses are characterized by an "extensive breach [*Durchbruch*] being made in the protective shield against stimuli [*Reizschutz*]" (Freud 1920g: 31) resulting in sheer fright and the incapacity to bind the incoming stimuli to representations of concrete danger. Defences against the influx of stimuli can only be established when these stimuli can be "bound" to representations of a danger the ego can effectively respond to. The notion of a conflict within the ego implies that the danger is already bound to representations. From this, we can understand why the ego conflict in the war neuroses can be seen as an "eased" traumatic neurosis. In such cases, the ego would be capable of mastering the incoming drive energy through binding it to representations – and this would result in an inner ego conflict.

This means that in order to gain insight in the aetiology of the war neuroses (as, or in so far as they attest to, a conflict within the ego), one has to understand the traumatic neuroses. This implies a return to the problem we have been discussing so far. Can the traumatic neuroses be understood from a theory of the sexual aetiology of the neuroses or are the traumatic neuroses "beyond" a sexual problematics? If "beyond", can a theory of the aetiology of the traumatic neuroses be formulated, such that it does not contradict or falsify a theory of the sexual aetiology of the psychoneuroses?

Repetition and binding

In Chapter 2 of *Beyond the Pleasure Principle*, Freud concludes from his analysis of the child's *fort-da* game that once the dominance of the pleasure principle through active mastery is assured, "what is unpleasurable in itself" can be made "into a subject to be recollected and worked over in the mind" (Freud 1920g: 17). This capacity to include unpleasurable experiences and feelings in memories, that is to say, to bind them to representations situated in space and time, shows that the repetitive activities we find in the child's re-enactment of the traumatic experience of being overwhelmed with excitation "give no evidence of the operation of tendencies *beyond* the pleasure principle, that is, of tendencies more primitive than it and independent of it" (Freud 1920g: 17; Freud's italics). The child's repetitions of a traumatic experience (the departure and absence of the mother) serve the aim of actively mastering a situation the child had first passively suffered as disrupting the relative stability of the usual course of events.

Here, Freud is thinking of a functional form of repetition that prepares for traumatic situations to be recollected and represented. To think of this repetition as "reparative" (Bernet 2020: 210; Soreanu 2023: 152) or "restitutive" (Lacan 1991: 66) can be somewhat misleading.[13] After all, it seems to suggest that this is a reparation of an original bond or unity preceding absence and lack.[14] This is not what Freud is telling us in his analysis of the child's play. The repetitions Freud finds in the play aim at and amount to a very first binding of excitation to representations, and to a network of representations that allows experiences to be part of a world of experiences.[15] In fact, play illustrates that this binding is indeed accomplished. The repetitions are no longer disparate repetitions of anxious situations manifesting themselves in helpless kicking and screaming, but they are repetitions through which objectal representations of the experience of disappearing and reappearing, absence and presence are created. The *fort-da* play illustrates that repetitions produce concatenations of representations and thus continuity and stability in psychic life – and this is what makes it possible to experience pleasure at what was previously an unpleasurable experience.

These repetitions are therefore not merely the unmediated manifestations of the drives as constant persisting forces pressuring the psychic systems. Freud does maintain that the drive for mastery, like any other drive, is "acting independently of whether the memory was in itself pleasurable or not" (Freud 1920g: 16), but this does not lead him to conclude that the child's play is "beyond" the pleasure principle. The child's repetitive activities are expedient repetitions that make use of drive energy to yield pleasure. In addition to the immediate pleasure of satisfaction at the expression of hostile impulses against the mother and father, the child's activities produce a variety of pleasures. There is, first, pleasure experienced at muscular activity; second, pleasure at the rhythmic character of re-experiencing something as always the same (*fort-da*) in the play itself (Freud 1920g: 36); third, at the repetitive staging of the mother's presence (*da*); and, lastly, at the mastery over the repetitive activity up to the point where the child can decide to end the game and stop protesting against the unpleasurable experience of the departure of the mother (Freud 1920g: 15–16).

Repeating and remembering

In the opening sections of Chapter 3 of *Beyond the Pleasure Principle*, Freud discusses another form of repetition, namely the repetitive acting out of "repressed material as a contemporary experience" in the "sphere of the transference, of the relation to the physician". In the relation with the analyst, the analysand repeats repressed drive representations that, according to Freud, "have as their subject some portion of infantile sexual life – of the

Oedipus complex, that is, and its derivatives" (Freud 1920g: 18). What we find in what Freud calls the transference neuroses is the re-enactment of what it "replaces", namely an earlier neurosis in which the repressed consists of drive impulses and their psychical representatives (*Triebrepräsentanz* – representations cathected with psychic energy produced by the drives) (see Freud 1915d: 152).[16] The fact that he explicitly refers to repressed portions of infantile sexual life is telling. For Freud, what is repressed always consists of aspects of sexuality, such as, for example, certain polymorphous perverse drive impulses, sexual activities or infantile sexual researches. Such drive impulses and activities at one point were experienced as pleasurable or at least could have been experienced as pleasurable.

Are there exceptions? One may want to argue perhaps that Emma Eckstein presents a case of an initial experience that was not pleasurable (see Freud 1914g: 149). After all, Freud assumes Emma's childhood asexuality; the problematics of pleasure/unpleasure is only introduced in the second scene. But this trauma theory becomes more complicated after Freud's inquiries into the polymorphous perverse character of infantile sexuality. In the Dora case – and in later cases such as the Rat Man and the Wolf Man – the question is no longer how and why sexual experiences in puberty can have a traumatic, that is, pathogenic effect. The question now becomes, what interactions between constitutional or dispositional factors, on the one hand, and accidental factors in earliest childhood, on the other, form the basis for later experiences to have a pathogenic effect. In the case of Dora, the traumatic impact of experiences in puberty cannot be understood if one does not consider her infantile sexual activities (such as masturbation) and subsequent reaction formations (such as disgust).[17] In this case study, Freud argues that hysteria is fundamentally characterized by a spontaneous rejection of sexuality that evokes only disgust: "I should without question consider a person hysterical in whom an occasion for sexual excitement elicited feelings that were preponderantly or exclusively unpleasurable" (Freud 1905e: 28). From this perspective, acquiring insight into hysteria first of all means understanding what exactly it is that caused this "reversal of affect" from a pleasurable sensation to disgust. Freud's analyses of Dora lead him to conclude that her traumatic experiences in puberty have no aetiological meaning in themselves, but in fact actualize and transform a previous hysterical disposition that is the very basis of hysteria. This disposition consists in the spontaneous reaction formation of disgust against an initially pleasurable sexual excitation.

This line of reasoning is continued in later writings. In the case of the repetition of traumatic sexual experiences, we are dealing with experiences that could only become traumatic because they were at an earlier stage associated with pleasure and unpleasure. For the transference neuroses, this means that the unpleasure the analysand tries to avoid remembering – and instead repeats – concerns repressed portions of infantile sexual life. For this reason, Freud refers to a formula that describes the relation between the ego and the repressed in terms of pleasure-unpleasure: "unpleasure for one system and simultaneously satisfaction for the other". Any part of "what is re-experienced under the compulsion to repeat must cause the ego unpleasure" (Freud 1920g: 20). The repetition in transference neuroses therefore does not contradict the pleasure principle. There is always one system that will find pleasure, such as the unconscious when repeating the initial pleasurable excitation, or the ego when repressing unpleasure (see also Freud 1915d: 147).[18] As long as there are conflicts between systems, the psychic apparatus can be said to be regulated by the pleasure principle.

The transference neuroses point towards a repetition that is first and foremost a mechanism of defence against and repression of sexual drive impulses. However, they do bring us closer to the problem Freud that wants to discuss. In the transference neuroses, Freud finds the analysand compulsively repeating repressed impulses and its derivatives.[19] This repetition causes the ego unpleasure "since it brings to light activities of repressed instinctual impulses". For this reason, Freud writes, "our efforts ... are directed towards procuring the toleration of that unpleasure by an appeal to the reality principle" (Freud 1920g: 20). The analyst should seek to convince the analysand "of the impossibility of conducting life on the pleasure principle" as long as he or she resists and repeats (Freud 1919a: 159). In order to reach the point where unpleasure is tolerated and pleasure assured, the analyst must allow the analysand to re-experience a "portion of his forgotten life", but should maintain a degree of superior aloofness. This should enable the analysand "to recognize that what appears to be reality is in fact only a reflection of a forgotten past [*vergessene Vergangenheit*]" (Freud 1920g: 19): "He [the patient, HW] is obliged to *repeat* the repressed material as a contemporary experience instead of, as the physician would prefer to see, *remembering* [*erinnern*] it as something belonging to the past" (Freud 1920g: 18; Freud's italics). Repetition here means that an experience (*Erlebnis*) from the past is not automatically assigned a place in a temporal linear order. The repetition (in acting-out) of repressed material indicates that an experience can be a past and a contemporary experience at the same time. According to Freud, a past experience can persist in such a way that it remains present or returns to the present as an experience in the here and now. This view of repetition in the transference neuroses is connected with earlier ideas such as those articulated in "Remembering, Repeating, and Working-Through". In this text, Freud states that the compulsion to repeat one finds in transference is a "way of remembering" (Freud 1914g: 150). Repeating is reproducing and reliving the past as present. He adds that repeating can therefore also be seen as replacing remembering, when we define remembering as carrying the past – the forgotten, the repressed – into the present "psychical field" (Freud 1914g: 151). Remembering is re-collecting the past, such that it can be expressed in thoughts through speech. That repeating replaces remembering indicates that a person is unable to recollect and cannot bring a past experience back into consciousness or, in other words, is unable to trace a contemporary forceful experience back to the past

(Freud 1914g: 152).[20] This means, on the one hand, that repeating is a way of repressing – it is a reaction formation against the becoming conscious through recollection. "We repeat because we repress" (Deleuze 2004: 18). On the other hand, the repetition replacing recollection can be seen as an attempt to integrate the repressed trauma into the subject's world of experience (Van Haute & Geyskens 2007: 13). Repetition in transference is an attempt at psychic repair. Regarding this repair, Freud argues that analysis works towards replacing repetitions of the repressed by memories of experiences in the past (Freud 1920g: 19). In and through analysis, the patient should become aware of his or her "actions" as repetitions of experiences that actually belong to a forgotten past.

However, we should note here that for Freud, remembering is not only a matter of bringing the past back into the present. It is not only bringing back to consciousness a past scene as significant for the onset of one's life trajectory and current state. For Freud, remembering is conditioned by a more fundamental psychic activity that he also refers to as *erinnern*. Remembering is the process of assigning a repeated scene in the present to its proper place in the past (Moyaert 2014: 37–38; Martínez Ruiz 2020). We have already encountered this in Freud's analysis of the child's play. The repetitive activities turn a traumatic situation into "a subject to be remembered" (*zum Gegenstand der Erinnerung machen*) (Freud 1920g: 17). Remembering is here a psychic activity through which the repeated can be recognized and understood as part of a past life.[21] Remembering thus produces distinction and distance between present and past. Remembering is not reconnecting a contemporary "state" (*Zustand*) to a past experience. It is assigning this state a place in the past such that it can become a past experience and, as such, can also become a memory. It is grouping the events in a certain order of succession (see Lacan 1991: 185). Remembering is historicizing, and, as such, precedes the recollection of the past in the present. It creates the archive from which memories can be retrieved. Remembering produces temporality. It serves as the very condition for organizing and stabilizing psychic life.[22]

What the traumatic neuroses show is that reparation and mastery through binding, and remembering as historicizing, are not self-evident. It cannot be assumed that these patients suffering from traumatic neuroses will repeat repressed material as contemporary experiences. These patients do not appear to be replacing repressed memories with repetitions. Also, these patients cannot be said to fail in integrating into their psychic life traumatic experiences that were originally given in a coherent way, i.e., that were already experiences of something at a certain moment and occasion. The traumatic neuroses point towards more fundamental problematics – namely the incapacity to produce memories, the inability to repress. This is what Freud finds in the dreams of traumatic neurotic patients: the compulsion to repeat the situation of the accident (*Situation des Unfalles*) (Freud 1920g: 13) as impossible to remember, that is, as impossible to assign a place belonging to the past. The compulsion to repeat concerns traumatic situations that are – as Lacan writes – "unassimilable" in the psychic economy; they cannot be assigned a place in a person's life history (Lacan 1998: 55; also Caruth 1996: 104–105).[23] Having no place in a personal history, the repeated traumatic situations are "beyond" history. The traumatic neurotic patient does not suffer from reminiscences but from repetitions; the patient is unable to give meaning to an experience afterwards (*nachträglich*). What thus makes the trauma truly traumatic is the fact of its meaningless repetition.

Freud adds an element that further distinguishes traumatic neuroses from transference neuroses:

> But we come now to a new and remarkable fact, namely that the compulsion to repeat also recalls [*wiederbringt*] from the past experiences which include no possibility of pleasure, and which can never, even long ago, have brought satisfaction even to instinctual impulses [*Triebregungen*] which have since been repressed.
>
> (Freud 1920g: 20)

The compulsion to repeat is situated "beyond" and independent of the pleasure principle and activities aimed at mastery. The compulsion to repeat does not repress, but to the contrary "carries into the present" (*wiederbringt*) the same "state" or "situation" again and again.[24] And since this state is highly unpleasurable, the compulsion to repeat can apparently over-ride the pleasure principle and repressive – and hence defensive – mechanisms.

For Freud, this means that the compulsion to repeat must be the expression of drive characteristics. Manifestations of the compulsion to repeat "exhibit to a high degree an instinctual [*triebhafter*] character" (Freud 1920g: 35). His argument runs as follows. Nothing in the nature of the drives or in the unconscious resists the becoming conscious and the actualization or discharge of drive energy (as evidenced in "acting out"). The resistance against this becoming conscious stems from the higher psychic functions, that is, from the ego and the secondary processes of binding drive excitation (*Erregung der Triebe*) to representations. Tendencies that are not part of the secondary processes or ego-functions must be assigned to primary processes in which the drive impulses are freely mobile (see Chapter 1). Since the compulsion to repeat found in traumatic neuroses is "independent" of the pleasure principle, it must be thought of as expression of unconscious drive impulses. The compulsion to repeat, Freud writes, is "more primitive, more elementary, more instinctual" than the pleasure principle (Freud 1920g: 23). The compulsion to repeat is a fundamental characteristic of the human as pulsional (*triebhafte*) living substance. Because of this pulsional character of repetition, the situation that is repeated cannot as yet be represented. For that to occur, the drives first need to be bound. In fright-dreams, patients repeat situations because they cannot yet represent experiences (also Zupančič 2017: 109; Ingala 2020: 582).

Anxiety dreams and fright-dreams

In the first version of *Beyond the Pleasure Principle* and in "Memorandum on the Electrical Treatment of War Neurotics" from February 1920, Freud argues that the recent study of the war neuroses confirms what he had already concluded in 1893. The cause of traumatic disorders cannot be attributed to "organic lesions of the nervous system brought about by mechanical force" (Freud 1920g: 12). These disorders must in fact be "traced back to disturbances of emotional life", despite the spectacular motor symptoms that at first sight seem to be the immediate effect of "concussions due to the explosions of a shell" (Freud 1955c: 212). The concrete disturbance he is referring to is fright. According to Freud, fright can be defined in terms of a "state" (*Zustand*) into which a person enters when he is caught by surprise and unprepared for a life-threatening danger (Freud 1920g: 12). In a further reflection on this causative factor, he writes that this fright corresponds to a breach in the protective shield against stimuli (Freud 1920g: 31). In this state, the psychic systems lack preparedness for anxiety, are overwhelmed by the sudden forceful influx of quanta of excitations, incapable of the economic processing of energy, and unable to bind these excitations to representations of an identifiable danger.[25]

According to Freud, the fright reactions due to amounts of excitation entering the psychic systems, and the attempts to produce preparedness for anxiety can best be studied through the study of the dreams of traumatic neurotic patients in which they relive the situation of the traumatizing accident (Freud 1920g: 13). At first sight, it may appear that these dreams such as one finds in *Unfallsneurotiker* confirm a trauma theory in which the trauma is caused by an external stimulus. He writes on this: "We describe as 'traumatic' any excitations *from outside* which are powerful enough to break through the protective shield" (Freud 1920g: 29; my italics). The result of this is that "such an event as an external trauma is bound to provoke a disturbance on a large scale in the functioning of the organism's energy and to set in motion every defensive measure" (Freud 1920g: 29). In this situation, the pleasure principle "is for the moment put out of action", and the psychic apparatus without any protective shield will be flooded with amounts of drive impulses. In other words, trauma cannot be defined merely in terms of the accidental impact of an external force. The accidental factor merely triggers – like an *agent provocateur* – a constitutional factor, that is, it evokes an increase of unbound amounts of drive energy that pressure the psychic apparatus from the inside. The result is permanent disturbances of the way in which this energy is dealt with or worked off (see Freud 1916–1917a: 275). The fright-dreams testify to this: the patient repeatedly responds with fright to the amounts of drive energy that overwhelm the psychic systems. The patient is haunted by the repetitive reality of a situation that is not only violent but also incomprehensible.[26] It cannot as yet be ascribed a specific meaning in a person's life history.

The puzzling question for Freud in *Beyond the Pleasure Principle* is therefore not how an external factor can damage the protective shield and cause internal disturbance. The question is rather why and how the psychic apparatus keeps being disrupted and disturbed by repeated incoming amounts of drive stimuli. What is characteristic of the drives such that they cause "repeated" interruptions? Freud thus confirms what he had been arguing since the late 1890s. Trauma is not caused by the impact of external accidental factors but must be understood from internal – constitutional and dispositional – factors. Trauma must be understood from pulsional sources. In order to understand trauma, one must ask what is "in the drives" that is or leads "beyond" the pleasure principle. It is for this reason that Freud calls the compulsion to repeat "malignant" and "daemonic" (Freud 1920g: 21, 36). The repetition cannot be explained from the accidental confrontation with life-threatening situations in the trenches, but only from internal processes that apparently do not care for the individual's psychic well-being. The fright-dreams are supposed to provide insight into these internal daemonic forces.

Of course, this is not the first time in Freud's work that dreams are key to gain insight into the aetiology and characteristics of neuroses. In the Dora case, for example, Freud argues that because "the dream is one of the roads along which consciousness can be reached by the psychical material which … has been cut off from consciousness and repressed" (Freud 1905e: 15), dreams make it possible to gain insight into the psychical mechanisms that determine the formation of neurotic symptoms (Freud 1905e: 114). In this case study, not only do Dora's dreams reveal infantile yet repressed sexual activities and sensations; they also function as defensive reactions against traumatic incidents (Freud 1905e: 64, 72; Van Haute & Geyskens 2012: 45–60; Westerink & Van Haute 2025: 51–71). In the case of the Wolf Man, the patient's repetitive mention of the anxiety dream of the wolves convinces Freud that a primal scene has been activated in this dream, which has a traumatizing effect *nachträglich*. This anxiety dream threatens to bring back the memory of an experience that can only now be understood, that is to say, after a number of accidental experiences interacting with constitutional factors in the period between the primal scene and the anxiety dream, which together serve as the condition for understanding the primal scene as sexual gratification, along with its implications (Freud 1918b: 29ff; Westerink & Van Haute 2025: 95–126). The fact that the Wolf Man in the therapeutic sessions repeatedly returns to the dream indicates that he – like other psychoneurotic patients – suffers from reminiscences. In this case, more concretely, this concerns the memory of the anxiety dream as traumatic experience in which an even earlier memory was activated.[27] Anxiety dreams like those of the Wolf Man, Freud writes, can be seen as replacing "the forbidden wish-fulfilment by the appropriate punishment for it" (Freud 1920g: 32). In the case of the Wolf Man, this forbidden wish-fulfilment is the desired sexual satisfaction from the father. In this case, the punishment for this satisfaction (namely castration) is the price to be paid for taking the position of his gratified mother (Freud 1918b: 46–47). In a section added in the 1919 fifth edition of *The Interpretation of Dreams*, Freud elaborates on anxiety dreams ("unpleasurable dreams") as wish-fulfilments along similar lines. In the anxiety dream, an unconscious and repressed wish meets the ego's reaction of "violent indignation" and "outburst of anxiety" (Freud 1900a: 557). The ego's reaction in such dreams is indeed a reaction of anxiety as defined in *Beyond the Pleasure Principle.* Anxiety describes "a particular state of expecting the danger [*Erwartung der Gefahr*] or preparing for it, even though it may be an unknown one" (Freud 1920g: 12). The ego anticipates an unconscious persisting wish as danger and reacts accordingly, in an outburst of anxiety that terminates the dream. In this sense, the anxiety dream can be seen as a defensive reflex, taking flight from approaching danger from the inside, in the form of a wish. The actual anxiety in the anxiety dreams is thus the defence against a drive impulse seeking repetition of an originally pleasurable experience. In line with this train of thought, in the 1920 edition of *Beyond the Pleasure Principle*, Freud adds a paragraph in which he confirms that anxiety dreams and punishment dreams can be seen as fulfilments of wishes.

In the dreams of traumatic neurotic patients, however, one finds neither a wish nor wish-fulfilment nor an ego capable of any effective reaction against incoming stimuli. The fright-dreams in traumatic neuroses "arise, rather, in obedience to the compulsion to repeat" (Freud 1920g: 32). As such, these dreams are characterized by a compulsion to repeat highly unpleasurable sensations that are not as yet regulated by the pleasure principle. These dreams show that "there was also *a time before* the purpose of dreams was the fulfilment of wishes" (Freud 1920g: 33; my italics). These fright-dreams point towards a "beyond" of the pleasure principle that is actually a chronological and logical "before" the pleasure principle (Lear 2000: 74; Malabou 2012: 196; Fletcher 2013: 300; Martinez Ruiz 2020). The dreams of traumatic neurotic patients thus provide insight into the conditions for the formation of the pleasure principle, memory and temporality, stable relations between representations, and consciousness and ego-formation. These dreams provide knowledge of the conditions for the principles and functions that organize psychic life in such a way that it is able to adequately and purposefully interact with the inner and outer world. With Deleuze we can agree that Freud's analysis of the fright-dreams is a transcendental exercise of thought, i.e., an inquiry into the conditions of the possibility of psychic life and the "conditions under which pleasure effectively becomes a principle" (Deleuze 2004: 120; see also 1991: 111ff).[28] Freud provides an account of the conditions for psychic life; the mastering of incoming drive stimuli; the binding of excitation to representations; and the situating and distinguishing of experiences in space and time.

The repetitions that Freud finds in the dreams of traumatic neurotic patients indicate that the "situation of the accident" is not automatically assigned a place in a temporal linear order. Freud confirms this in his discussion of Kant's necessary forms of thought: "We have learnt that unconscious mental processes are in themselves 'timeless' [*zeitlos*]." The unconscious is the domain of excitations not as yet bound to a network of representations and hence not organized in a linear temporal order, not modified through *a priori* ideas of time or corrected by actual experiences of and in time. In fact, the unconscious can be said to have no relation to time whatsoever (Freud 1920g: 28; also 1915e: 187). The fright-dreams as attempts to produce preparedness for anxiety as a first act of binding excitations to representations can therefore be said to provide insight into the very conditions under which a sense of time and a distinction between present and past will be established. The fright-dreams are attempts to produce and willingly accept anxiety.[29] Here, Freud aligns with Hume: it is only through repetition of identical impressions that these impressions can be bound to representations, become ideas and be assigned a place in a temporal order.

How, then, is the sense of time as the condition for the possibility to have experiences situated in time established? What is the condition for remembering? We recall here that Freud defines anxiety as a "state of expecting the danger". This state of expecting – as he had already argued in "Project" (Freud 1950c: 369) – can be described in terms of a state of anticipating a danger situation to happen or appear in the near future.[30] Such a state of expecting (*erwarten*) describes an active mode rather than a passive awaiting (*abwarten*) (also Lacan 2019: 125). Expecting is the psychic activity of relating to the possibility of a certain future experience. The preparedness for anxiety can be seen as the condition of possibility for the expectation of a future experience, hence, for the very possibility of a future in which something can be experienced.[31] This means, first, that the expectation can take the form of a wish. The dreams of traumatic neurotic patients can be seen as attempts to produce wishes and wish-fulfilments (Lear 2000: 72–73). Second, the possibility of future experience implies the notion of a preceding state (the state of expectation). The anticipation of danger thus implies a distinction between the past, the present and the future.[32] It is from the expectation of a future event that a past state becomes conceivable. What is expected is something that "reminds" and calls into memory past traumatic experiences. And with this, the past as such and as a sequence of experiences becomes conceivable.

Repetition and preparedness for anxiety

According to Freud, "before" the pleasure principle is a situation in which quantities of drive energy flow into the psychic systems in such a way that these systems and their associated functions are "breached", become paralyzed and incapable of reacting in an appropriate manner.[33] These systems and functions are "unprepared" for the sudden overwhelming impact of quantities of excitations. The accompanying dreams are not characterized by anxiety, but by fright as a "state" of unpreparedness for danger and as a defining factor of the "situation" of the accident (Freud 1920g: 12–13). These dreams manifest unanticipated "disturbing impulses" that are not yet bound to representations. These dreams, Freud writes, obey the compulsion to repeat (Freud 1920g: 33). The compulsion to repeat is seen here as the immediate expression of drives persisting in – or as Lacan would rather say, "insisting" on[34] – prolonging and maintaining their intensity and movement. For Freud, this pulsional compulsion to repeat produces repetitions for the sake of repetition, and hence without any consideration of the feelings of pleasure and unpleasure they may produce. The compulsion to repeat thus points towards the drives as seen from the physiological perspective we discussed earlier. They are constant forces that only change direction when opposed by other (reactive) forces. The fright-dreams indicate a lack of such opposing forces and capacities.

And yet, according to Freud, these fright-dreams unfold not simply in obedience to a pulsional compulsion to repeat. These dreams also have a "function" or "task" (Freud 1920g: 32). The fright-dreams are attempts at transforming the dreams into anxiety dreams, that is eventually, into wish-fulfilments,[35] and thereby mastering them. In the situation of large-scale disruptions by incoming drive energy, the psychic apparatus will, Freud argues, still be able to react according to its most primary reflex function which can be witnessed in dreams. It will use all the available energy to produce defensive measures. According to Freud:

> these dreams are endeavouring to master the stimulus [*Reizbewältigung*] retrospectively [*nachzuholen*], by developing the anxiety [*Angstentwicklung*] whose omission was the cause of the traumatic neurosis. They thus afford us a view of a function of the mental apparatus which, though it does not contradict the pleasure principle, is nevertheless independent of it and seems to be more primitive than the purpose of gaining pleasure and avoiding unpleasure.
>
> (Freud 1920g: 32)[36]

The production of anxiety or what Freud calls the "preparedness for anxiety" is the most primitive protective shield through which a psychic system is able to receive and start mastering stimuli. It is the first and crucial step in the "transformation" of unbound drive energy into an affect that can be bound to representations (Freud 1915d: 153). Through anxiety the psychic apparatus is able to establish a first binding (of drive energy to something conceived as danger) that will serve as the condition for any further binding and mastering of excitations (Freud 1920g: 35).[37] This explains Freud's notion of binding as a "preparatory act" that "occurs on *behalf* of the pleasure principle" and "introduces and assures the dominance of the pleasure principle" (Freud 1920g: 62; Freud's italics). The preparedness for anxiety as first protection against incoming flows of drive stimuli does not stand in opposition to the pleasure principle, does not suspend the pleasure principle, but precedes the dominance of the pleasure principle.

But if the development of the preparedness for anxiety is a first preparatory act that occurs on behalf of the pleasure principle, can one maintain that the dreams of traumatic-neurotic patients have a function or task "independent" of the pleasure principle? In the final sentences of the 1919 text, Freud writes that his inquiries into the "beyond" of the pleasure principle "reach what is at bottom no very simple conclusion" (Freud 1920g: 63). The reference to "the pleasure drive, which governs all psychic life" (Freud 2024: 78) indicates that beyond a more assured dominance of the pleasure principle in the secondary process, the primary process is also dominated by the urge to eliminate erupting unpleasure. The primary process which in order of time precedes the secondary processes, shows that "at the beginning of psychic life" the pleasure principle is already "operative" in the aim of the pleasure drive. Freud's analyses of fright-dreams developing into anxiety dreams can be seen as an inquiry into the transition from the primary to the secondary process. In the traumatic neurotic's dreams the felt unpleasure due to amounts of excitation sets in motion an intense striving for pleasure as a motor force for the production of the first defensive measures (preparedness for anxiety). Yet, the compulsion to repeat one finds in these fright-dreams also indicates that the transition towards a (more or less) stable psychic organization is far from self-evident. The fright-dreams are repeated, and repeatedly failing, attempts to produce the first productive shield against the influx of excitations.[38]

The compulsion to repeat we find in these dreams would then – as others have also noted[39] – consist of two distinct forms of repetition. On the one hand, the compulsion to repeat is the immediate manifestation of drive impulses and amounts of excitation that constantly or repeatedly flow into the psychic apparatus, interrupting and disrupting psychic life such that there can be no experience of time, space and the self (Caruth 1996: 3). Such repetitions do not produce or insist on psychic change and development. On the other hand, the compulsion to repeat has a reparative character. The repetitions of the "state" of fright are meant to retrospectively produce anxiety. Such anxiety implies a first identification of a danger situated in another time and space – a danger back then and there. If the repeated content can be assigned its proper place in the past, the present can – possibly and eventually – become the site of pleasurable experiences again.[40] Reparative repetitions thus go hand in hand with remembering, i.e., with binding drive energy to representations.[41]

If the fright-dreams give an insight into the conditions of psychic life, however, the repetitions cannot be exclusively reparative. They are productive. It is only through repetitions that the basic organization of psychic life can be (re-)established in the first place. But in what sense can the compulsion to repeat be productive? How can the repetitions that Freud calls "daemonic" produce psychic life? Freud's answer to this question can be traced back to earlier writings, such as "Project" and *Three Essays*. The repeated influx and reception of drive stimuli produce reactive formations (*seelische Reaktion* or *Reaktionsbildung*) (Freud 1920g: 11, 42, 51).[42] Freud considers such formations as spontaneous formations in the terms of mechanistic reasoning – action is reaction. Repetitions are productive because they spontaneously trigger organic and psychic reactions in the form of organizations and structures capable of managing the influx of excitation.

It is telling in this context that Freud does not refer to the ego, but to dreams as endeavouring to master stimuli. The dreams point towards a psychic process "before" proper ego functions are operative. We can here recall Freud's definition of the ego from "Project" as the totality of the ψ cathexes (Freud 1950c: 323). In that text, he argued that the ego is the effect of the binding of excitation in a network of stable and facilitating cathexes (Freud 1950c: 322–323). This process of binding and facilitating can be described in terms of repetition, that is, the regularly repeated reception of endogenous excitation. Repetition and the possibility of reception are the condition for the facilitation and thus for the organization of psychic life that becomes formative for the ego. The ego results from repetition and reception of excitation.[43] In his inquiries into the "before" of the pleasure principle, Freud returns to the ideas voiced in "Project". The binding of excitation through repeated receptions of excitation precedes the ego as an organization or agency capable of repressing and resisting while operating "under the sway of the [*im Dienste des*] pleasure principle" (Freud 1920g: 19, 20).

What is repeated in these fright-dreams is also not an experience of the ego, but a "state" in which amounts of stimuli and excitation create "breaches".[44] Contrary to his discussion of the *fort-da* game and transference neuroses, Freud does not focus on the repetition of a repressed or re-enacted experience (*Erlebnis*), but on the repetition of a "situation" or "state" of fright that was registered in the unconscious in reaction to the "strength" of an impression (*Stärke des Eindrucks*), i.e., the unexpected influx of quanta of energy and excitation (Freud 1920g: 13). This state – the breaching of the defensive shields and the reaction of fright (Freud 1920g: 29) – is what defines the trauma. The repetition thus concerns a state – or what Walter Benjamin has called an "occurrence" (*Vorfall*) (Benjamin 1991: 615) – that was never lived as an experience (*Erlebnis*).[45] For, if the trauma had been consciously experienced, it would have already been bound to representations by an ego capable of perceiving, receiving and processing stimuli. The trauma is a psychic wound, an "interruption" or disturbance to which the psychic reflex apparatus spontaneously responds "with every possible defensive measure" (Freud 1920g: 29) but without an efficient agency or psychic mechanism capable of adequately mastering the stimuli. The major difference between the child's *fort-da* game and the traumatic neurotic's dreams is that the child is able to actively assure pleasure while managing – with pleasure – the experiences of departure, absence, return and presence. And the difference between traumatic neuroses and transference neuroses lies in the fact that, in the latter, a repressive ego is allowing repetitions. In the dreams of traumatic-neurotic patients, we find attempts, through repetition, to turn the traumatic state into an experience; but these attempts repeatedly fail because there is as yet no functional ego that could be said to have experiences and be able to organize these experiences.

Because of their tragic character – the failing endeavours to produce a first protective shield – the fright-dreams can be compared to the psychotic's projections to which Freud briefly refers in this text. These projections are, he argues, another primitive form of bringing "the shield against stimuli in operation as a means of defence against them" (Freud 1920g: 29). Projections are attempts to put the influx of overwhelming amounts of drive stimuli at a distance in the external world. We can think here of Schreber's "internal catastrophe" that is projected onto the outside world as an envisioned "end of the world", and the subsequent delusional formation which according to Freud, "*is in reality an attempt at recovery, a process of reconstruction*" (Freud 1911c: 71; Freud's italics). The traumatic neurotic's attempts to produce anxiety through dreams and the psychotic's attempts to re-establish a relation with reality through delusions appear to be two tragic variants of failures in mastering internal drive stimuli. And yet, there is a limit to this comparison as well. After all, despite Schreber's "general detachment of the libido from the external world", the ego-cathexes remain in existence and are able to maintain a relation to the outside world. Schreber's ego is not paralyzed – it is still able to meet self-preservative needs (Freud 1911c: 74, 75). However, this cannot be said of patients who are suffering severe shell shock and displaying stuporose and catatonic symptoms.

The daemonic character of repetition

This tragic failing to produce something new and act differently (instead of repeating the same) is highlighted in a section at the end of Chapter 3 of *Beyond the Pleasure Principle*, where Freud associates the daemonic character of the compulsion to repeat with concrete examples of a gruesome and tragic fate (Freud 1920g: 20–21). The examples he mentions underscore the tragic aspects of repetition. In this context, Freud uses the term "compulsion of destiny" (*Schicksalzwang*). Freud's mention of Nietzsche's "eternal recurrence" (*ewige Wiederkehr des Gleichen*) in this context is meant to underscore the uncanny character of repetition. This reference is an uncanny twist. For Nietzsche in *The Gay Science* and *Thus Spoke Zarathustra*, the notion of the eternal return concerns the question whether one is actively willing to affirm life as struggle for domination and maximization of the will to power. The eternal return is not the "repetition of the same", but the welcoming of life, including all possible suffering and pleasure, such that one is willing live life again and again (Nietzsche 1882: 570; 1887: 274). But for Freud, it is the eternal recurrence of the same that is of interest. This does not point towards a will to power and the affirmation of life. It underscores instead the person's active involvement in apparent passive suffering of the reality of fate. This involvement does not so much consist of subjection or adaptation to external circumstances, but indicates that what appears as activity follows from what Freud refers to as the "exigencies of life" (*Not des Lebens* or *Ανάγκη*). Activity is in fact reactivity. With this concept he refers to the pressure from inner constant forces (drives), the phylogenetically inherited constitutional characteristics and tendencies, and the acquired disposition that determine an individual's reactions (Freud 1900a: 565; 1916–1917a: 355; 1950c: 297). In other words, the exigencies of life are a concept that refers to the "fate" resulting from inner "daemonic" forces theatrically staged in object relations. In the example mentioned by Freud, there was no "decision" that stopped the woman from the daemonic compulsion to marry three successive husbands, each of whom fell ill soon after, and had to be nursed on their deathbeds. And there was no "act" that prevented Tancred in Tasso's *Gerusalemme Liberata* from killing his beloved Clorinda twice and thus repeats the same fatality through similar acts of violence. Although Freud uses the notion of eternal recurrence in a non-Nietzschean way, at the heart of the matter, he expresses an idea that is profoundly Nietzschean: the critique of a view of life as organized progression and improvement, as rising to higher forms. Both Nietzsche and Freud voice an idea of life as characterized by necessary yet inexpedient repetitions that include the possibility of suffering and death (Nietzsche 1882: 468).

What then exactly makes repetition "daemonic"?[46] The daemonic character of repetition does not manifest itself in extraordinary individual fates and tragedies – it is not based on anomalies, coincidence or choice. The daemonic, on the contrary, is exactly that which eternally recurs in every human being, independently of whether this recurrence produces pleasure or unpleasure. The compulsion to repeat is daemonic because it signifies repeatedly finding oneself again (*Wiederfinden*) in the same situation (Freud 1920g: 36).[47] Freud speaks of repetition in these terms in order to indicate that the compulsion to repeat does not result in meaningful experiences. On the contrary, these repeated situations are deadly repetitions in the sense that they stifle all psychic activity and creativity. The daemonic character of the repetition resides in repetition for the sake of repetition, that is to say, a repetition which is not aimed at a result other than to persist in the repetition, to continue the same trajectory of that or those that came before. The daemonic repetition is neither functional or meaningful, nor aimed at adaptation to circumstances, acquiring capacities or contributing to well-being. It is not aimed at completion of a movement or an activity. Instead, it will persist unless it finds opposition or resistance in another force or obstacle. As repetition for the sake of repetition, daemonic repetition is not motivated by anything other than its own pulsional character as inherited constitutional force. Therefore, another way to the define the daemonic character of repetition is that each individual repeats the life trajectory of its evolutionary lineage – ontogeny repeats phylogeny (see Chapter 3).

Sexual excitation and traumatic neuroses

We should not be surprised to find no references to sexuality in Freud's discussion of the traumatic neuroses and the fright-dreams in the first edition of *Beyond the Pleasure Principle*. The reasons for this absence of references to sexual drives or infantile sexual pleasures experienced at sensitive and excitable erogenous zones are seemingly obvious. In the traumatic neuroses, highly unpleasurable situations are repeated as contemporary states. And these situations have never been and will never be a source of pleasure. Contrary to the various psychoneuroses, there is no repressed sexual drive impulse or sexual activity involved in the aetiology of the traumatic neuroses. This also indicates that the trauma we find here is structured differently than the sexual traumas Freud had studied and theorized so far. The traumatic neuroses are "beyond" the sexual. In the compulsion to repeat frightful situations, there is no temporality of trauma. Emma's fright – or, in retrospect, better, her anxiety – was the effect of her understanding a previous experience that came back to memory in a second experience. The Wolf Man's anxiety was the effect of his understanding the implications of the primal scene. But this is not the case in the war neuroses. The fright one finds here has nothing to do with a retrospective understanding of a previous scene. What is repeated is fright felt at the sudden and unexpected impact of, for example, the explosion of a shell. This state of fright is not associated with any experience in the domain of sexuality nor is it structured through stages of sexual development. The minor reference that the "conflicts in the ego" between the old "peaceful ego" and its newly formed parasitic "warlike ego" (Freud 1919d) in the final sentence of the 1919 version of Chapter 4 indicates that Freud cannot as yet answer the question whether the traumatic neuroses can be fully understood as mere variants of the narcissistic neuroses.

At the end of Chapter 4 of the 1920 edition of *Beyond the Pleasure Principle*, however, Freud adds a paragraph in which he does suggest a direct relation between "the mechanical violence of the trauma" one finds in traumatic neuroses, on the one hand, and "a quantity of sexual excitation which, owing to the lack of preparation for anxiety, would have a traumatic effect", on the other (Freud 1920g: 33). Freud's argument for this suggestion derives from a reference to *Three Essays* in which he had stated that mechanical agitation of the body such as the rhythmic shaking during railway travels produces sexual excitation (*Sexualerregung*) similar to the way in which muscular activity is pleasurable. He writes: "A compulsive link of this kind between railway-travel and sexuality is clearly derived from the pleasurable character of the sensations of movement" (Freud 1905d: 202). He adds that, although psychoanalysis has not yet been able to chart the aetiology of traumatic neuroses, it may be assumed the excitations from movement "lead to a profound disorder in the sexual mechanism or chemistry if they operate with exaggerated force" (Freud 1905d: 202). There is continuity between the rhythmic vibrations that evoke moderate sexual excitation and the severe mechanical violence produced by a huge quantity of sexual excitation. This suggestion is based on the fact that Freud does not make qualitative distinctions between forms of excitation but primarily takes into account quantitative differences. This makes his statement at least decidedly speculative and not very convincing. From the fact that the shaking of a train could lead to sexual excitation, it is hard to gather that a train accident would produce sexual excitation to an extreme degree.

This raises the obvious question as to why Freud adds this suggestion to the 1920 edition of the text. A preliminary answer to this question can be formulated with reference to the major innovations in the 1920 edition of *Beyond the Pleasure Principle*. These concern the idea of the life drives as the internal source of pleasurable and unpleasurable tensions and excitations. According to Freud, it is the life drives – which include the sexual drives – that produce excitation in all organs and body parts. If all neuroses, including the traumatic neuroses, have to be understood as stemming from internal causes, it seems obvious and maybe even necessary to assume that all neuroses can be traced back to this constitutional factor of the life drives producing excitation in organs and body tissue. This reasoning allows Freud to make the suggestions in the 1920 passage in Chapter 4. It implies an argument for the integration of the traumatic neuroses into a general theory of the sexual aetiology of the neuroses.

But what makes excitation "sexual" when this excitation can be traced back to the life drives? The answer Freud gives to this question can be found in *Three Essays* in a section rewritten in 1915. He argues that there are two kinds of excitations arising "from the somatic organs, based upon differences of a chemical nature".[48] "One of these kinds of excitation we describe as being specifically sexual, and we speak of the organ concerned as the 'erotogenic zone' [*erogene Zone*] of the sexual component instinct [*Partialtrieb*] arising from it" (Freud 1905d: 168). The other kind of excitation would be the one associated with hunger and the need for nutrition – the paradigmatic manifestation of the self-preservative drives. For Freud, excitations associated with the need for nutrition are limited to digestive organs. In the case of sexual excitation, however, any excitable organ or part of the body surface can become an erogenous zone (Freud 1905d: 183–184) and hence can produce sexual excitation. According to Freud, in short, all excitation is sexual when this excitation arises from peripheral erogenous zones susceptible to stimuli. Because of its source – including the susceptible surface and composition (skin, mucous membranes), every erogenous zone can produce a kind of excitation that can be said to be sexual. This explains why Freud can claim that the mechanical agitation and rhythmic vibrations of the body during railway travel produce sexual excitations. In this case, the whole body is one erogenous zone, as it were, receiving stimuli. Excitation and pleasure occur simultaneously only when the susceptible erogenous zones are stimulated in a certain manner – with rhythmic repetitions and moderate intensity of stimuli.

However, according to Freud, these zones are equally susceptible to "mechanical violence" disturbing chemical and physiological processes and thereby liberating a quantity of "sexual excitation" experienced as highly unpleasurable (Freud 1920g: 33).

The vicissitudes of traumatic neurosis

In Chapter 6 of the 1920 version of *Beyond the Pleasure Principle*, there is not a single reference to traumatic neuroses or war neuroses. The clinical cases that lead Freud to explore the question of the "beyond" of the pleasure principle suddenly seem irrelevant for his formulations of a new drive theory. We will later discuss in more detail what questions and problems lead to Freud's decision not to publish the first version of the text. For now, it suffices to say that these questions and problems were not related to issues concerning the aetiology of the traumatic neuroses. Rather, they concerned the implications of his reflections on the compulsion to repeat and its pulsional character, on the one hand, and of his ideas on the conservative and restorative character of all drives, on the other. The theory of life and death drives introduced in the 1920 version of the text is supposed to rearticulate the drives in such a way that not all phenomena of life need to be viewed through the lens of repetitive and restorative tendencies in reaction to external disturbing influences. In Chapter 6, Freud will argue that the sexual drives cannot be understood in terms of repetition: "But we still feel our line of thought appreciably hampered by the fact that *we cannot ascribe to the sexual instinct the characteristic of a compulsion to repeat* which first put us on the track of the death instincts" (Freud 1920g: 56; my italics). Regarding the compulsion to repeat, Freud then concludes that since not all drives have a "regressive character", the significance of the compulsion to repeat and hence of the traumatic neuroses as a clinical point of reference may have been "over-estimated" (Freud 1920g: 59).

Is Chapter 6, then, the end of Freud's discussions of traumatic neuroses? It is a striking fact that in later texts, such as *The Ego and the Id* and *Civilization and Its Discontents* (Freud 1923b; 1930a), in which he further discusses the life and death drives, Freud makes no reference to the traumatic neuroses. Trauma and repetition are – if at all – marginal issues in these texts. At the same time, texts in which the life and death drives play only a secondary role such as an *Inhibitions, Symptoms and Anxiety* (Freud 1926d: 124–125), or no role at all such as in *Moses and Monotheism* (Freud 1939a), are texts in which Freud returns to the problematic of the traumatic neuroses while emphasizing the significance of repetition.

Notably in *Inhibitions, Symptoms and Anxiety*, Freud once again investigates the aetiology of traumatic neurosis.[49] Although these neuroses often follow a life-threatening situation, Freud writes, it does not suffice to exclusively seek out the aetiology in "a fear of death (or fear *for* life)" (Freud 1926d: 129; Freud's italics).

He had already provided an argument for this contention in "Thoughts for the Times on War and Death" (Freud 1915b). In the unconscious, there is no knowledge of negativity and hence no knowledge of one's own death.[50] So, if fear of death does not play a role in the aetiology, may one assume that "deeper levels of the mental apparatus" are involved (Freud 1926d: 129)? As in *Beyond the Pleasure Principle*, Freud here refers to "excessive amounts of excitation" that impinge upon the psychic apparatus (Freud 1926d: 130). But he now adds that an actual life-threatening situation – such as a soldier's situation in the trenches – can only produce traumatic neurosis because it puts the person in a state of helplessness (*Hilflosigkeit*). This is a state with which everyone is familiar, since it defines the earliest biological-physical and psychical state of the newborn baby. After all, this baby is not only helpless in the sense that it needs others to provide for the satisfaction of basic needs, but more importantly, it is helpless against its own drive impulses in a state in which psychic life is not yet organized (Freud 1926d: 142). The baby is as yet without any efficient protective measurements against its own drive impulses. This traumatic situation of helplessness defines the constitutional factor in the aetiology of the traumatic neuroses.[51] Helplessness is the traumatic situation that threatens to repeat itself in every later situation of life-threatening danger (Freud 1926d: 150).[52]

According to Freud, the original trauma – the helplessness against massive influx of excitation – is modified and reinterpreted in successive stages of life. For example, castration anxiety would be a modification of anxiety for the separation from the mother and the first helplessness (Freud 1926d: 138–139, 145–148). Does this lead Freud to conclude that an original traumatic situation becomes sexualized in a second moment? Is the original helplessness perhaps *nachträglich* reinterpreted as sexual trauma? Again, Freud is determined to defend the sexual aetiology of the neuroses. He does this by arguing that the foetus is already aware of disturbances in the economy of its narcissistic libido and has feelings of unpleasure due to rising sums of excitation (Freud 1926d: 135). The newborn's helplessness can thus, according to Freud, already be described in terms of quantities of excitation and disturbances in libidinal investments.

Final remarks

We should not conclude from the previous that the First World War suddenly confronts Freud with the problematics of trauma, forcing him to return to and reconsider his initial trauma theory – the seduction theory – he had supposedly abandoned in 1897 in favour of an oedipal theory of phantasy life. Such a conclusion would have been in line with the dominant account of the development of Freudian theory, but should be seriously contested when we consider the fact that the oedipalization of Freudian theory only began after the introduction of the concept of the Oedipus complex in 1910, and reached its zenith in several publications from the 1920s. A reading of the major case studies and key metapsychological texts in fact shows that at the heart of Freud's thinking – from the seduction theory to his last writings – one finds a systematic inquiry into the relation between accidental and constitutional (and hereditary) factors that contribute to trauma and its pathogenic effects (Westerink & Van Haute 2025). Freud's study of the traumatic neuroses in *Beyond the Pleasure Principle* can be seen as a contribution to the further development of his trauma theory. The focus on the inner forces that produce trauma and conflict, the economic problem of unpleasure and pleasure, the issue of repetition and (lack of) memory, the question of the relation of the traumatic neuroses to the other neuroses (including the relation to sexuality) all point in this direction. But, most importantly, the traumatic neuroses provide Freud with a unique opportunity to speculate on the significance of trauma in the evolution of species and for thinking about the human physiological constitution and elementary psychical principles, mechanisms and organization. We will further explore this in Chapter 3. We end this chapter with the minor remark that in Freud's reflections on trauma in *Beyond the Pleasure Principle* no attempt is made at oedipalization of the traumatic neuroses.

Notes

1 For more detailed discussions of the traumatic neuroses, see Fischer-Homberger (1975), Micale (1995), Micale and Lerner (2010), Fletcher (2013) and Westerink and Van Haute (2025).
2 The many references to railway accidents in discussions of what Oppenheim names "traumatic neuroses" is typical of the body of literature we are discussing here, including Freud's discussions of traumatic neuroses (see also, e.g., Freud 1896c: 193; 1939a: 67). These references can be understood in the context of the discussions on the traumatic effects of shock and fright, which can be traced to the studies of the English surgeon John Erichsen from the 1870s on the effects of railway accidents, categorized as "railway-spine" or "concussion of the spine" (Harrington 2010).
3 Such an interpretation could draw upon Joseph Babinski's view of hysteria as caused by self-suggestion (pithiatism).
4 In their contributions to the Budapest conference, Ferenczi and Jones both refer to Freud's notion of the "complemental series" (*Ergänzungsreihe*), that is, the reciprocal relation between accidental factors, such as an actual traumatic experience, on the one hand, and constitutional and dispositional factors, on the other.
5 The relation between the two scenes cannot be translated in simple causal terms: the second scene is not the causal effect of the first. Instead, one could say that the first scene only becomes the "cause" (of trauma) because of the effect of the second scene on the first scene: The second scene adds meaning (sexuality) and affect (fright) to the first scene.
6 Laplanche has concluded from this that neither of the two events is in itself traumatic; it is the nachträgliche arousal of a memory that is traumatic (1985: 41–42).
7 Deleuze and Guattari associate this notion of *Nachträglichkeit* in puberty with a conversion of autoerotic activities ("desiring-production") into a reactive signification of sexuality within an oedipal framework (Deleuze & Guattari 1997: 73–74, 129). Traumatization is thus inherently linked to oedipalization.

8 As early as the 1905 edition of *Three Essays*, Freud is puzzled by the question of the "unknown origin" of a compulsion to repeat, which he articulates in terms of a "pertinacity or susceptibility to fixation" in both neuroses and perversions (Freud 1905d: 242).
9 From this, Jung had concluded that the distinction between the ego and the sexual drives was purely artificial and that in fact one had to assume one fundamental drive impulse: the primal libido (Jung 1912: 133–141). On the debate between Freud and Jung on the drive theory, on sexuality and psychoses, see Vandermeersch (1991).
10 On this issue, see also Malabou (2012: 11ff).
11 Freud's intuition that fright and anxiety are key when answering the question of the relation of the traumatic neuroses to other neuroses can be traced back to earlier writings in which he stated that "neurotic anxiety is transformed sexual libido" (Freud 1897b: 251). If this is also the case for fright or anxiety in the traumatic neuroses, these neuroses can be integrated into a theory of all neuroses.
12 The notion of "preparedness for anxiety" (*Angstbereitschaft*) is already mentioned in "On the Grounds for Detaching a Particular Syndrome from Neurasthenia under the Description 'Anxiety Neurosis'", in the context of a discussion of the psychic processing of fright (Freud 1895b: 107).
13 In his discussion of repetition in Freud's work, Jonathan Lear has argued that the compulsion to repeat one finds in the (traumatic) neuroses "is actually a failure to repeat", since repetition is always productive and liberating. This productivity, he argues, is apparent in all forms of repetition that lead to an increase of capacities that stimulate meaningful engagement in emotional and ethical life (Lear 2022: 54ff). We note here that whereas Freud discusses repetition from a pathoanalytical perspective, Lear seems to take repetition in teaching and knowledge acquisition as the starting point for a sharp distinction between healthy and unhealthy forms of repetition.
14 Even as early as 1895, in "Project", we find the idea that the repetition of impressions contributes to the creation of "facilitations", "cathexes" and "contact-barriers" that are the conditions for the genesis of the higher psychic systems such as memory (Freud 1950c: 300). In his reading of the "Project", Derrida highlighted the notion that repetition in this text not only "reproduces the same impression" over and over again, but in doing so has the power of generating *Bahnung* and is thus the condition for the creation of memory traces that in their turn serve the protection of life from immediate threatening situations (Derrida 1978: 200–202). Derrida thus highlights the productive character of repetition as the condition for the creation of memory.
15 My interpretation of the fort-da game builds on the reading of the *Three Essays* as a text in which Freud gives primacy to non-objectal polymorphous-perverse drives (Van Haute & Westerink 2021). From this perspective, the child's game can be seen as an illustration of a first object finding. This reading of the game is in line with, for example, Jean-François Lyotard's comments on this game in *Libidinal Economy* (2022: 38–41).
16 Lacan will take the repetition as the return to something that has been repressed as the starting point for his reflections on repetition as insistence (see Lacan 1991: 171). Lacan is not concerned with the clinical problem that puzzles Freud: the repetition of unpleasurable situations that were never repressed and cannot be repressed. For Lacan, the problematics of traumatic neuroses are beyond the limits of psychoanalysis.
17 For a more detailed discussion, see Westerink and Van Haute (2025).
18 In a footnote added to the 1920 edition of *Three Essays*, Freud writes: "Neurotic symptoms are based on the one hand on the demands of the libidinal instincts and

on the other hand on those made by the ego by way of reaction against them" (Freud 1905d: 163).

19 Because of the compulsory character of the repetition, Freud highlights the role of the analyst in the process of transforming the repetitions in recollections (Freud 1920g: 19).

20 In fact, Freud seems to be arguing that wherever we find "acting out", there is repetition of what is not fully "psychical" and hence unconscious. This idea paves the way for the next step: "repetitive action" is an immediate manifestation of the "untamed drives" (compare Freud 1914g: 154). See also, Hock and Scarfone (2024).

21 *Erinnern* is derived from the German *innern*, which means "to make something inner". *Innern* is related to words like *inne werden* ("to become aware", "to perceive") and inne haben ("to possess", "to have at one's disposal", "to understand").

22 From this we can understand Freud writing that it is not the repression of libido that produces anxiety (as he had maintained until *Beyond the Pleasure Principle*), but on the contrary, it is anxiety that produces repression (Freud 1926d: 108–109). Without anxiety and the identification of a danger, there can be no repression of the dangerous.

23 It is a remarkable fact that Charcot's student Pierre Janet – who throughout his career focused on the study of hysteria, trauma and dissociation – in *Les médications psychologiques* from 1919 (sic!) voices ideas quite similar to Freud's. In traumatized patients, one finds the "repetition" of a traumatic "situation" and the incapacity to turn the situation into a "memory", i.e., into an experience assimilated in a series of experiences (Janet 1919: 274–275; see also Van der Kolk & Van der Hart 1995). In this text, Janet formulates his views on trauma and repetition in the context of a critique of the Freudian theory of sexual trauma, arguing that this theory ignores the immediacy of trauma as a result of shock and fright (Janet 1919: 214ff).

24 This is what Deleuze will describe as Freud's "materialistic" account of repetition of and regression to a fixated traumatic state. That is, a repetition – similar in the way matter can move unchanged through space and time – indicates that what is repeated always remains the same (Deleuze 2004: 128).

25 This also explains why patients with wounds and physical injuries seldom develop a traumatic neurosis (Freud 1920g: 12). In these cases, the danger is already bound to a representation, namely what it was that caused the injured organ (Freud 1920g: 33). What about the factor of "hypercathexis of the injured organ"? "Fleeing into illness" implies that the excitation is "bound" to the representation of a physical injury.

26 Cathy Caruth has argued that "incomprehensibility" is key to the repetition of trauma. What is incomprehensible is not only the intensity of the violence and the confrontation with one's own death (in war situations), but also the fact of survival and "awakening" to life (Caruth 1996: 6, 66–67).

27 The dream introduces new meaning to the coitus a tergo that the Wolf Man had witnessed a few years earlier:

> What was essentially new for him in his observation of his parents' intercourse was the conviction of the reality of castration – a possibility with which his thoughts had already been occupied previously … For now he saw with his own eyes the wound of which his Nanya had spoken, and understood that its presence was a necessary condition of intercourse with his father.
>
> (Freud 1918b: 45–46)

28 See also Schuster (2016), Somers-Hall (2017), and Ingala (2020).

29 Angstbereitschaft in *Beyond the Pleasure Principle* does not describe anxiety as preparedness (for danger) or preparedness through anxiety. It indicates the willingness or readiness (*Bereitschaft*) to be or become a person experiencing anxiety (*Angst*).

30 On this issue, see also Freud's discussion of *Erwartung* and "anxious expectation" in *Introductory Lectures* and *Inhibitions, Symptoms and Anxiety* (Freud 1916–1917a: 398; 1926d: 164–168).

31 In his seminar on anxiety, Lacan directs attention to this notion of "expectation". He describes *Erwartung* as "the first line of recourse beyond *Hilflosigkeit*" (Lacan 2004: 75). We should note here that for Lacan, Freud's view of anxiety as expectation of and preparation for danger does not suffice to define anxiety proper. Anxiety arises at the unexpected "appearance" of an object which cannot be symbolized or imagined. Lacan contrasts this anxiety with fear, the latter being defined as the response to an identifiable object (see Freud 1920g: 12). It seems as if Lacan's conceptualization of anxiety is in fact a reconceptualization of Freud's concept of fright. We should note, however, that Lacan's concepts of fear and anxiety are situated in the domain of object-relations from the onset. His elaborations of anxiety can be seen, to a large extent, as reflections on Freud's *Hilflosigkeit* (see below) in the face of separation (loss, lack) from the mother. This approach differs from that of Freud's: in *Beyond the Pleasure Principle*, Freud situates fright "beyond" (e.g., "before") object-relations, relating fright to a traumatic "situation" of being overwhelmed by amounts of excitation. In his view of trauma and anxiety, Lacan redefines Freud's notion of an unexpected overwhelming endogenous drive energy in terms of an intrusion of an unrepresentable dimension of the subject's own desire.

32 Deleuze explores this issue at length in the second chapter of *Différence et répétition*. This chapter can be seen as a reflection on Freud's repetition in traumatic neuroses in which the compulsory repetitions in the present are the starting point for considering anticipation and memory, that is to say, the constitution of memory as a reflexive mental act, situating an experience in the past, and the possibility of anticipation as a condition for a reflexive act of prediction (Deleuze 2004: 91ff).

33 See also the following statement from *New Introductory Lectures*: "It is only the magnitude of the sum of excitation that turns an impression into a traumatic moment, paralyses the function of the pleasure principle and gives the situation of danger its significance" (Freud 1933a: 94; my italics).

34 In Seminar II, Lacan introduces the concept of "insistence" (*insistance*) as translation of *Wiederholungszwang*. He emphasizes this concept in order to distinguish repetitive insistence situated beyond the pleasure principle (and, as such, identified with the death drive) from restitutive (reparative) repetition that operates in the service of the pleasure principle and the principle of constancy (Lacan 1991: 61; Bernet 2020: 208–210).

35 Compare Freud's statements in *New Introductory Lectures*:

> With the traumatic neuroses things are different … We should not, I think, be afraid to admit that here the function of the dream has failed … We say that the dream is a fulfilment of a wish; but if you want to take these latter objections into account, you can say nevertheless that a dream is an attempt at the fulfilment of a wish … Unconscious fixation to a trauma seems to be foremost among these obstacles to the function of dreaming.
>
> (Freud 1933a: 29; Freud's italics)

36 The use of the word nachholen is, as Hock has suggested, a key word, since it combines nachträglich und wiederholen: it is through repetition that only "afterwards" stimuli will be mastered (Hock 2000: 258).
37 In *Beyond the Pleasure Principle*, Freud does not associate "danger" with "castration" – as he will later do in *Inhibitions, Symptoms and Anxiety* (Freud 1926d). This is not a surprise, given Freud's clinical material of the traumatic neuroses.
38 As early as 1895, in "Project", Freud states that the analysis of dreams provide insight into the primary processes, that is, into processes in which the secondary processes are temporarily paralyzed (Freud 1950c: 336, 338).
39 In Seminar II on the ego in Freud's theory we find Lefèbvre-Pontalis and Lacan arguing for a distinction between repetition as function and repetition as mechanism. The function could be described as "restitutive" in the service of establishing the dominance of the pleasure principle as manifest in homeostasis and "the cycles that life consists of, cycles of need and satisfaction". The mechanism points towards the death drive (Lacan 1991: 22–23, 66). In later seminars, this distinction is further elaborated (e.g., Lacan 1998: 48ff; 2007: 16, 45–46). See also Bernet (2020: 196 ff).
40 Ferenczi had paved the way for this perspective on the "reparative" compulsion to repeat. In his Budapest paper, he argues that the grave symptoms one finds in patients suffering from war neuroses should not be interpreted as direct expressions of trauma, but, on the contrary, as manifestations of self-protective tendencies (*Sicherungstendenz*) against the repetition of unpleasurable experiences. The disturbing fright-dreams of these patients should be seen as "spontaneous attempts at cure" (*selbsttätige Heilungsversuche*) in which fright is drained off with each repetition (Ferenczi 1919a: 22, 29).
41 Already in "Project" Freud argues that repetition of the release of unpleasure (*Unlustentbindung*) simultaneously means a decrease in the intensity of unpleasure (Freud 1950c: 359).
42 In Three Essays, Freud defines reaction formations in terms of spontaneous and "organically determined" psychic counter-forces constructed to repress the unpleasure (excitation) produced by the drives (Freud 1905d: 177–178).
43 At other moments in "Project", Freud seems to suggest that the ego produces and maintains the cathexes, which would imply that the ego precedes the process of binding (Freud 1950c: 369). On this issue, see also Strachey's "Appendix C" to "Project" in the *Standard Edition* (Freud 1950c: 392–397).
44 On this issue, see also Ray Brassier's discussion of trauma in Freud's views of traumatic neurosis (Brassier 2007: 234ff). See also, Zupančič (2017: 106ff).
45 This marks an important shift in Freud's discussions of trauma in earlier (and later) writings. In the Wolf Man case, for example, Freud is primarily concerned with identifying the actual experiences (primal scene as historical fact) vis-à-vis the phantasies (primal phantasy) in the aetiology of the Wolf Man's later complex neurosis. The focus is on the distinction between two different kinds of experiences. The dreams of traumatic neurotic patients are situated "beyond" this distinction (Westerink & Van Haute 2025: 150).
46 On this question, see also Moyaert (2014: 45ff) and Bernet (2020: 199ff).
47 Strachey translates *Wiederfinden* as "re-experiencing". In my view, it can better be translated as "finding oneself in a certain situation again".
48 We note here that already in "Project" Freud argues that "endogenous stimuli" – which he will later refer to as drive energy or simply drive – "consist of chemical products, of which there may a considerable number" (Freud 1950c: 321).

49 See also for what follows, Van Haute and Geyskens (2007: 18ff); Westerink and Van Haute (2025: 172–178).

50 In "Thoughts for the Times on War and Death", Freud writes:

> It is indeed impossible to imagine our own death; and whenever we attempt to do so we can perceive that we are in fact still present as spectators. Hence the psycho-analytic school could venture on the assertion that at bottom no one believes in his own death, or, to put the same thing in another way, that in the unconscious every one of us is convinced of his own immortality.
>
> (Freud 1915b: 289)

According to Freud, fear of death is the outcome of guilt because of death wishes against another person (1915b: 299).

51 The very fact that Otto Rank ignores the general constitutional factor of helplessness in his theory of "the trauma of birth" (Rank 1924) is Freud's main argument for dismissing Rank's theory in which the intensity of this trauma and the subsequent anxiety reaction determine whether a person will ever be able to control the anxiety and whether it will become neurotic or normal (Freud 1926d: 151–152).

52 At this point, Freud makes a distinction between the infant's helplessness as a "traumatic situation" (*traumatische Situation*), on the one hand, and "danger situation" (*Gefahrsituation*), on the other. Whereas in the traumatic situation (of helplessness), the individual experiences the trauma passively, the danger situation can be defined in terms of the recognizing, remembering and expecting of a situation of helplessness (Freud 1926d: 166). In such a case, the ego repeats the traumatic situation actively in order to be able to direct its course, that is, to master the situation. Freud again refers to children's play as attempts to master psychical experiences (Freud 1926d: 167).

Chapter 3

Pathoanalysis and bioanalysis

Psychoanalysis as pathoanalysis

In the opening section of the first chapter of *Beyond the Pleasure Principle*, Freud states that his "speculative assumptions" on the pleasure principle automatically regulating psychic life have been arrived at "in an attempt to describe and to account for *the facts of daily observation in our field of study*" (Freud 1920g: 7; my italics). The study of the psychopathologies is the starting point for a text in which Freud seeks to gain insight into the fundamental properties and functions of psychic life. *Beyond the Pleasure Principle* explores the possibilities and limits of the contention that the fundamental characteristics of all organic life can be studied from the perspective of the various psychopathologies. But what are Freud's arguments for such bold undertaking? In answering this question, we will consider the status and significance of Freud's many references to (evolutionary) biology in particular. Are these references merely part of a metaphorical or mythological manner of speaking (compare Lacan 1991: 75–76; Laplanche 2015b)? Or do these references form significant parts of Freud's argumentations and aims?

After the alleged abandonment of his seduction theory in 1897, Freud will systematically consider hereditary and constitutional factors in his aetiology of the psychoneuroses. The trauma theory of seduction (*Verführung*) is supplemented with a theory of constitution.[1] The first major contribution to this new line of inquiry – the 1905 *Three Essays on the Theory of Sexuality* – consists of an inventory of the physiological processes that define the general human sexual constitution. This study concludes that the "theory of the 'sexual constitution'" had taken "the place of a 'general neuropathic disposition'" (Freud 1906a: 275–276). This turn towards hereditary and constitutional factors goes hand in hand with the introduction of certain physiological and psychic characteristics defining human existence.

Contrary to his predecessors' functional approaches to sexuality and the subsequent pathologization of non-functional perversions, Freud's starts from the assumption that the general human sexual constitution and infantile sexual life cannot be defined in functional terms.[2] Instead, he argues that the

DOI: 10.4324/9781003680413-3

study of the perversions provides insight in polymorphous perverse, autoerotic, and non-objectal pleasurable sexual activities and the need for variations that define infantile sexual life (Davidson 2001; Van Haute & Westerink 2021). In other words, it is from the study of the perversions that one can gain insight into the general human sexual constitution and its various components (Freud 1905d: 171; also Geyskens 2005: 20). And not only the perversions, also their "negative" – the neuroses – provide insight into the general human sexual constitution and the physiological processes that characterize infantile sexual life (Freud 1905d: 165). In *Three Essays*, it is hysteria that provides the model for the further study of infantile sexuality. According to Freud, hysteria displays an exaggerated sexual need and an overly powerful formation of the sexual drive; yet "the character of hysterics shows a degree of sexual repression in excess of the normal quantity, an intensification of resistance against the sexual instinct" (Freud 1905d: 164–165). Hysteria shows in a magnified and caricatured way the general human physiological processes that define sexuality, the organic repression of sexual urges, and the symptom formations that result from the unresolved conflict between the sexual drives and repression (Van Haute & Westerink 2021: 18).

The "pathological" approach to perversions and psychopathologies is thus replaced by an "anthropological" approach.[3] Freud's psychoanalysis turns into what can be called the pathoanalysis of human existence.[4] From now on, psychoanalysis can be considered clinical anthropology. If the perversions and psychopathologies are characterized by (quantitative) exaggerations, magnifications and intensifications of normal psychic and physiological processes, forces and tendencies that may or may not have been increased by external influences, the study of these perversions and pathologies has philosophical-anthropological implications. Various aspects of human existence can best – and maybe even only – be studied from the pathological variations. The psychopathologies give insight in generally human physiological processes and psychic dynamics and complexes.[5]

In *Beyond the Pleasure Principle*, it is particularly in the study of the fright-dreams of traumatic neurotic patients that Freud finds the most elementary tendencies and functions of psychic life in general (Freud 1920g: 32).[6] Not only do these dreams provide insight into the preparedness for anxiety as the first protective shield against drive stimuli, and into the elementary architecture of psychic life. They also prompt Freud to consider a general human tendency to repeat, and to elaborate the "pulsional character" of the compulsion to repeat: "At this point we cannot escape a suspicion that we may have come upon the track of a universal attribute of instincts and perhaps of organic life in general which has not hitherto been clearly recognized" (Freud 1920g: 36).

The traumatic neuroses, Freud claims, provide insight into the elementary characteristics of human life, as well as all organic life. The analysis of fright-dreams does not lead Freud to focus on the exceptional psychic states of traumatized patients; instead, it paves the way for speculations on the receptive cortical layer of the first living vesicles. The traumatic neuroses thus shed light on specific aspects of all organic life, namely the most elementary tendencies and mechanisms involved in the formation of the first protective shield against the influx of stimuli.[7] These neuroses provide a unique insight into processes unfolding at a time "before" there is any efficient psychic functioning.

This train of thought is also apparent in other texts from the period during which Freud completed the first version of *Beyond the Pleasure Principle.* In "The Uncanny", Freud applies his findings from the study of traumatic neuroses to the uncanny (*das Unheimliche*) as a subject "undoubtedly related to what is frightening". "Uncanny" refers to a state of feeling in response to something that suddenly appears as alive and dangerous when it should have remained inanimate, secret and hidden (Freud 1919h: 219, 224–226). Analyzing the uncanny in cultural representations, Freud argues that the study of pathological psychic phenomena has shown that feelings of uncanniness can be traced back to sensations accompanying a very early psychic stage in which the ego was not yet fully formed and hence easily disturbed. This stage is further characterized by a "sense of helplessness", and by involuntary repetitions of situations that appear "inescapable" (Freud 1919h: 236–237). The analyses of neurotic patients make it "possible to recognize the dominance in the unconscious mind of a 'compulsion to repeat' proceeding from instinctual impulses and probably inherent in the very nature of the instincts". And Freud concludes: "All these considerations prepare us for the discovery that whatever reminds us of this inner 'compulsion to repeat' is perceived as uncanny" (Freud 1919h: 238). The feeling of uncanniness points towards a fateful recurrence of a situation of helplessness vis-à-vis the daemonic, unbound character of the drives. The uncanny is the manifestation of a momentary breach or collapse of stable and consistent temporal and spatial representations.

In the 1919 version of *Beyond the Pleasure Principle*, it is not only the traumatic neuroses that provide knowledge of general human psychic structures and principles. Although there is only one minor reference to hypochondria and melancholia (Freud 1920g: 12), it can be argued that it is especially the study of these pathologies that first made Freud doubt the dominance of the pleasure principle in psychic life. In "On Narcissism", it was hypochondria that had raised the question "why the damming-up of libido in the ego should have to be experienced as unpleasure" (Freud 1914c: 85). After all, one would expect the psychic apparatus and "a strong egoism" to direct the surplus quantity of libido to objects in order not to fall ill.[8] And melancholia had confronted Freud with the puzzling question as to how to explain in economic terms the remarkable fact that people cling to lost objects, experience this as "painful unpleasure", and yet find it difficult or impossible to detach themselves from such objects (Freud 1917e: 245). Why do people cling to lost objects when alternative objects providing the possibility of pleasure are available? If the sexual drive aims at pleasure, as Freud had been insisting, and if the object is the most variable aspect of the drive (Freud 1915c: 122–123), how can we understand that the drive apparently has a hard time giving up the objects in which it was invested? In "On Transience", Freud states:

> But why it is that this detachment of libido from its objects should be such painful process is a mystery to us and we have not hitherto been able to frame any hypothesis to account for it. We only see that the libido clings to its objects and will not renounce those that are lost even when a substitute lies ready to hand.
>
> (1916a: 306–307)

Although Freud focuses on narcissistic object choice, identification and the ambivalence of feelings of love and hate as the main factors in the aetiology of melancholia, the remarks on the "attachments" of the libido (see also Freud 1917e: 244; Moyaert 2022: 25–31) are significant for the his further reflections on the "conservative" character of the drives in *Beyond the Pleasure Principle*. Melancholia shows in an exaggerated form that the drives (libido) are "tenacious" and "adhesive". Apparently, drives resist change and progress. Melancholia shows Freud that it is not the severity of the traumatic impact (the shock of the loss of a beloved object), but a constitutional (pulsional) factor that determines the continuation of attachments felt as unpleasure. There is something in the drives that resists the pleasure principle.[9]

Throughout Freud's writings, the pathoanalytical perspective is undermined by a developmental approach to psychopathology (Van Haute & Geyskens 2012: 18–19; Van Haute & Westerink 2021). In fact, the latter approach comes to dominate the later editions of *Three Essays* from 1915 onwards, through sections devoted to the phases in the sexual organization, the sexual researches of children, and the narcissistic libido (Freud 1905d: 194–200, 217–219; Van Haute & Westerink 2021: 49–83). In line with this approach, Freud starts to consider psychopathologies as developmental disorders. The psychopathologies are increasingly seen as resulting from the interplay between constitutional and accidental factors, such that the choice of neurosis is determined by the "point of fixation" of the sexual drive relative to a certain phase of sexual development. The psychopathologies are being understood as "inhibitions in development" characterized by regression to the point of fixation (Freud 1913d: 318). The order in which psychopathologies "are usually enumerated" corresponds to the constitutionally determined order of phases in the normal sexual development. This implies that the psychopathologies can again be defined in opposition to normality – they are deviations from the progressive development towards normal adulthood. Instead of providing insight into general human psychic structures and processes, the psychopathologies merely shed light on specific disturbances in a developmental process. In this context, Freud argues that the point of fixation in paranoia and psychosis has to be sought "in a stage of development *before* object-choice has been established" (Freud 1913d: 318; Freud's italics). His analyses of the traumatic neuroses in *Beyond the Pleasure Principle* follow a similar train of thought. The point of fixation concerns a traumatic situation "before" any adequate and efficient organization of psychic life.

The question arises as to which approach is dominant in *Beyond the Pleasure Principle* – the pathoanalytical or the developmental one. For the latter to be the case, there would have to be some notion of "normal" development and its aberrations. Yet, this not what Freud is positing in the text or concluding from his elaborations on the conservative character of the drives and the evolution of organic life. On the contrary: if the evolution of organic life can, from its very beginning, be described in terms of being "disturbed" by external influences (see below), and in terms of "diverging" from an initial inorganic state, there is no such thing as an ideal "normal" progressive development. The emergence of life is the first distortion and diversion. What we call "normal" development is the sum of physiological and psychic reactions to the numerous traumatic impacts of external influences. The normal development of an organism is nothing but the repetition of the always-already derailed evolution of the species.

Freud can be said to give priority of the pathoanalytical over the developmental approach in *Beyond the Pleasure Principle.* The traumatic neuroses are the model from which to understand the most elementary characteristics of all organic life. This raises the obvious question what Freud's arguments are for this application of the pathoanalytical perspective on all organic life. If this approach is based on clinical observations and the assumption of quantitative differences between pathological and normal human psychic life, what is the argument for making claims about all living substances? Is such inquiry not irrelevant when clinical practice only asks for a theoretical reflection on constitutional and accidental factors in the aetiology (Freud 1905d: 131, 239)? Should psychoanalysis not limit itself to the analysis of memories, impressions and experiences in an intersubjective sphere? What is it, then, that prompted Freud to inquire into phylogeny?

Towards the study of phylogeny

Evolutionary biological perspectives were never absent from Freud's writings, but they gain in importance when he finds himself compelled to reconsider hereditary and constitutional factors in the aetiology of the psychoneuroses. In this context, he will rely on a body of knowledge with which he had been familiar since his student days and his first zoological researches.[10] In *Three Essays* and other texts, he maintains that the various aspects of infantile sexuality, such as, for example, organic repression and reaction formations, can be understood from an evolutionary perspective. Evolution from animals to human beings is accompanied by physical changes such as a clear distinction between excretory and reproductive organs. In walking upright, the role of smell changed, giving rise to disgust felt at trails of excrements and dirt on the ground (Freud 1985c: 269; 1916–1917a: 354–355). While the reaction formations of disgust and shame are typically human and can be traced to the organization of the erogenous zones and the senses, these formations relate to perverse aspects of sexuality that are a "continuation" of the "perverse" sexuality of animals.[11] There is no discontinuity between animal and human life. The continuity between the two is in fact the very starting point of *Three Essays*. In the first paragraph of the text, Freud introduces the concept of drive to indicate the fundamental significance of motive forces and needs found in both human and animal life (Freud 1905d: 135). For Freud, the human sexual constitution is merely a variation within a realm of animal sexual constitutions.[12] What interests Freud is the distinction between infantile sexual life as continuous with the perverse sexual life of other animals, on the one hand, and the transformations of sexual life in puberty after a period of latency, on the other.[13] And yet, the focus of his discussions of the transformations in puberty is not on individual preferences or internalized cultural norms, but once again on physiological (e.g., chemical) processes. The transformation and integration of polymorphous-perverse sexual activities into a functional sexuality aimed at reproduction are presented as a delayed manifestation of the instinct for the preservation of the species that one finds in all organic life (Freud 1905d: 207ff).

Contrary to post-Freudians such as Lacan and Laplanche, Freud is not concerned with a systematic distinction between animal instincts and human drives (Lacan 1998: 49, 102; 2006: 88; Laplanche 1989; 2015b; also Johnston 2005: 156ff; Bernet 2020: 211).[14] Like animal life, human life is largely organized according to biological principles such as "the pressure of vital needs" and "the predetermined course of development" (Freud 1916–1917a: 355). For Freud, human life, as regulated by cultural norms and the moral organization of object relations, is not the "radical other" of nature. He does not argue that human psychic life should be exclusively defined in relation to a symbolic order (culture, language, valuable and meaningful objects). In fact, these norms and regulations are built on psychic "patterns" and "dams" – reaction formations of shame and disgust formed before interaction with objects and culture. The cultural norms merely give specific content to what originally were organic processes (Freud 1905d: 178–179; Van Haute & Westerink 2021: 15, 35). Culture maintains and complicates structures and dynamics that are organic and natural.

Freud's growing interest in phylogeny and the historical acquisitions of what will determine the "hereditary and constitutional factors" in the aetiology of the psychoneuroses run parallel to two developments in Freud's work: the introduction of the Oedipus complex and the emergence of applied psychoanalysis from about 1910 onwards.[15] The pathoanalytical approach that we have already discussed can be seen as the condition for these developments in

Freudian theory. After all, if the psychopathologies inform us about aspects of general human psychic life, these pathologies may also shed light on cultural phenomena that, after all, can be seen as resulting from psychic motives. In certain cultural phenomena, the psychic conflicts that characterize the psychopathologies find preferred opportunities in which these conflicts can become manifest without posing a direct threat to individual life and social life (Van Haute & Geyskens 2012: 16).[16]

The most important study from this period is *Totem and Taboo*. In this text, Freud raises the question as to how the traumatic event of primordial murder, and especially prehistoric man's initial reactions to this act – namely those of mourning and guilt – can influence later generations in such a way that these initial reactions persist in religion, social organization and morality throughout cultural history. How is continuity of psychic life possible – between generations over a period of thousands of years? According to Freud, we cannot assume that such continuity is based on oral and scriptural transmissions only: "A part of the problem seems to be met by the inheritance of psychical dispositions which, however, need to be given some sort of impetus in the life of the individual before they can be roused into actual operation" (Freud 1912–1913a: 158). At the heart of these inherited psychical dispositions Freud identifies the fear of castration, ambivalence of feelings, and sense of guilt (Freud 1912–1913a: 157); but also the "schemata" that converge in the associated network of representations and affects called the "Oedipus complex" and that can be said to form "the nucleus of all neuroses" (Freud 1912–1913a: 157). The inquiry into phylogeny can be seen as a decisive step in the gradual oedipalization of Freudian theory.[17]

The case study of the Wolf Man offers a clinical illustration of these developments in Freud's thinking. For the most part, this study consists of a reconstruction of the various accidental moments in the earliest stages of sexual development, which together form an associated complex of distorting and diverting experiences. Taken together, these experiences have a traumatic effect only *nachträglich* – in the Wolf Man's anxiety dream at the age of 4. In this anxiety dream, the little boy unconsciously realizes the implications of his object choice: in order to have intercourse with the father, the boy would have to be castrated (Freud 1918b: 28, 43ff).[18] However, this interpretation of the anxiety dream is not without its problems that Freud finds difficult to resolve. The most pressing of these concern the Wolf Man's identification of the father as the castrator of his infantile sexuality, when in fact all actual castration threats were uttered by women in the boy's social surrounds. Freud tackles this problem by assuming "phylogenetically inherited schemata, which, like the categories of philosophy, are concerned with the business of 'placing' the impressions derived from actual experience" (Freud 1918b: 119).[19] These schemata do not automatically organize impressions and experiences. Like all constitutional factors, they first need to be activated by an actual experience. In this case, it is the anxiety dream that activates a phylogenetically inherited Oedipal scheme in which the father is presented as castrator.[20]

Ontogeny as recapitulation of phylogeny

Totem and Taboo (1913) is the first major contribution to the study of the historical development of the general human psychic constitution. The mention of inherited acquired psychical characteristics is a reference to the psycho-Lamarckian theories with which Freud was familiar. In the following years, he will continue these trains of thought, arguing that the human somatic and psychical constitution needs to be seen as the result of series of "complemental series", that is, series of interactions between constitutional and accidental factors from which a new disposition emerges (e.g., Freud 1916–1917a: 346). In this period, we also find explicit references to Ernst Haeckel's biogenetic law – "ontogeny is the abbreviated (*kurze*) and accelerated (*schnelle*) repetition (*Recapitulation*) of phylogeny" (Haeckel 1866, vol. 2: 300) – as a principle "applicable to psychic life" (Freud 1913j: 184). This law or "recapitulation theory" will play a crucial role in Freud's arguments in the 1919 version of *Beyond the Pleasure Principle.*

Why is Freud keen to integrate this law into his metapsychology in general and into *Beyond the Pleasure Principle* in particular? The first thing to note here is that Haeckel was generally considered an authority in the field, a scholar who had played a crucial role in the reception of Darwin's ideas in the German-speaking countries. His recapitulation theory was widely accepted and was considered "Darwinian" – among others by Fechner and Weismann.[21] This theory plays a crucial role in Freud's arguments as it allows him to expand the pathoanalytical scope to speculations on the evolution of all organic life. After all, the biogenetic law states that the development of each individual – from embryo to adult – repeats in an abbreviated and accelerated form the evolution of the species. For Freud, this means that the individual (including its embryonic life) repeats the complete history of interactions between constitutional factors and newly acquired characteristics that together produce the elementary physiological properties and psychological organizations defining each individual. However, not only does the biogenetic law express that each individual organism must repeat the history of the species; it also expresses the idea that at each stage of development, a previous stage is abandoned and will nevertheless persist, and can even be re-established (through regression) (Freud 1915b: 285–286). Haeckel thus offers a theory in which progress and the appearance of new species in evolution do not cancel out the remainders of the most primitive forms and associated tendencies (Ansell-Pearson 1999: 108).

This includes trauma. We have already mentioned Freud's seduction theory and the idea of trauma in two phases, that is, of the return or repetition of a first experience in a second one. The recapitulation theory provides Freud with the possibility of articulating the human constitution as a disposition for pathogenesis in an analogous way. Phylogenetically inherited traces can be individually repeated with pathogenic effects. For Freud, the recapitulation theory underpins his seduction theory, and marks the shift from a focus on contingent accidents in individual lives to a notion of trauma as co-determined by historically acquired dispositions.

Furthermore, the biogenetic law implies that since each individual repeats the development of an entire evolutionary lineage, all regulatory mechanisms, functions and tendencies valid for all organisms in that lineage must also apply to the individual. And vice versa, all fundamental (constitutional) regulatory mechanisms and functions found in the individual organism must also be present in all organisms in the same lineage up to the point in evolution where these mechanisms or functions were first formed or acquired. In other words, not only does phylogeny provide insight in ontogeny, but the law also allows for the reverse: the study of individual physiological and psychic characteristics provides knowledge of the evolutionary lineage. The recapitulation theory thus provides a crucial argument for extending the pathoanalytical study of the fundamental aspects of human beings to all organic life.[22]

In the first version of *Beyond the Pleasure Principle*, Freud refers to Haeckel's biogenetic law at a crucial point in the text. Having argued that the compulsion to repeat has a "pulsional character", he states that "we cannot escape the suspicion that we may have come upon the track of a universal attribute of instincts and perhaps of all organic life in general" (Freud 1920g: 36). What follows is the definition of drive as an "*urge inherent in organic life to restore an earlier state of things*". Freud defines "drive" not as a "factor impelling towards change and development", but as an "expression of the *conservative* nature of living substance" (Freud 1920g: 36; Freud's italics). The argument for this claim about the characteristics of all organic life does not depend so much on concrete examples of the migration of certain fish (such as salmon) to their spawn grounds, or the yearly migratory flights of birds. His main argument centres on the biogenetic law:

> we are quickly relieved of the necessity for seeking for further examples by the reflection that the most impressive proofs of there being an organic compulsion to repeat lie in the phenomena of heredity and the facts of embryology. We see how the germ of a living animal is obliged in the course of its development to recapitulate (even if only in a transient and abbreviated fashion) the structures of all the forms from which it is sprung, instead of proceeding quickly by the shortest path to its final shape.
>
> (Freud 1920g: 37)[23]

We should note here that Freud's reference to the recapitulation theory undeniably comes with a twist. In Haeckel's writings, one finds a firm belief in progressive natural development – a belief rooted in German idealist thought more than in Darwin's writings. According to Haeckel, the study of the evolution of the species does not only show the emergence of an abundance of species through external forces demanding adaptation to new circumstances.

The fact of recapitulation of an evolutionary development in each individual organism also gives evidence of a powerful factor inherent in all organic life forms. Haeckel refers to this inner factor as the formative drive (*Bildungstrieb*), but unlike his predecessors does not give any spiritual or metaphysical meaning to this concept. It denotes the forces that emerge from physico-chemical processes. It is from these processes that one can understand the natural development and completion (*Vervollkommnung*) of the individual and of nature as a whole (Haeckel 1866, vol. 1: 154; also Kleeberg 2005; Richards 2008).

In the 1919 version of *Beyond the Pleasure Principle*, Freud decidedly denies the drives any progressive formative capacity. His explicit abandonment of the belief in a "drive towards perfection" (*Trieb zur Vervollkommnung*) entails a strong critique of Haeckel's theories, among others (Freud 1920g: 42).[24] This also implies that he distances himself from the kind of cultural and political *Weltanschauung* represented by Haeckel – a worldview in which a clear distinction between the pathological (as degeneration and inhibited development) and the normal underpins notions of race and eugenics (Willner 2022; 2024a; 2024b). This is made explicit in Freud's critique of the idea of the "development into supermen" (*Entwicklung zum Übermenschen*) which he classifies as a "benevolent illusion" that "cannot be preserved".

Against Haeckel's and others' views on progressive development towards *Vervollkommnung* of individuals and species, Freud introduces a radical different teleology in the 1919 version of *Beyond the Pleasure Principle*. The drives are not urges impelling humans to change and perfection, but aim to restore an earlier state. The drives are regressive forces. The *telos* of the drives is a state that precedes life. The fact that, according to Freud, life aims at death, does not mean that the drives aim at death in the future. For Freud, death does not come after life. Death precedes life and haunts life from its very beginning.[25] The fact that organic life forms have a certain life span results from life-prolonging enforced modifications and adaptations to external life-threatening circumstances. These create "detours" that enable species to resist the urge to return to the inanimate as rapidly as possible (see Alfandary 2019). For Freud, this means that life is in the first place survival – that is, not only survival in a hostile environment, but more importantly, the survival vis-à-vis the drives as forces that pressure life from the inside without concern for the individual's well-being, on the one hand, and as the innate tendency towards the inanimate, on the other. The organic does not want to coincide with its very own instinctive core that is at the same time alien and hostile. All living substances strive to rid themselves of that which essentially characterizes them.

This view of life as that which seeks to return to the inanimate indicates Freud's pathoanalytical – and, at the same time, mechanistic – perspective on the emergence of life as a "traumatic" event: "The attributes of life were at some time evoked [*erweckt*] in inanimate matter [*unbelebter Materie*] by the action of a force of whose nature we can form no conception [*unvorstellbare Krafteinwirkung*]" (Freud 1920g: 38). He elaborates:

> The tension [*Spannung*] which then arose in what had hitherto been an inanimate substance [*unbelebter Stoff*] endeavoured to cancel itself out. In this way the first instinct [*erste Trieb*] came into being: the instinct to return [*zurückzukehren*] to the inanimate [*leblose*] state.
>
> (Freud 1920g: 38)

Freud describes this incomprehensible force in terms of "the pressure of external *disturbing* forces [*Störungskräfte*]" (Freud 1920g: 36; my italics). The reference to forces as being "disturbing" reveals Freud's pathoanalytical perspective on this issue. The creation of life from inanimate matter can be described in terms of a violent mechanical shock that produces effects and reactions analogous to the traumatic neuroses.[26]

It is the biogenetic law that provides Freud with a justification for his speculative reflections on the remaining influence and significance of the traumatic character of the origin of life. The first impact of a force that created the first living substance is the first disturbance in an endless series of disturbances. Freud's statement that "decisive external influences" altered the first living substance in such a way "as to oblige the still surviving substance to diverge [*Ablenkungen*] ever more widely from its original course of life and to make ever more complicated *détours* [*Umwege*] before reaching its aim of death" (Freud 1920g: 38–39), shows that the development of organic life towards ever more complicated life forms can be described from the perspective of, and in analogy to, the psychopathologies. The use of the terms *Ablenkungen* and *Umwege* is significant here: it connects *Beyond the Pleasure Principle* to the seduction theory (*Verführungstheorie*) which Freud never really abandoned but in fact expanded, including constitutional factors in the aetiology of the psychoneuroses. It is significant, in this context, that *Ablenkung* (*ablenken*) is regularly used throughout Freud's writings as the definition of *Verführung* (*verführen*). Even in the period of the seduction theory, the word *verführen* did not refer exclusively to seduction and abuse by other persons; rather, it described the effect of every traumatic experience or impression. Such experiences produce derailment, diversion and deflection from a "normal" course (see, e.g., Freud 1918b: 108; also Laplanche 1980: 87; Westerink & Van Haute 2025: 36, 105–106). For Freud, life is disturbed and derailed matter. Life is survival of the traumatized, of those who only apparently got away unharmed and were able to postpone death.

The vesicle and its differentiations

The biogenetic law allows Freud to introduce the picture of "a living organism in its most simplified possible form as an undifferentiated vesicle [*undifferenziertes Bläschen*] of a substance that is susceptible to stimulation [*reizbarer Substanz*]" as the starting point for inquiring into the conditions for and elementary organization of psychic life (Freud 1920g: 26).[27] It is not the first time Freud refers to the significance of the most primitive life forms for human psychic life. From the moment he engages in a more systematic study of phylogenetic factors contributing to the human constitution, we find occasional references to the most primitive life forms scattered throughout his various writings (Freud 1914c: 75; 1916–1917a: 139; 1923b: 57). These references can be traced back to his earlier pre-psychoanalytical research. His mentors in Vienna, including Ernst Brücke and Ernst Mach, showed a great interest in *Elementarorganismen* and their "irritability" and "susceptibility" or "excitability".[28] For these and other scholars, the cell was the first and most simple form of life, i.e., an elementary organism (Schloegel & Schmidgen 2002). Given the properties of irritability and response (movement, change) to stimuli, the study of cells promised insight into the most elementary physiological and psychological characteristics of all organic life forms. These elementary organisms were hence supposed to manifest psychological properties also found in human beings. The study of these cells or organisms also promised insight into the processes of natural selection, i.e., the first appearance of variations that were either favourable or injurious (compare Darwin 1859: 63).

For Freud, the impact of the incomprehensible force that produced the first living substance has not only an immediate (disturbance, excitation) but also a delayed – *nachträglich* – effect:

> It was still an easy matter at that time for a living substance to die; the course of its life was probably only a brief one … For a long time, perhaps, living substance was thus being constantly created afresh and easily dying …
>
> (Freud 1920g: 38)

Freud suggests that the earliest history of organic life is characterized by constant extinction and re-creation – a process unhindered neither by self-preservative instincts or an inclination towards the preservation of the species, nor by any self-regulatory principles and functions. The plasmatic vesicle is in a constant state of becoming extinct due to its constitutional irritability and vulnerability in an environment replete with stimuli.[29] It is, Freud writes, "undifferentiated". This means, first of all, that the vesicle, apart from the distinction between its surface (an irritable membrane) and its interiority (plasm) initially lacks any functional organization or structure that would enable it to actively respond to incoming stimuli. In this situation, the vesicle lacks any form of agency, striving or intentionality. It is as yet unable to perceive, receive, inhibit, absorb, internalize and process stimuli. Or more precisely, perception equals reflex. As such, the vesicle is in a state prior to perceiving and distinguishing pleasure or unpleasure (pain). It has only a short life-span because it cannot experience something outside – or inside – as life-threatening or unpleasurable. The vesicle's life is prone to death and dying. It is in a state of primal helplessness. It is merely an irritable or excitable substance effected (destroyed, modified) by external stimuli.

The undifferentiated vesicle changes after endless and habitual repetitions of "easy dying" when external influences oblige the "still surviving" living substance to abandon the organic membrane that is its external structure, and to diverge further from its original easy-dying-mode. This second development can be seen as a kind of delayed reaction to the traumatizing impact of the first incomprehensible force repeated in later external forces that act on the living substance, destroying the vesicle. According to Freud, the susceptible vesicle that is exposed to ceaseless external influences will develop a crust, an "inorganic" shield composed of chalk and minerals, a siliceous external skeleton (Freud 1920g: 26–28).[30] This shield is the product of secretion, as it were.[31] The vesicle is now able protect itself against external stimuli (*Reizschutz*) and to receive stimuli in such way that these do not further modify – that is, destroy – the living substance. This living substance no longer dies easily; it prolongs its life through a process as "dying" at its surface. It can live in the face of life-threatening stimuli. It can fend off and postpone death through the formation of a dead surface. The surface modifications – that is, solidifications – thus go hand in hand with internal stabilization. The first differentiations are the condition for the first detour from the trajectory towards death, and the prolongation of – what now can properly be called – individual life. From here, Freud assumes, further internal differentiation will proceed. The differentiated vesicle is a unit with an elementary internal organization such that it can sustain itself and resist the external world. It is a living substance that will be able to "die in its own fashion"; it has a certain temporality. It can delay reactions to perceptions, and it can associate present sensations with past experiences. What Freud thus adds to a theory of natural selection is an explanation of the production of variations from the notions of trauma and the reactive formations that produce new, more complicated detours (*Umwege*).[32] Since the reaction formations imply conflict instead of the immediate discharge of excitation (that would result in death), for Freud, life (as detour) is the result of inner conflicting forces – and not the other way around.

In his conceptualization of these processes such as the creation of the vesicle's inorganic crust and the "organic elasticity" that characterizes the drives, Freud remains close to concepts Haeckel and Fechner use to describe characteristics of the most primitive life forms: the capacities for crystallization (*Krystallisation*) and elasticity (*Elasticität*) (Haeckel 1866, vol. 1: 115, 129; Fechner 1873: 13ff).[33] But whereas for these authors, these characteristics define the progressive interaction between the building blocks and aspects of variability, plasticity and stability inherent in all organic life, Freud regards both aspects – crystallization and elasticity – as reaction formations to external disturbing influences. When Freud writes that the drives are "elastic", he does not – as Catherine Malabou has correctly argued (2022: 275–286) – indicate an innate capacity to produce new forms and amalgamations. On the contrary, elasticity means the urge to return to the inorganic, to retreat to the initial form, and hence to undo change and development. The drives seek to undo the effects of trauma.

Why and how does Freud relate the introduction of the undifferentiated vesicle in the first version of *Beyond the Pleasure Principle* to his clinical observations and metapsychological claims? The vesicle makes its appearance in Chapter 4 – the chapter that famously opens with the words "What follows is speculation" (Freud 1920g: 24). This speculation concerns the origins and early evolution of psychic life, that is, of its elementary systems and their topography, functions and regulating principles. In this chapter, Freud refers back to the main psychic systems that he says he had already charted in *The Interpretation of Dreams* and in "A Metapsychological Supplement of the Theory of Dreams", among other writings. The assumption in those texts was that the psychic apparatus could be defined in terms of two major distinct systems (Freud 1900a: 536ff; 1917d; 1920g: 24–26). First, there is "the system *Pcpt.-Cs.*" which has the function of giving orientation to the individual by differentiating the internal from the external. This system has a receptive capacity for perceptions of excitatory stimuli, but is also characterized by the fact that these impressions leave no trace in the system. Second, there is the mnemic (*Mnem.*) system (*Gedächtnis*) in which the perceived excitation leaves traces; in this system, excitation is stored without being conscious. For this reason, these two systems are said to be "mutually exclusive". In *The Interpretation of Dreams*, Freud had further argued that the memory traces stored in the *Mnem.* system can subsequently be made conscious. In *Beyond the Pleasure Principle*, Freud boils this train of thought down to the following formula: "*consciousness arises instead of a memory-trace*" (Freud 1920g: 25; Freud's italics). Consciousness would thus largely be the effect of unconscious memory-traces becoming conscious. Consciousness is an epiphenomenon of the unconscious. The speculations on the origins of the system *Pcpt.-Cs.* are now meant to shed light on the order of appearance of the two main systems and their functions. What Freud seeks to explain is the position of the system *Pcpt.-Cs.* on the borderline between the internal and the external world, and, second, its incapacity to be modified by incoming stimuli and to store traces. What also needs to be explained are the conditions of possibility for the formation of the *Mnem.* system, its capacity to undergo modification, to store traces and to produce and reproduce memories.[34] From the speculations on the vesicle's first differentiations, Freud concludes that consciousness first arises in the perceptual system as a "layer" that is in fact part of the first protective shield established against incoming external stimuli. The formation of memory-traces and the foundation of the mnemic system are the next steps in a development that goes hand in hand with the capacity of the temporal and spatial organization of representations.[35]

Let us take a closer look. Freud's starting point in Chapter 4 is the idea that "the system *Pcpt.-Cs.*" can be assigned "a position in space" on the "border between outside and inside" – and hence not safely housed somewhere in the brain's inmost interior (Freud 1920g: 24; see also 1917d: 232–233). The undifferentiated living substance is introduced to account for this specific topographical organization of psychic systems starting from the surface – the outer membrane – of the living substance. The differentiations within the psychic apparatus must be understood from processes prior to – i.e., "beyond" – this apparatus, namely the modifications of the vesicle as originally undifferentiated living matter. That this bold speculative idea derives from Freud's use of the biogenetic law, is confirmed in the following passage:

> Indeed embryology, in its capacity as recapitulation [*Wiederholung*] of developmental history, actually shows us that the central nervous system originates from the ectoderm; the grey matter of the cortex remains a derivative of the primitive superficial layer of the organism and may have inherited [*durch Erbschaft übernommen*] some of its essential properties.
>
> (Freud 1920g: 26)

What Freud finds in the earliest modifications of the living substance is a first topographical and functional differentiation: the formation of an inorganic protective shield and an inner cortical layer "which is later to become the system *Cs.*" adjacent to the shield that is able to receive stimuli from the outside and inside (Freud 1920g: 28). Although not explicitly mentioned, we can add that these first topographical differentiations also include – or at least make possible – a first elementary mnemic system in which memory-traces can be stored permanently. "Beyond" these protective-functional layers there are the inner sources and constant flows of drives ("disturbances").

The first reaction formations of the living organism against the influx of stimuli from the outside and inside provide Freud with an evolutionary argument for identifying three conditions for all later modifications that will determine the actual advancement and development towards more complex organisms. First, the protective shield is still vulnerable to breaches and therefore to possible traumatization from the outside (Freud 1920g: 29). Second, the formation of the protective shield or crust explains why consciousness is relatively unprotected from the amounts of drive stimuli that act upon the system *Cs.* from the inside. Third, the fact that the system *Cs.* develops from a first crust (the surface of the vesicle, modified through the impact of external stimuli) would explain why, in this system, there can be no "permanent change" through storage of perceptions: the crust and the first attributes of the system *Pcpt.-Cs.* are formed at an early stage in evolution (and embryonic life) such that they cannot be further modified by passages of excitations. It cannot develop new "facilitations" for the storage of traces. Freud further speculates that in the earliest life forms the system *Cs.* must have been constantly flooded with amounts of excitation coming from within, without this living substance being able to adequately process ("bind") these excitations (Freud 1920g: 29). According to Freud, this must have given rise to feelings of pleasure and unpleasure as an "index" of what is going on in the interior of the organism. The organism is able to register excitations. The first primitive defence mechanism against the increase of unpleasure finds its origin here: the projection of inner sensations into the outside world, "an externalization of inner processes" (Freud 1917d: 223).[36] Projection is a mechanism through which excitation can be bound to representations of external danger.

Freud's speculations serve the purpose of defining the fundamental concepts and processes that define psychic life. What distinguishes his ideas from other contemporary reflections on the origin and evolution of life derives from his pathoanalytical perspective. The traumatic neuroses provide insight into the relation between a first shock that creates permanent inner disturbance and first – yet delayed – urges and mechanisms that seek to eliminate this disturbance. The "traumatized" living substance uses its inner energetic resources to create a new organ (crust) – a process that Freud associates with hysteria. The shielded vesicle can also be said to behave in a paranoid way – retreating behind a largely inorganic shield against the threatening external world while projecting inner sensations into the external world. The living substance treats excitation from the inside "as though they were acting … from the outside, so that it may be possible to bring the shield against stimuli into operation as a means of defence against them" (Freud 1920g: 29; also Willner 2024a: 246). It creates delusions – and hence representations – of external dangers.[37]

The vesicle also allows Freud to associate the organization of the psychic apparatus with the location of somatic organs (brain, nervous system, sense organs). According to Freud, the question of the relation between psychic systems and somatic organs had always remained unanswered (Freud 1920g: 31; see also Kistner 2024). In the "The Unconscious", Freud writes that the psychic topography and the distinctions between the various systems (*Ucs.*, *Cs.*, *Pcs.*) raise a question that goes "beyond pure psychology", namely the question how the psychic topography relates to anatomy (Freud 1915e: 174). This relation must exist, Freud writes, and yet

> every attempt to go on from there to discover a localization of mental processes, every endeavour to think of ideas as stored up in nerve-cells and of stimuli as travelling along nerve-fibres, has miscarried completely. The same fate would await any theory which attempted to recognize, let us say, the anatomical position of the system *Cs.*—conscious mental activity—as being the cortex, and to localize unconscious processes in the subcortical parts of the brain. There is a hiatus here which at present cannot be filled, nor is it one of the tasks of psychology to fill it. Our psychical topography has *for the present* nothing to do with anatomy; it has reference not to anatomical localities, but to regions in the mental apparatus, wherever they may be situated in the body.
>
> (Freud 1915e: 174–175; Freud's italics)

The vesicle and its first differentiations present the opportunity to describe the relation between psychic topography and anatomy in terms of an original structural and functional correspondence between anatomy and psychic topography. The later modifications and complexities in higher developed organisms such as human beings make it more difficult to relate and trace the "transformations" of energy and excitation that enter the sense organs, the processing of excitation in the "receptive cortical layer", and the transition to the psychic systems (Freud 1920g: 26–28). The differentiated vesicle provides a model – a simplification of the complexity found in human beings – that shows an initial congruence of anatomy and psychic functions.

Freud's speculations on the first transformations of the vesicle are presented as the phylogenetic analogy to the processes one can witness in the dreams of traumatic neurotic patients. More precisely, in these dreams, one finds processes that repeat phylogenetic processes on an ontogenetic level. Freud's speculations on the vesicle and the origins of defensive shields, perception and consciousness thus shed light on the most elementary reaction to incoming amounts of stimuli, namely attempts to produce preparedness for anxiety as the first protective measure. It is only through the formation of the surface crust that the system *Pcpt.-Cs.* becomes operative and can develop awareness of situatedness in space and time. It is this system that allows localization of oneself in this world, of objects in the outside world, and of oneself vis-à-vis the constant excitations that arise from within, that is, from the unconscious as another *topos* – *ein anderer Schauplatz*. In other words, it is only through the erection of protective shields that the living organism and the human individual can create a distinction between the incoming amounts of drive stimuli and the processing psychic functions, between oneself (ego) and an external world of objects, and between present and past.

The combination of ontogenetic and phylogenetic inquiries shows that Freud does not take for granted psychic life as situated life. Psychic life originates in a environment in which an organic substance is susceptible to stimuli without being able to perceive their source or direction and without being able to protect itself against their destructive effects.[38] The first living organism is not yet an organization of functional elements and not yet dominated by regulatory principles or habits. Freud can thus be seen as distancing himself from any (previous or later) position that takes its starting point either in the interactive situatedness of an organism in, and vis-à-vis, a differentiated surrounding world in which various bodies and forces can be identified, or in any form of self-consciousness, self-awareness and self-relatedness.[39]

The undifferentiated vesicle provides insight into the situation (and lacking situatedness) of the shell-shocked patient and his compulsory repetitions. This patient repeatedly returns to a situation in which he is exposed to and surrounded by life-threatening forces he cannot keep at bay. Life in the trenches is being surrounded by death. Instead of the possibility of fleeing death, there is the certainty of rushing forward towards death. In a sense, this life is dead since the past of more or less stable and peaceful life has ended. Like the life of the vesicle, the life of the soldiers in the trenches is a life of "dying easily".

Psycho-Lamarckism

In the years following the publication of *Totem and Taboo*, Sándor Ferenczi was to become his companion, paving some of the ways for Freud's further inquiries into the history of the human constitution.[40] A metapsychological paper on this topic was written in the summer of 1915, "Overview of the Transference Neuroses" – a text which Freud sent to Ferenczi but decided not to publish. The central thesis in this text is that the psychoneuroses are repetitions of the developmental history of human beings (Freud 1985a: 11–12). The psychopathologies are the starting point for a reconstruction of the evolutionary origins of those neuroses, their precipitation in the constitution and temporal sequence. That primal history of the hominids is structured and characterized by a number of primordial geological catastrophes, life-threatening hardships, and systemic violence. Primal history is seen as a sequence of traumatic – sexual and non-sexual – experiences, triggering a number of organic and psychic reaction formations that will then be transmitted to future generations as (part of the) constitution in the form of fixations. Certain characteristics of the drives – notably the diphasic relation between the sexual and the genital drives (Van Haute & Westerink 2021) – can be said to result from sequences of prehistoric traumatic experiences. In this way, Freud can relate his trauma theory to his drive theory in a double bind: traumas modify drives; drives produce trauma (see also Grubrich-Simitis 2007).[41]

This text shows that Freud ventures – albeit hesitantly – into what Ferenczi will call "metabiology" and "bioanalysis" (Freud & Ferenczi 1996a: 84, 92; also Willner 2022; 2023; 2024a; 2024b). From their study of Lamarckism, Freud and Ferenczi expect to gain insight into the processes of acquisition and inheritance of physical and psychological traits, and of the (interaction between) modifications by external factors and internal unconscious motives (Freud & Ferenczi 1996a: 166–167, 171, passim). Regarding the latter, Freud remarks in a letter (November 1917) to Karl Abraham:

> The idea is to put Lamarck entirely on our ground and to show that his 'need', which creates and transforms organs, is nothing but the power of *Ucs.* ideas over one's own body, of which we see remnants in hysteria.
> (Freud & Abraham 2002: 361–362)

The 1919 version of *Beyond the Pleasure Principle* can be seen as Freud's major contribution to this Lamarckian bioanalytical project. Why and how is Lamarckism important in this text? In whatever form and interpretation, Lamarckism was a widely accepted approach in biology at the time. Haeckel, for example, saw Lamarck's insights as a substantial part of the theory of evolution and the progression of species.[42] In his *Geschichte des Lamarckismus* – a book Freud owned and studied – Adolf Wagner mentions an important reason for the favourable reception of Lamarckism at the time. Lamarck's theories offer a way out of Darwinian reasoning in which the development of organic life is considered in terms of coincidental circumstances determining natural selection (Wagner 1909: vi–viii; Butzer & Burkholz 1991: 39). Lamarck offers an alternative to a theory prioritizing chance and coincidence. But, for his part, Freud had different reasons for turning his attention to Lamarckism. If all drives are conservative and aim to return to a previous state, a theory of the inheritance of acquired characteristics is needed in order to explain why the detours towards death become longer and more complicated in the course of evolution and the processes of natural selection. Freud's Lamarckism holds that all characteristics are indeed acquired. Change and development should not be explained on the basis of an innate principle or tendency that directs organisms to a predetermined end. Change and progress must be considered as responses to repeated or continuous pressure from external forces or challenging circumstances (see also Simanke 2020). What we call "progress" is nothing but the unintended side-effect of enforced reaction formations and defensive mechanisms.

Having said this, the letter to Abraham shows that Freud does not readily agree with classical Lamarckism. This is understandable, considering that Lamarck, in his *Philosophie zoologique* (1809), had articulated the acquisition of physiological characteristics as the effect of functional, expedient and intensive use (or non-use) of organs and body parts during the life of a certain number of generations (Lamarck 1910: 73). Lamarck associates this functional and expedient use with perception, knowledge, and intention respectively. An organism perceives its environment, "understands" what it needs to access food, and proceeds to adapt to circumstances on the basis of this "knowledge" and a desire to improve.[43] In other words, Lamarckism presupposes a certain "consciousness" and inclination towards improvement of qualities. But Freud cannot accept such premises. We have already seen in our brief discussion of psychophysics that Freud, notably in "Project" and *Beyond the Pleasure Principle*, is guided by theories on the physiological (material) origins of gradually developed psychic complexity. What needs to be explained are the very origins and evolution of perception, memory, knowledge, expedient action, etc. Precisely at this point, the psycho-physical work of scholars such as Fechner, Hering and Mach intersects with the contemporary psycho-Lamarckian literature.

Indeed, what clearly interested Freud more than Lamarck's functional theory was the psycho-Lamarckism of August Pauly (Freud & Ferenczi 1996a: 179; Butzer & Burkholz 1991: 40–44), who in 1905 had published a book entitled *Darwinismus und Lamarckismus*. In the work of this and other contemporary authors, attention shifts from the functional use of body parts and organs to a study of the various psychological processes and functions that, in addition to mechanistic causes, create the conditions for somatic and psychical modifications (Pauly 1905: 8–14, 20; Sulloway 1979: 274–275; Willner 2024b: 194–195). These psychic conditions cannot be defined in terms of *a priori* formative progressive tendencies but have to be considered in relation and as responses to a concrete context of externally and internally modifying influences. Whereas Lamarck's theory of evolution has an optimistic character with its focus on gradual progression without regression or extinction, Pauly notes that organisms often behave in a "conservative" manner, preferring to return to earlier stages in order to escape the intensification and complication entailed by the "processing" of modifying influences. There is no drive that aims at development and change, but the drives do present the organism with a workload and force the organism to action, change and development (Pauly 1905: 19).

This is what would explain Freud's reluctance to continue with the Lamarck project (Grubrich-Simitis 1985: 94; May 2024: 149–150). In the first version of *Beyond the Pleasure Principle*, Freud articulates his own subverted version of Lamarckism and the inheritance of acquired of characteristics:

> Let us suppose, then, that all the organic instincts are conservative [*konservativ*], are acquired [*erworben*] historically and tend towards the restoration [*Wiederherstellung*] of an earlier state of things. It follows that all phenomena of organic development must be attributed to external disturbing and diverting [*störender und ablenkender*] influences. The elementary living entity would from its very beginning have had no wish to change; if conditions remained the same, it would do no more than constantly repeat [*wiederholt*] the same course of life … Every modification [*Abänderung*] which is thus imposed upon the course of the organism's life is accepted by [*aufgenommen*] the conservative organic instincts and stored up [*aufbewahrt*] for further repetition.
>
> (Freud 1920g: 37–38)

In the 1919 version of *Beyond the Pleasure Principle*, Freud decides against the classical Lamarckian notion of functional, expedient and progressive self-modification and autoplasticity (compare Freud & Abraham 2002: 362: see also Willner 2024b: 190–191). All acquired modifications (characteristics) are seen as reactive formations following external "traumatizing" influences. In principle, organisms behave passively, conservatively and reactively. And yet, the reactive capacities of living substances are productive and, as such, contribute to the survival and prolongation of life. Constitution, then, is the totality of stored and repeated acquired characteristics. This includes the drives which, according to Freud, conservatively seek the reduction of tension, even in the enforced modifications:

> Both higher development and involution might well be the consequences of adaptation to the pressure of external forces; and in both cases the part played by instincts might be limited to the retention [*festzuhalten*] (in the form of an internal source of pleasure) of an obligatory modification.
>
> (Freud 1920g: 41)

We should note here that the main and unresolved problem in the contemporary Lamarckian theory is not addressed in the first version of *Beyond the Pleasure Principle*: how to theorize the inheritance of memory-traces, reaction formations and psychic contents acquired by previous generations? How and where can these traces and formations be stored and transmitted to a next generation in such a way that they can be reproduced when activated by new experiences and impressions?[44] Although Freud remains silent on these questions, we do know that he was influenced by Ewald Hering's 1870 lecture "Über das Gedächtnis als eine allgemeine Funktion der organisierten Materie", in which recapitulation of the species' evolution is defined in terms of transmitted "unconscious memory" (*unbewußtes Gedächtnis*) of impressions and experiences that modified and organized organic life in the course of the species' history (Hering 1870; also Gould 1977: 96–97).[45] Every new individual's psychic life is the product of transmitted unconscious memories that determine its organization and capacities.[46] This implies that memory cannot be limited to human beings. All organic life – from the differentiated living substance onwards – has the capacity to add received sensations and affect responses to lived situations.[47] What is inherited, more concretely, are the reactive patterns to external and internal stimuli. If a similar situation or experience appears, the new individual will respond in ways similar to those of its predecessors. But, again, it remains a riddle as to how information acquired by one generation can be transmitted to the next one.[48]

While Jones is correct in stating that Freud's references to Haeckel and Lamarck found only little enthusiasm among his followers (Jones 1957: 302–314), this does not mean that the issue of heredity, the influence of previous generations on individual life, and ontogeny as the effect of repetition were dismissed in post-Freudian psychoanalysis. Psychoanalysis' tragic view of human life, including the compulsion to repeat the reactions of previous generations, was no longer seen as embedded in the evolution of organic life as the totality of detours and derailments due to traumatic impressions. Individual trauma should no longer be understood (partly) from an inherited history of traumatic events and the biological – quasi-mechanical – laws involved in this inheritance. Notably in Lacan's work, these aspects of Freudian thought will be redefined in terms of an "inheritance" of a "discourse of the circuit in which a subject is integrated". It is this discourse of the other which structures the unconscious such that every subject is "condemned to reproduce" its possibilities and limitations (Lacan 1991: 89; also Godley 2018). The inevitable entrance into the symbolic order implies that the subject cannot but articulate and position himself vis-à-vis objects in a shared language in which significations represent the desires of past and present others, and in which "inherited" cultural constraints determine and shape subjectivity. In his first seminar, for example, commenting on Freud's Wolf Man case (Lacan 1988: 189–191), Lacan avers that the traumatic concerns a powerful impression that cannot attain signification and cannot be integrated into the symbolic order in which experiences are historicized. In the eleventh seminar, Lacan argues that trauma is that which cannot be assimilated in the *automaton*, the chain of signifiers with its "insisting" (repetitive), regulatory and law-abiding character (Lacan 1998: 52–64). For Lacan, the tragic dimension of being human is thus situated in an intersubjective, linguistic and cultural context in which manifest desires and aggressive impulses are limited by the law (of the father) that defines the symbolic order, while traumatic scenes beyond the subject's control haunt psychic life and insist on satisfaction. Lacan moves in this track when he points out – in his reading of Sophocles' *Antigone* (Lacan 1992: 243–287), for instance – that the tragic and the traumatic are pre-eminently contained in the structure of desire as essentially transgressive – as limitless and boundless, and therefore (self-)destructive. In short, whereas for Freud, the tragic character of human life is inscribed in the evolution and the tragic fate of all living organisms, for Lacan and others, the tragic aspect associated with life in culture is what distinguishes human beings from animals.[49]

Towards clinical metaphysics

Having introduced the biogenetic law in his reflections on the restorative and conservative character of all drives, Freud writes (in the 1919 version of *Beyond the Pleasure Principle*): "This behaviour [the recapitulation of the structures of all the forms of previous generations, HW] is only to a very slight degree attributable to mechanical causes, and the historical explanation cannot accordingly be neglected" (Freud 1920g: 37). With this remark, he recalls previous writings in which he complemented "physiological" with "biological" perspectives of the drives (Freud 1915c: 118–123); but he also situates his ideas within the contemporary discussions of his time.[50] Freud can be said to stand in a mechanistic (that is, dynamic) materialist tradition when it comes to applying concepts from physics to psychoanalytic theory. From the statement quoted above we learn, however, that when it comes the phylogenetic factor and the question of the origin and organization of the human constitution, mechanistic theories fall short and need to be supplemented with theories from evolutionary biology. This echoes a broad contemporary literature in biology that seeks to steer between the Scylla of strict mechanistic approaches, and the Charybdis of vitalist approaches. The path in between consists of the idea that the human constitution and notably the drives are the accumulation and prolongation of the past in the present.

In some respects, influential figures like Haeckel had paved the way for this trend in late nineteenth- and early twentieth-century biology. In his *Generelle Morphologie der Organismen*, Haeckel had argued that his morphological theory aimed at a monistic evolutionary theory was based on mechanical laws. But he had also assumed inner principles (based on physical-chemical processes) that would account for progressive development and completion. But can such a formative tendency really be seen as originating from mechanical principles or chemical processes, August Pauly asks (1905: 144–145). In proposing a mechanical approach, Pauly and others seek alternatives for references to a formative principle that still echoes the notion of *Bildungstrieb*, and dismiss any form of vitalism. On the contrary, Haeckel's contemporaries acknowledge the rise of "neo-Lamarckian" psycho-biological theories in which mechanical approaches are supplemented with theories of psychic properties, such as sensitivity, perception, volition, etc. These theories fully accept the fundamental mechanical laws (such as the Newtonian laws of motion and the thermodynamic laws), but complement them with psychological factors that can account for active (including reactive) motive forces and capacities interacting with external factors and with each other in the development of species and individuals.[51] In other words, not all change, development or modification can be explained by reference to mechanical principles of cause and effect. Organisms can actively relate and respond to the forces acting on them (Pauly 1905: 134–161; Wagner 1909: 169–212). When Freud writes that the recapitulation of forms and structures in organisms cannot be fully explained by mechanical principles, the reference to the "historical explanation" is meant to cover the acquisitions and the further development of organic and psychological properties, functions and processes involved – protective measures, reaction formations, fixations, various psychic capacities, tendencies and aims (notably the aim of pleasure and satisfaction).[52]

Both Pauly and Wagner propose psycho-biological theories as alternatives to mechanical approaches that fall short in accounting for the developments and capacities of living beings. Also, they steer away from vitalist approaches in which life is the expression of an active spiritual (non-material) and creative life force that constantly produces new forms, change and development in matter which, as such, is passive, inert and resistant to change. They explicitly distance themselves from the kind of vitalism of Hans Driesch's *Naturbegriffe und Natururteile* (1904). Driesch's concept of *Entelechie* indicates a spiritual force arranging and composing matter, reminiscent of quasi-mystical and metaphysical speculations on a *Bildungstrieb* in German Idealism (Pauly 1905: 192; see also Holt 1967; Bennett 2010: 62–81). Instead, Pauly and others propose psycho-biological perspective as an alternative "vitalism" in which psychological properties and forces are inherent to and characteristic of organic life (e.g., Pauly 1905: 148–149; Binet 1910: iii).[53]

This psycho-biological literature tells us about the bioanalytical project that Freud and Ferenczi tried to develop in the years preceding *Beyond the*

Pleasure Principle. In *Thalassa* (drafted in 1914–1915 and published in 1924), Ferenczi will argue in line with Pauly, Wagner and others that the mechanistic approaches in biology fall short in explaining all phenomena of life. Turning to psychology, they argue that psychological knowledge can help solve "problems" that the existing biological science is unable to solve. These problems mainly concern the principles involved in the development of organisms, and the question as to whether this development is expedient and conducive to the formation of a cohesive and functional whole. What Freud and Ferenczi add from their pathoanalytic perspective is a critique, not only of purely mechanistic and vitalist approaches. More specifically, they reject any reference to a "formative drive" in the tradition of Blumenbach's and Kant's *Bildungstrieb*. [54] Such a formative drive was not considered a historical acquisition, but as an expedient impetus or supra-organismic force directing life and organisms towards a predetermined set of ends. Freud, in contrast, will prioritize trauma, the non-functionality of infantile sexuality and aggression, the initial general human "helplessness", and a notion of psychic conflict.

Now we can understand why Ferenczi writes that "solely and exclusively psychoanalysis" can provide the psychological knowledge to the field of biology: it does not rely on a notion of progressive striving towards perfection, a life force that acts on inert matter or a concept of the organism as a cohesive functional whole (Ferenczi 1924: 81). Hence, the bioanalytical project should not be understood as the introduction of biological theory into psychoanalytic studies. The references to biology and evolutionary theory do not indicate biologism, i.e., the reduction of psychoanalytic theory to biological paradigms. The aim of the Lamarck project was not to found psychoanalysis on valid and solid scientific ground. On the contrary, the aim of the project was to transfer psychoanalytic concepts to organic phenomena and to identify the psychic principles and processes manifest in all organic matter and their development/evolution. Biology is not the model for metapsychology; the primitive cell is not the model for a theory of the traumatic neuroses. It is rather the other way round. Psychoanalysis is in the unique position to rethink biology and evolutionary theory (Willner 2022; 2023; 2024a; 2024b). The implications become apparent in the first version of *Beyond the Pleasure Principle*: Freud's clinical anthropology is turned into a clinical metaphysics, that is to say, a systematic and "speculative" reflection from a clinical (pathoanalytical) perspective on the fundamental concepts and principles that define life.

But doesn't Freud oppose metapsychology to metaphysics, dismissing the latter as yet another – quasi-psychotic, quasi-animistic – "system of thought" that seeks to develop a coherent and consistent worldview out of the need to control the world without considering facts and necessities of life (Freud 1912–1913a: 75ff)? Clearly, Freud stands in a tradition that distances itself from a metaphysics with *a priori* propositions and concepts adducing reason outside of and apart from the domain of the explanatory sciences (Freud 1915c: 117). And yet, in *Beyond the Pleasure Principle*, Freud states that his discussion of death and immortality in terms of biological theory has "unwittingly steered our course into the harbour of Schopenhauer's philosophy" (Freud 1920g: 49–50; see also 1917a: 143–144). Freud regarded Schopenhauer as a materialist philosopher who explicitly considered the natural sciences capable of reaching an understanding of the fundamental principles of nature (Assoun 1976: 206–213; compare also Schopenhauer 1854: 1–3). Also, Freud recognized that Schopenhauer was the philosopher who had convincingly dismantled the idea that man is a rational being, when arguing that all psychic representations and physical expression must be traced back to a "will" that can be defined in terms of unconscious force, energy or drive.[55] His philosophy had paved the way for a style of metaphysics that, according to Wagner, can be seen as "Aristotelian". In this tradition, metaphysics, seen as the systematic reflection of fundamental concepts that define being, is a continuation of the knowledge of nature and reality based on observation, and merely seeks to systematize this knowledge without any "mystical" references to transcendence or "dogmatic" principles. Metaphysics is thus always situated in a context in which certain sets of observable natural phenomena give impetus to systematizing thought (Wagner 1909: 192–195). Given the nature of a clinical practice in which various psychopathologies and unique case histories are the starting point for such systematizing thought, it is hardly surprising that Freud insists that reflection on basic concepts "does not tolerate any rigidity even in definitions" but, on the contrary, implies that "definitions are constantly being altered in their content" (Freud 1915c: 117). The various psychopathologies represent different models or "complexes" that lead to different theoretical and hence also bioanalytical constructs.

Freud's metapsychology in general, and drive theories in particular, inevitably enter into discussion with a tradition in metaphysics in which, from Aristotle onwards, the fundamental principles of being, movement and change have been articulated (Bernet 2020; Westerink & Van Haute 2025: 213ff). More concretely, this is evidenced by the fact that Freud's metapsychology can be situated in the scientific debates of his time between mechanistic and vitalist paradigms and perspectives on the principles of ontogenetic development and phylogenetic evolution. The classical metaphysical questions of cause, purpose and telos of what exists and moves occupy a central place in those debates. What defines Freud's own unique position in the reflection on the fundamental principles that define life, movement and change is the clinical perspective. It is the study of the psychopathologies, the significance of trauma and inner conflict, and the non-functionality of infantile sexuality that are the heart of Freud's critical thinking vis-à-vis a tradition in which, from Aristotle onwards, the predominant assumption has been that the fundamental principles that characterize life and movement are of an unfolding, progressive nature aimed at growth, integration and/or perfection. In this tradition, nothing in life works fundamentally against life, i.e., against the progression of species and individuals. Yet in his clinical practice, Freud is confronted with patients in whom psychic life is seriously disturbed by memories, regressions, fixations and repetitions that undermine life from within and give it a profound tragic character. What he highlights is the negativity of the drives in various ways: as forces that strain life or push it beyond its limits, as "surplus" energy that cannot be functionalized, as urges that attack psychic unity, such that it leads to auto-destruction or introduces aggression and violence into relationships with fellow human beings, as nihilistic-entropic "urges" that seek to dissolve all sources of inner tension and thus lead life towards death, or as the viscosity and adhesiveness that is inherent to the libido. And yet, these various conceptualizations of negativity cannot be considered without references to positivity, to the ongoing evolutionary processes of change and development. With the concept of the life drives, Freud will indicate that this positivity cannot be reduced to natural selection or enforced adaptations. They are to be considered as fundamental forces pressuring cells and bodies to the creation of new life forms independent of external circumstances. But this creative capacity can again not unambiguously be associated with growth or progress; the life drives' pressuring produces tension that – if excessive – can have pathological (traumatic) effects. We will return to these issues in Chapter 4.

Chemical substances

In Chapter 6 of the 1920 edition of *Beyond the Pleasure Principle*, Freud, while moving away from the 1919 trains of thought, investigates the constitutional factors involved in organic and psychic change and development. In this context, he suggests that the processes involved in the life and death drives include chemical and metabolic processes. Whereas the death drives insisting on reduction of excitation lead to "an abolition of chemical tensions", the life drives continuously produce new tensions when initiating new chemical reactions and metabolisms in the process of "binding" compounds into unities (Freud 1920g: 55). In fact, Freud argues, one cannot understand the life drives if one does not take into consideration that in these drives "the chemical affinity of inanimate matter" persists (Freud 1920g: 58). Even before matter is "disturbed" and life exists, and before there are life drives seeking to bind components in larger unities, there is chemical intermixture and compounding of substances. The constitution of matter is complementary to the aim of the life drives. Freud's mention of Jacob Loeb's "celebrated experiment" with chemical stimuli induced in sea urchins producing processes of conjugation, segmentation and coalescence supports his intuitions that the activities of the life drives appear to coincide with chemical processes that are part of inanimate matter's "constitution" (Freud 1920g: 48). Freud's references to Hering's concepts of "assimilation" and "dissimilation" also fit into this context. Hering discusses these as chemical and metabolic processes produced in sensitive and excitable substances. What is reproduced in sensations and feelings in psychic life (consciousness) are not so much the external objects, but the internal assimilative and dissimilative processes (Hering 1878: 77–87). Freud aligns himself with Hering's argument that the effects of impressions and accompanying sensations evoked by external forces are largely determined by internal physical-chemical and psychological processes producing tensions and excitation. These various references to chemical processes producing fresh tensions and interactions (fusions, defusions) with other substances are important for the arguments that Freud is developing in Chapter 6 of *Beyond the Pleasure Principle*. Change and progress need to be considered from inner causes, without appealing to a spiritual vitalist principle; fresh tensions and excitations need to be explained without having to call upon external modifying forces.

References to chemical processes are certainly not new. In the "Project", Freud argues that "endogenous stimuli" – which he will later refer to as "drive energy" or simply "drives" – "consist of chemical products, of which there may a considerable number" (Freud 1950c: 321).[56] And in the 1905 *Three Essays*, Freud includes a section on chemical substances in an attempt to answer, first, the question of the origin of sexual excitation, and second, the causes for the transformations in puberty. During the period in which Freud was working on his new drive theory, he revised the paragraphs on chemical substances in *Three Essays* (Freud 1905d: 215–216). That is no coincidence. In the 1905 edition of that text, Freud had to admit that he was completely "in the dark" when it came to the question of the origin of excitation and tension. His best hypothesis at time was that the sex-glands (or the thyroid gland) played a crucial role (Freud 1905d: 216).[57] After reading Alexander Lipschütz's *Die Pubertätsdrüse und ihre Wirkungen*, which was published in 1919 (May 2024: 88), Freud finds a convincing theory on the puberty glands, which provides an answer to the question of the origin of sexual excitation in early infancy. Moreover, it is a theory that matches his views on the diphasic development of sexuality. Lipschütz had argued that the maturation of sexual characteristics in puberty was only an acceleration of a process that begins much earlier in time, namely during intrauterine life. Lipschütz's theory of the puberty gland as the source of the production of sexual excitation thus provides Freud with an explanation, in chemical terms, of the origins of sexual excitation in both infancy and puberty (Freud 1905d: 177). Freud's exploration of the origins of sexual excitation in *Three Essays* leads him to highlight the role played by chemical substances that not only "cause particular parts of the nervous system to be charged with sexual tension" but also produce the metabolism (*Sexualstoffwechsel*) stimulating the production and accumulation of sexual substances (Freud 1905d: 215, 216). The references in the 1920 version of *Three Essays* to Eugen Steinach's experimental research on the possibility of changing the manifest sexual characteristics of animals and human beings through transplanting testicles and ovaries attest to Freud's interest in the decisive role of chemical substances in the transformations in sexuality and sexes.[58]

The references to chemical substances and processes are meant to solve the riddle of the constitutional elements involved in causing fresh tensions and amalgamating different components into compounds. The production of "new forms" needs to be explained "beyond" a theory of the conservative drives.[59] The introduction of references to chemistry is in line with what we have seen and discussed so far. In Chapter 1, we briefly mentioned Fechner's ideas about the tendency towards stability being disrupted repeatedly by chemical and metabolic processes in molecules and cells producing "fusions" and "defusions" in organs and bodies, and by the incorporation of air and food as elementary for the continuation of life. And Fechner is likely not the only source of inspiration. In the psycho-biological literature with which Freud is familiar, references to chemistry are common in attempts to avoid either references to adaptation in order to explain change and development, or references to a spiritual life force as in vitalism (Wagner 1909: 172). Teachers and influential predecessors such as Ernst Brücke and Émil du Bois-Reymond had accepted only physical-chemical forces as the active forces in organisms with which to explain attraction and repulsion, development and organization (Sulloway 1979: 14).

The embryologist Wilhelm Roux,[60] for instance, had put forward a theory of the body and its functions as the harmonious result of reciprocal expedient interactions between cells, organs and tissues (Pauly 1905: 69–86; Wagner 1909: 142–144). His theories are characterized by a strong mechanistic approach to the development of embryonic life forms. This approach is supplemented with a notion of a psychical "regulatory formative factor" that insists on establishing an expedient and functional unity capable of optimal adaptation to circumstances. This unity is established through internal natural selection, i.e., the struggle for survival between molecules, cells, tissues and organs with different capacities and characteristics. What is decisive in this "struggle" are the various assimilative and dissimilative metabolic and chemical processes, and the unequal distribution of nutritive materials and stimuli in the body (Roux 1881; also Ritvo 1990: 63; Burkholz 1995: 70, 112; Churchill 2015: 265–270).[61] Freud follows neither Roux's Darwinian views on internal natural selection, nor his ideas on goal-directed developments towards an adaptive unity. He rejects the aspects of purposiveness in Roux's thought that Pauly and Wagner also criticize. But in the 1920 version of *Beyond the Pleasure Principle*, Freud does agree with the idea that the unity of the body should be understood on the basis of the interaction and differentiations between cells, communities of cells (cell state – *Zellenstaat*), organs and tissues, and that, ultimately, the metabolic and chemical processes define the organic constitution.[62] On this point, Freud stands in the tradition of his predecessors, such as Virchow, Brücke, du Bois-Reymond, Fechner, and Roux, arguing that the final explanation for organic phenomena had to be "physical-chemical".[63]

Our reference to Roux's experimental embryology sheds light on another aspect of the turn to biochemistry in the 1920 edition of *Beyond the Pleasure Principle*. Roux discards the biogenetic law, arguing that the development of the embryo cannot be seen as a mere repetition of the morphology of ancestors and that progress and the appearance of new life forms in evolution cannot be reduced to the mere acquisition and inheritance of characteristics in processes of adaptation. Instead, change and development should be explained by physical-chemical transformations in cellular processes, which determine their functions and chances of survival in interaction with other cells (Gould 1977: 194–197; Gilbert & Sarkar 2000). Whereas the biogenetic law presents a major argument for the definition of the repetitive and conservative character of the drives in the first version of Freud's text, this law hardly plays a role in Freud's argumentations in Chapter 6 of *Beyond the Pleasure Principle*. Freud shifts attention to the endogenous forces that define the properties of cells, their interactions, and the variety of forms that are produced as a result of these interactions. But Freud does not follow Roux in applying the theory of natural selection to the interaction between cells, tissues and organs. He rather opts for another "Darwinian" train of thought.

From repetition to reproduction

We have already suggested that from his speculations on the first differentiations of the vesicle, Freud articulates his ideas in Chapters 4 and 5 of *Beyond the Pleasure Principle* within a broader framework of considering natural selection and the recapitulation of acquired characteristics. The notion of trauma is employed to provide insight into the emergence of variations that "die less easily" and are more likely to prolong life and pass on their acquired traits. Survival is survival of the traumatized. The surviving living organisms take more and more complicated and longer detours before reaching their aim of death (Freud 1920g: 38–39). We must assume, Freud argues, that the tendency towards the composition of complicated bodies depends on the capacity of germ cells – i.e., cells that retain the original structure of living matter – to meet with other yet different germ cells. It must be assumed, Freud writes, that quite early in the evolution of life, cells were formed that could not sustain themselves independently. In these germ cells an as yet "completely incomprehensible"[64] tendency arose to seek contact and merge (*Verschmelzung*) with other germ cells (Freud 1920g: 40). From this first coalescence, cells would form multicellular organisms in which the fragile germ cells are surrounded by greater numbers of protective cells – the body. According to Freud, the coalescence of germ cells of different sexes capable of producing a next generation of organisms is "watched over" by those drives that can now be properly considered "sexual drives". This coalescence of germ cells is the condition for recapitulation proper. Each new multicellular organism develops from the coalescence of two germ cells into one cell that will then re-envelop itself in a mortal body. It is from the coalescence of germ cells that one can explain the composition of bodies that act like "a safe shelter" against external stimuli. While these bodies "die in their own fashion",[65] the germ cells can "separate themselves from the organism as a whole" and repeat the same process of development (Freud 1920g: 40). This repetition of a return to earlier states of the living substance, and the subsequent development of a new generation, show that the germ cells are the carriers of life. They facilitate the repetition and continuity of previous states into the next generations. In the context of speculations on the relation between the urge to the inanimate and the sexual drives, Freud's brief elaboration of the coalescence of cells echoes Sabina Spielrein's views on this issue. According to her, the creation of a new life and the production of a next generation imply the "destruction" or "annihilation" of the germ cells as individual units (Spielrein 1912: 100–101). Since in fact this annihilation is the condition for the continuation of life in a new individual, the sexual drives (reproductive drives) can be said to aim at death. In line with this train of thought, Freud argues that a portion of the germ cells dies in the process of coalescence while from another portion, a "residual germ" (*Keimrest*), a new individual will begin its development. The sexual drives seek coalescence; coalescence implies death. It is the residue of the coalescence that survives this death. And yet, this residue answers to the inevitable repetitions characteristic of the evolution of the species. Every new individual is from the onset on a course towards its death.

In this discussion on the coalescence of cells, Freud does not explicitly refer to Weismann's theory of the inheritance of the properties of germ cells but still privileges a Lamarckian perspective on external pressure that provokes developments, such as the coalescence of sexually differentiated germ cells and the formation of protective bodies. There is a brief reference to Weismann's notion of the "potential immortality" of the germ cells. Yet, concerning this immortality, Freud remarks that this "may mean no more than a lengthening of the road to death" (Freud 1920g: 40). The fact that there is life, despite the urge to return to the inanimate, and that life has gradually developed into more complex organisms is still predominantly seen as the effect of an endless series of imposed modifications and adaptations to circumstances. These acquired characteristics determine the life cycle of organisms and are repeated in subsequent generations. Reproduction is seen as repetition, i.e., the repetition of trajectories towards death.

This passage in Chapter 5 on the coalescences of germ cells in the context of arguments in favour of recapitulation and the inheritance of acquired characteristics can be said to be the starting point for a new train of thought in Chapter 6 in the 1920 version of *Beyond the Pleasure Principle*. In fact, from the opening paragraph of this chapter Freud moves towards a Weismannian perspective on evolution and the variety of species. In *Die Bedeutung der sexuellen Fortpflanzung für die Selektions-Theorie* from 1886 and *Das Keimplasma* from 1892 – copies of which books Freud had in his personal library

(Davies & Fichtner 2006) – Weismann had raised the question of how to explain the variety of species and individuals when one rejects both the Lamarckian theory of inheritance of acquired characteristics (see below) and a theory of an inner formative and purposeful principle (Weismann 1886: 13).[66] In order to answer this question, he had turned to Darwin's notion of sexual selection, arguing that variation can only be explained with reference to the "form of reproduction".[67] More concretely, he refers to the coalescence (*Verschmelzung*) of two sexually differentiated cells – and with different inherited properties – as the condition for new variations (Weismann 1886: 28; 1892: 30). This is most apparent in multicellular organisms, but also in unicellular organisms that multiply through fission (*Teilung*) or conjugation (*Konjugation*). In short, the appearance of new variations can be explained by a theory of the inheritance of properties of germ cells in combination with the form of reproduction. One only needs to assume a minimum of (acquired) differences between germ cells in order to account for both continuity of characteristics and the production of new forms and combinations. Ontogeny can thus be understood from the fusion of the properties of parental germ cells.

Freud opens Chapter 6 with the contention – contrary to the argument of Chapter 5 – that only the self-preservative drives can be properly considered conservative. On the sexual drives, however, Freud writes:

> though it is true that they reproduce primitive states of the organism, what they are clearly aiming at by every possible means is the coalescence [*Verschmelzung*] of two germ cells which are differentiated in a particular way ... It is only on this condition that the sexual function can prolong the cell's life and lend it the appearance of immortality.
>
> (1920g: 44)[68]

According to Freud, following Weismann, this coalescence involves differentiated germ cells and is particularly characteristic for the reproduction in sexually differentiated species. But this is only one form of reproduction; it can be traced back to older forms such as the conjugation of two protista (Freud 1920g: 44)[69] and fission (Freud 1920g: 56). Indeed, in the opening sections of Chapter 6, Freud sides with Weismann who had stated that the fundamental forces of life (*Grundkräfte des Lebens*) manifest in the various forms of reproduction are assimilation, growth and multiplication (Weismann 1892: 53). In this context, Freud appears to distance himself from Spielrein's view on reproduction and death: the union (*Vereinigung*) of cells is the condition for the prolongation of life; if this union is not effected, the germ cells die, along with the rest of multicellular organism. It is the absence of union, of coalescence, that Freud now associates with death.

In this opening passage, Freud does not give credit to Weismann for his views on the fundamental forces of life. The fact that he does not explicitly refer to Weismann and his views on sexual reproduction and inheritance of the properties of germ cells in Chapter 5 and notably also in the opening passages of Chapter 6 is undoubtedly related to the fact that he is critical of Weismann's theory of the potential immortality of germ plasm and the late acquisition of mortality. Also, an explicit affirmative reference to Weismann's texts would immediately reveal a fundamental problem in *Beyond the Pleasure Principle* since Weismann's theory of inheritance is explicitly anti-Lamarckian. He had introduced the principle of non-transmissibility of acquired somatic characteristics (the "Weismann barrier") in order to support his ideas on the germ plasm as the potentially immortal and unalterable carriers of properties continued throughout generations. The germ plasm is immune to modifying environmental influences. Its transmission (via germ cells) through generations implies that heredity can be defined in terms of an unbroken repetitive chain of inherent properties.[70] The external intrusions that modify bodies have no effect on the evolution of species.[71] And this Freud cannot accept.

Death and life

The question Freud raises in the opening section of Chapter 6 is what decisive event in the development of the first living substance is "repeated" in the coalescence of sexually differentiated germ cells and its forerunner, the conjugation of two protista. Clearly, what the sexual drives repeat is not the restoration of the inanimate, but a primitive state that, as such, is the starting point for the development of a new living substance. If, indeed, then the prolongation of life is a fundamental characteristic of organic life, the idea articulated in Chapter 5 that all drives are conservative and have a character corresponding to a compulsion to repeat "would no longer possess the importance we have ascribed to it" (Freud 1920g: 44).

In order to answer this question, Freud enters in a critical discussion with Weismann and his views on the potential immortality of the germ plasm and the acquisition of mortality. According to Freud, the distinction between ego-drives and sexual drives "and the view that the former exercise pressure towards death and the latter towards a prolongation of life" (Freud 1920g: 44)[72] may find support in Weismann's biological writings on the duration of life and the death of organisms.[73] He writes:

> What strikes us in this is the unexpected analogy with our own view, which was arrived at along such a different path. Weismann, regarding living substance morphologically, sees in it one portion which is destined to die – the soma, the body apart from the substance concerned with sex and inheritance – and an immortal portion – the germ plasm, which is concerned with the survival of the species, with reproduction. We, on the other hand, dealing not with the living substance but with the forces

> operating in it, have been led to distinguish two kinds of instincts: those which seek to lead what is living to death, and others, the sexual instincts, which are perpetually attempting and achieving a renewal of life. This sounds like a dynamic corollary to Weismann's morphological theory.
> (Freud 1920g: 46)

Can this corollary be confirmed and sustained? And, if so, what are its consequences? According to Freud, the correspondence between his and Weismann's ideas dissipates when one considers that the latter's distinction between germ plasm and soma only relates to multicellular organisms. Weismann considers the unicellular organism potentially immortal since its development is open-ended (Weismann 1884: 5). It multiplies through fission, and thus endlessly repeats (recapitulates) itself; this is the foundation for any germ line and the unbroken transmission of inherited properties and characteristics. In his view, death is acquired with the appearance of multicellular organisms, that is, with the appearance of complex metabolic processes and differentiations between organs, functions, etc., which imply internal processes eventually leading to natural death. Death appears with the appearance of the soma as a functional carrier of the germ cells. In other words, death is not a universal attribute of organic life (Weismann 1882: 33). It does not belong to the essential properties of life. It is merely a biological function to eliminate weakened and worn-out bodies (Simanke 2020).

For Freud, the theoretical problem here is not Weismann's view of the mortality of the soma as "a matter of expediency, a manifestation of adaptation to the external conditions of life" (Freud 1920g: 46).[74] The theoretical problem is that, in Weismann's view, the capacities to die and to reproduce through the conjugation or coalescence of cells are acquired in the course of evolution. This would mean that the ego-drives and sexual drives would also have to be considered late acquisitions.[75] After all, why would a potentially immortal unicellular organism have a drive for the prolongation of life through coalescence? And, if unicellular organisms remain the same and lose nothing of their original vitality, and if death is a late acquisition of organisms, what would be the argument for assuming there must have been "death instincts from the very beginning of life on this earth" (Freud 1920g: 47)? The problem that Weismann's theory poses is how to consider the fundamental characteristics of the drives.[76] Or, in other words, if Freud follows Weismann in considering assimilation, growth and multiplication as the fundamental forces in life – hence, as characteristics of the sexual drives or life drives – what, then, are the arguments for the death drives?

The solution to this problem is articulated several pages later when Freud argues that processes tending towards death may already have been present, yet "their effects may be so completely concealed by the life-preserving forces that it may be very hard to find any direct evidence of their presence" (Freud 1920g: 49). In other words: "even if protista turned out to be immortal in

Weismann's sense, his assertion that death is a late acquisition would apply only to its *manifest* phenomena and would not make impossible the assumption of processes *tending* towards it" (Freud 1920g: 49; Freud's italics).

Freud concludes that when death (here: the appearance of a corpse) is the manifestation of an already existing tendency, "our expectation that biology would flatly contradict the recognition of death drives has not been fulfilled" (Freud 1920g. 49). This means that the correspondence between his and Weismann's theories remains significant and does not as yet force Freud to reconsider his views of the first characteristics of life.

Freud returns once more to Weismann in the course of the chapter, arguing that what has been said about the tendency towards and manifestation of death is, *mutatis mutandis*, also true for the life drives. On this point, Weismann (following Darwin) was right, Freud argues, in surmising that reproduction through the coalescence of two sexually different cells appeared relatively late in evolution, that it occurred by chance and proved to be advantageous. This fact does not contradict the notion of drives striving to hold together or assimilate portions of the living substance in earlier forms of reproduction. The tendency towards coalescence, like the tendency towards dissolution, appears from the onset of life. The death drives and life drives can thus be assumed to be constitutional tendencies present in the first and simplest life forms (Freud 1920g: 56–57, 60 n.).

Between the references to Weismann's theories and these conclusions, Freud engages in presenting the state of discussions in biology on life, death and immortality. The text part of *Beyond the Pleasure Principle* mentions a range of authors. Besides Weismann's relevant works, Freud's main sources for discussions in (popular) biology are Max Hartmann's *Tod und Fortpflanzung* (1906), Alexander Lipschütz's *Warum wir sterben* (1914) (which Freud probably already studied in 1918)[77] and Franz Doflein's *Das Problem des Todes und der Unsterblichkeit* (1919).[78] The main issue in these discussions concerns the alleged immortality of unicellular organisms. In their studies, Hartmann, Lipschütz and Doflein refer to Weismann and other important scholars mentioned by Freud (such as Götte, Loeb, Hertwig and Maupas), as well as to Woodruff's experiments on unicellular organisms. To the latter's research, Freud pays special attention (Freud 1920g: 47). Lorande L. Woodruff had shown that unicellular organisms do not show any signs of loss of vitality or ageing if – and only if – every new generation is immersed in fresh water. At first sight, this experiment seems to give proof of immortality and processes of rejuvenation. Yet, as others have experimentally demonstrated, organisms are harmed by the metabolic products which they themselves extrude into the surrounding water. This shows that, like multicellular organism, unicellular organisms also die from products of their own metabolism (Freud 1920g: 48). This would contradict the idea that death is a late acquisition, and that unicellular organisms also "die a natural death as a result of their own vital processes", even though they do not leave behind a corpse (Freud 1920g: 48).

This implies a rejection of Weismann's theory of the potential immortality of germ plasm. There is no immortality in the sense of "an unchanging persistence of the cell", Lipschütz argues. Since "life is change", the definition of death does not depend on the notion of a "corpse", but on the fact that every change, for example, through cell division, implies the discontinuation, the death, of the unicellular organism and the appearance of new substances (Lipschütz 1914: 29; also Simanke 2020).[79] In short, there is no immortal and unchanging – endlessly recapitulated – essence in living organisms that is immune to any form of influence and modification. The implication of this conclusion is that Weismann's theory of inheritance cannot be maintained in its strict definition. This provides room again for a Lamarckian notion of inheritance of acquired characteristics. More important is the fact that, for Freud, the interactions between cells and the formation of cell states, organs and bodies need not be reduced to properties inherent to the germ line. As we will explore in Chapter 4, Freud will introduce the libido theory in order to account for coalescence, growth and variation.

From this preliminary conclusion on Weismann's theory of the potential immortality of germ cells, Freud moves forward in a new direction. A reference to Ewald Hering's *Zur Lehre vom Lichtsinn* (1878) and his views on the two fundamental processes of construction-assimilation and destruction-dissimilation at work in living substances, serves as introduction to a new formulation of the drives in terms of life drives and death drives. We should note here that until this point in the text, the concept of "death drives" still refers to the ego-drives or self-preservative drives that Freud mentions in the first sentences of Chapter 6 as the truly conservative drives. And the life drives he mentions in the reference to Hering still refer to the sexual drives which Freud had referred to as "the true life drives" in the 1919 version of the text (Freud 1920g: 40). This is confirmed by the reference to Schopenhauer, for whom, Freud writes, "death is the 'true result and to that extent the purpose of life', while the sexual instinct is the embodiment of the will to live" (Freud 1920g: 50).[80]

From the discussions of the contemporary biological literature on death and immortality, Freud draws the conclusion that the death drives and life drives can be said to be present in the first living substance. Biology does not contradict this speculative assumption. He writes that there is little agreement on the subject of natural death and immortality in the literature (Freud 1920g: 59), which gives rise to the impression that biology is "a land of unlimited possibilities" (Freud 1920g: 60). We should note here that the whole argumentation, through the discussion of Weismann's work up to the introduction of Hering's theory of assimilation and dissimilation, is moving away from the biological theories on which Freud relied in the first version of *Beyond the Pleasure Principle*. The speculative idea finally established in this chapter is that of the life drives and death drives operating in the living substance from the beginning of life. This new drive theory undermines Haeckel's recapitulation theory and nuances the Lamarckian concepts that played a significant part in Freud's overall argumentation so far. It was the biogenetic law that provided a phylogenetic correlate for the compulsion to repeat which Freud observed in several clinical and everyday phenomena. Lamarckism was introduced to account for the undeniable change and development of organic life due to external circumstances enforcing adaptation. Yet with the introduction of Weismann as an authority in the field, Lamarckism automatically loses its credibility. Despite Freud's criticism of Weismann's theory of the potential immortality of the germ plasm, he sides with Weismann's ideas on the fundamental forces and processes that define life and reproduction. And this marks the shift from the focus on external (accidental) traumatizing influences towards the inner constitutional factors on the level of cells that contribute to the variety of life forms. Life and its evolution can be considered on the basis of the principles of reproduction and the vicissitudes of cells (assimilation, growth and multiplication). Freud is well aware of this fundamental shift when he writes: "It is true that my assertion of the regressive character of drives also rests upon observed material – namely on the facts of the compulsion to repeat. It may be, however, that I have over-estimated their significance" (Freud 1920g: 59). This also entails a reconsideration of trauma. In the 1920 version of the text, not only Lamarckism and the biogenetic law are largely absent from the argumentation, also the traumatic neuroses and trauma hardly feature. This should not come as a surprise, since Freud's version of Lamarckism deals with modification through external factors in terms of sequences of reactions to traumatic events. In the 1919 version of *Beyond the Pleasure Principle*, Freud can be said to develop a clinical metaphysics based on the concepts of trauma and repetition. The new drive theory, in contrast, will focus on the endogenous forces that push life towards further variation, and the accompanying counter-forces. Instead of a biogenetic law that defines life in terms of the repetition – the eternal return – of the same forms, the new drive theory defines life by forces that produce new forms. In the first version of *Beyond the Pleasure Principle*, Freud shows himself to be a thinker of catastrophes; in Chapter 6, however, he introduces a new perspective based on a critique of the potential immortality and immutability of germ plasm, and the application of the libido theory to the creative interactions between cells (Freud 1920g: 50).

The life of plasm

In his letter to Abraham from November 1917 (see p. 83), Freud suggests that psychoanalysis may be able to shed light on how and why unconscious ideas can create and transform organs. This statement is in line with his earlier ideas on hysterical conversion and hypochondriacal libidinal investment in organs. For Freud, conversion is indeed a phenomenon in which psychic processes can transform organs and body parts disregarding strict anatomical rules. It is, Freud writes in the Dora case, "the translation of a purely psychical excitation into physical terms" (Freud 1905e: 53). He adds that the production of symptoms through conversion is not possible without "somatic compliance" (*somatisches Entgegenkommen*), that is, without certain preferred "channels" for discharge (*Abfuhrwege*) already present in the bodily organs and tissue. Dora's hysterical cough – one of her most prominent symptoms, for example – is not caused by a conversion from an unconscious idea into a random part of the body; instead, repressed thoughts use the irritability of the throat to make themselves known, to give the cough another meaning and make it "exaggerate" the irritability (Freud 1905e: 40; 1910i: 218). Dora's cough facilitates repressed sexual gratification *per os*, because of the throat's sensitivity to stimulation (Freud 1905e: 48). Hysterical symptoms require "the participation of *both* sides", Freud concluded (Freud 1905e: 40; also Wilson 2004: 11ff). Something similar can be found in hypochondria, as characterized by organic changes resulting from concentrated libidinal investments in sensitive – excitable, erotogenic – organs or body parts (Freud 1914c: 83–85; 1916–1917a: 390–391).

With the return of the problematics of traumatic neuroses with a symptomatic picture similar to that of hysteria – hence the term *Kriegshysterie* – the question of the interaction between psychic processes and organic symptoms becomes urgent again. After all, war-neurotic patients suffer symptoms – such as aphasia, tics and paralyses – similar to those of Charcot's hysterics. From late 1917 onwards, it is notably Ferenczi who becomes interested in the problem of what he calls "hysterical materialization phenomena" (Freud & Ferenczi 1996a: 247; see also Wilson 2015: 45–67; Soreanu 2023). Ferenczi credits Freud's studies of hysteria and notably *Three Essays* with having paved the way for further reflections on the creative interactions between the psychical and the physical (Ferenczi 1915: 209). In a text written in 1918, he falls in line with Freud's earlier observation that such materialization processes can, first of all, be seen as the effect of a repressed wish (idea). From here, Ferenczi takes a more radical and speculative step in considering materialization in the most primitive organisms. Here one finds life forms that are not yet modified through functional and expedient adaptations to the outside world and not yet imbued with proper psychic organization, yet nonetheless already capable of "autoplastic" self-modifications. For Ferenczi, such autoplasticity must be understood as being motivated by internal factors, notably the sensitivity of organs and the experience of pleasure. Hysterical materializations inform us about, first, the proto-psychic capacity of all organic life and of somatic processes to be sensitive to stimulation, and, second, the tendency in all organic life and somatic processes to seek pleasure.[81] Autoplasticity derives from autoeroticism. It consists of fabrications (condensations, cooperations, displacements, movements through stimulations, etc.) motivated by the pursuit of pleasurable physiological activities and interactions (Ferenczi 1919b).

Beyond the Pleasure Principle can be read as Freud's contribution to the inventorization of the constitutional factors involved in such "materialization" processes. It is an inquiry into the "somatic compliances" that facilitate new organic and psychic formations. In the 1919 version of *Beyond the Pleasure Principle*, the starting point for Freud's speculations on materializations is the undifferentiated plasma vesicle. Its first defensive modifications in the form of solidification, transforming its former sensitive membrane into an inorganic crust, indicate that Freud is thinking of the human constitution as the sum of reactive-defensive structures set in place to fend off incoming stimuli and to receive and discharge surplus drive energy. His remark in the 1919 version of the text that "the power of regenerating a lost organ by growing afresh a precisely similar one" (e.g., in lizards that have lost their tails), points towards a drive to restore a previous state of better adaptation in a hostile environment. The added suggestion that there may be drives that "push life forward towards progress and the production of new forms" is not further elaborated on in a context in which new forms are merely modifications prompted by external influences (Freud 1920g: 37).

But this changes in the 1920 version of the text: here Freud argues that the interactions and coalescences between cells and organs are to be understood as effects of the libidinal character of the life drives. Again, the plasmatic unicellular organism is the starting point. But instead of turning attention to the process of stabilization and solidification, Freud focuses on the "protista" and their fluidity which allows them to take different shapes (Freud 1920g: 44, 47ff, 56, 58).[82] These excursions on protista echo earlier references to protoplasmatic amoebae in the context of discussions of narcissism. On two occasions in earlier texts, Freud draws an analogy between the libidinal cathexis of the ego and the subsequent libidinal investment in objects, and amoebae and their capacity to stretch out pseudopodia in order to explore and connect to the immediate surrounding objects. Also, he underscores their capacity to withdraw these protrusions into themselves and return to their state of globule, on the other hand. Amoebae are adduced to illustrate the oscillations between narcissistic ego-libido and object-libido, and the associated plasticity and potential for the generation of new forms (Freud 1914c: 75–76; 1916–1917a: 416).[83] This idea is taken up again in *Beyond the Pleasure Principle*. Protista are homogeneous cells that can behave in a "narcissistic fashion", retaining libido in their own ego, but – pressured by the life drives – they can also spontaneously seek to interact with their environment (Freud 1920g: 50). Freud seeks confirmation of this idea in pointing to the protista's capacity to take different forms and interactively engage with the fluid space in which they are situated and of which they are a part.[84] Yet, while the life drives manifest themselves in plasticity, the death drives do so in elasticity, withdrawing the pseudopodia and returning to the former narcissistic state in which the cell lives for itself and dies in its own fashion. The protoplasm's plasticity and elasticity thus show that the life and death drives are already operative in the earliest life forms. This also explains how the amoebae can come to serve as a model for understanding the fundamental drive tendencies in psychic operations, such as libidinal object cathexis and withdrawal of libido, projection, and introjection.

Freud's interest in protoplasmatic living substances in a fluid space parallels the introduction of the libido theory and its application to the mutual relationship of cells (Freud 1920g: 50). In *Three Essays*, there is a strong tendency in Freud's thinking to associate the libido (sexual drives) with "flows" and "streams" that need to be contained, "dammed" and – as rivers flowing to the sea – directed towards the external world.[85] On the constitutional disposition of neurotic patients, for instance, Freud writes: "The libido behaves like a stream [*Strom*] whose main bed has become blocked. It proceeds to fill up collateral channels which may hitherto have been empty" (Freud 1905d: 170). And on sexual inhibitions, he writes that psychic forces "impede the course of the sexual instinct and, like dams, restrict its flow" (Freud 1905d: 177). And it is moisture (mucous membranes) and flows ("the warm flow of milk") that arouse sexual pleasure and excitation (Freud 1905d: 179–182). These associations of drives and the excitations they produce are developed further in *Beyond the Pleasure Principle*, with references to the "flowing" (*strömende*) character of Breuer's free mobile cathexes and the amounts of drive energy "flowing" into (*zuströmende, einströmende*) the psychic apparatus. Drives are "fluid", moving through bodies and pressuring organs and systems. To consider life through plasma is to consider the fluidity of the drives (see also Malabou 2022: 282–283).

To consider life starting from plasm is also to view life as plastic and indeterminate. This means, first, to consider the elementary living substance and its life drives as radically "unbound", not channelled, not confronted with any form of resistance in a fluid environment. Freud's protoplasmatic vesicles and protists are not as yet solidified in any way, and do not (as yet) stand in opposition ("shielded") to their environment and the world of objects. Their plasmatic character makes them almost indistinguishable from their environment. The protoplasm consists of a content similar to its environment. Freud's excursion on the protista, which are said to be dying from their own metabolic processes after having excreted these in their environment, illustrates exactly this point: they live and die as part of the fluid space in which they are situated (and hence leave no corpse). Second, the protoplasm is radically plastic, that is to say, it has no original form, and is in constant flux, transforming its shape through its capacity to send out and retract pseudopodia. It can thus be said to be autoplastic; one could also say it has the capacity to absorb and be transformed by the "flows" and movements in the fluid space, and by absorbing and being absorbed by other protoplasms.[86] The immersion in a liquid environment, the fluidity and mobility of form, and the ability to absorb and being absorbed, define its situatedness in an environment. The protoplasm's relation to this environment is one of "indifference": the fluid space is neither conceived of as "hostile" nor as the world of objects. And, third, the plasmatic life substances have the capacity to merge (*verschmelzen*), to "conjugate" (*kopulieren*) and separate again (*auseinandergehen*), and by doing so, to become "rejuvenated" (*verjüngt*). They thus have the capacity to resist death by continuous and spontaneous (or artificially enforced) processes of recuperation (Freud 1920g: 48). This is entailed by their plasticity, and by their situatedness in a space of alterations in the "composition", "temperature", or "movements" of the fluid.[87]

Having said this, Freud's view of the conservative character of all drives, and his concept of the death drives, indicate those forces that act against the initial plasmatic character of life. The solidification of the vesicle's surface remains the model for all later organizations and structures, systems and distinct functions, that define individual organisms as distinct from their environment and other objects. The vesicle's first surface differentiations in a "crust" is the condition for a self-positioning – eventually the system *Pcpt.-Cs.* – vis-à-vis a world of identifiable objects. For Freud, this appearance of an external world with objects finds its origin in the living substance, that is, in its capacity to secrete metabolic products that are either used for the creation of the inorganic "crust"' or excreted into the environment. Also, it has the ability to "project" internal excitation into the outside world, and to "force away" the death drives towards external things, such that they become hostile objects (Freud 1920g: 29, 48, 54).

Final remarks

In the reception history, Freud's phylogenetic speculations in *Beyond the Pleasure Principle* have often been considered as highly problematic. Frank Sulloway had a point when arguing that, in psychoanalytic orthodoxy, Freud was largely presented as having formulated psychological theories of trauma, representation, Oedipal phantasies, object relations, etc., and that there was a certain embarrassment with his apparent reductionist biologism (Sulloway 1979). But can it be maintained that Freud is a biologist seeking to base his psychological theories on the firm ground of natural sciences in general and biology in particular? To the contrary: *Beyond the Pleasure Principle* is Freud's major contribution to the joint bioanalytical project he and Ferenczi initiated in the years preceding the publication of the text. The aim of this bioanalytical project was to transfer and apply psychoanalytic concepts to organic processes, and to identify the psychic principles and dynamics manifest in phylogeny and ontogeny. This project was the most radical consequence of the pathoanalytical perspective Freud had developed in earlier writings: human existence – the physiological processes, psychical dynamics and structures, and their cultural expressions – can best be studied from the psychopathological exaggerations and intensifications. It is notably the study of the traumatic neuroses and the compulsion to repeat that not only leads

Freud to speculate "beyond" the pleasure principle on the fundamental characteristics and attributes of organic life, but also "beyond" what several commentators of the text – such as Lacan and Laplanche – considered the limits of psychoanalysis.[88]

In *Beyond the Pleasure Principle*, Freud insists again on the continuity between human psychic life and other forms of organic life. From the very first systematic introduction of the concept of *Trieb* in the 1905 *Three Essays*, the drives are defined as fundamental urges in both animals and humans (Freud 1905d: 135). This means that reflections on the drives cannot be limited to an inventory of the components of the human constitution. The specific manifestations of drives (as instincts) in a variety of species show that each species has its own – often more purposeful – drive constitution. Whereas, for example, Lacan and Laplanche will prefer to make a sharp distinction between drive and instinct (Lacan 2006: 851–854; Laplanche & Pontalis 1973: 216; Laplanche 1989), such a distinction cannot be found in Freud's metapsychology. He clearly considers the drive to be an urge inherent in all organic life forms (Freud 1920g: 36). The specific manifestations of the drives in human beings indicate that man is one variation among the variety of species, one possible trajectory – or detour – among many others.

Notes

1 The central thesis – contra classical interpretations of the development of Freudian thought – in the joint project with Philippe Van Haute, the monograph *Seduction, Drive and Repetition*, is that Freud did not abandon his seduction theory in 1897, but instead extended his trauma theory to constitutional factors (Westerink & Van Haute 2025).

2 It is only from puberty onwards that sexuality will be organized around the primacy of the genitals and functionally aimed at reproduction (Freud 1905d: 207; Van Haute & Westerink 2021).

3 See Freud's statement on inversion: "The pathological approach to the study of inversion has been displaced by the anthropological" (Freud 1905d: 139 n.).

4 The term pathoanalysis was introduced by Jacques Schotte (1990: 147–148) and has been identified as a fundamental heuristic and ethical principle in Freudian thought in, among others, Van Haute and Geyskens (2012); Van Haute and Westerink (2021), and Westerink (2020).

5 In his *New Introductory Lectures*, Freud introduces the image of a broken crystal to define his pathoanalytic perspective:

> we are familiar with the position that pathology, by making things larger and coarser, can draw our attention to normal conditions which would otherwise have escaped us. Where it points to a breach or a rent, there may normally be an articulation present. If we throw a crystal to the floor, it breaks; but not into haphazard pieces. It comes apart along its lines of cleavage into fragments whose boundaries, though they were invisible, were predetermined by the crystal's structure. Mental patients are split and broken structures of this same kind.
>
> (Freud 1933a: 58–59)

6 In this context, it is not without significance that Freud associates the traumatic neuroses with the other well-studied psychoneuroses, such as hysteria and melancholia (Freud 1920g: 12). By referring to hysteria and melancholia, Freud suggests that, like these psychopathologies, the traumatic neuroses can shed light on the "fixations to the experience which started the illness" and which "have long been familiar to us in hysteria" (Freud 1920g: 13). For the case of the perversions, Freud notes a fixation of pleasurable activities; in the traumatic neuroses, on the other hand, Freud finds a fixation and repetition of unpleasurable sensations that cannot be repressed and otherwise processed. This issue is also briefly addressed in "A Child Is Being Beaten" – a text that Freud completed while writing the first version of *Beyond the Pleasure Principle* (Freud 1919e: 182).

7 Other psychopathologies also play a part in Freud's analyses in *Beyond the Pleasure Principle.* For example, Freud refers to the mechanism of projection, which he had discovered through the study of paranoia as a tendency to deal with internal excitations "as though they were acting, not from the inside, but from the outside" (Freud 1920g: 29). Yet, according to Freud, this mechanism not only appears in paranoia (or only in psychopathologies), but in fact "has a regular share assigned to it in our attitude towards the external world" (Freud 1911c: 66). Projection is common in normal and in pathological psychic life as a "defensive procedure" and "primitive mechanism" in the perception of relations and coherence in the external world, that is, in the formation of a *Weltanschauung* (Freud 1912–1913a: 61, 64–65). Projection is not a mechanism that defines an aspect of psychopathologies, but in fact plays a role in every perception and interpretation of the external world.

8 In "On Narcissism", Freud briefly discusses hypochondria in relation to psychosis and paranoia, that is, as characterized by the withdrawal of libido from the external world, and – in this case – an overinvestment of libido in a specific organ. This "damming-up of libido" is then experienced as pain. In his discussion of hypochondria, Freud mainly focuses on the issue of libidinal investment in the ego; but he also raises the question as to why the hypochondriac would seek to maintain or repeat sensations of unpleasure (painful bodily sensations) (Freud 1914c: 83–86).

9 In Freud's later reflections on the death drive, melancholia will explicitly play a crucial role (De Vleminck 2013: 137–187). In *Group Psychology and the Analysis of the Ego,* Freud highlights melancholia as the psychopathology demonstrating that identification with and introjection of a lost beloved object lead to a breaking of the ego into two pieces, one of which will cruelly and relentlessly rage against the other (Freud 1921c: 109, 132–133). It is this characteristic aspect of melancholia that leads Freud to formulate his ideas on the ego and superego in *The Ego and the Id* (Van Haute & Westerink 2021: 94–100). The "conflict" between the ego and the lost love object is replaced by a continuous inner conflict between the ego and an aggressive critical agency producing severe self-reproaches (Freud 1917e: 248; 1923b: 28ff). In this context, Freud refers to melancholia as "a pure culture of the death instinct" (Freud 1923b: 53). Melancholia is presented here as the clinical material par excellence that attests to the death drive as the "drive of destruction" (Freud 1923b: 41).

10 Freud's first published article is a zoological study on the development of the sexual organs of eels, "Beobachtungen über Gestaltung und feineren Bau der als Hoden beschriebenen Lappenorgane des Aals" (1877), in which he shows that, in eels, a "transitional form" in the evolution of the reproductive organs becomes visible. See also Ritvo (1990: 125–131).

11 In a series of letters to Fliess written in 1897, Freud argues that the earliest sexual period of the child, in which disgust and shame are not yet formed, has an "animal character" (Freud 1985c: 241, 269).

12 What distinguishes humans from animals has to be understood from the specific reaction formations that are "organically determined and fixed by heredity" (Freud 1905d: 177). Infantile sexuality can be described in terms of physiological processes not yet organized through object relations and cultural norms. It is not based on a distinction between human life in culture and animal life in nature, as Lacan will argue (Van Haute & Westerink 2021: 25).

13 In "A Child Is Being Beaten", Freud confirms what he had been arguing since the late 1890s: what distinguishes man from animals is the fact that only a human being "begins his sexual life twice over, first like all other creatures in his early childhood, and then after a long interruption once more at the age of puberty" (Freud 1919e: 193).

14 For Laplanche, instincts denote goal-directed predetermined behaviour. Whereas these instincts are inherited, drives are acquired and thus vary from individual to individual, depending on the particularities of one's history (Laplanche 2015b: 121).

15 One trigger for this engagement with phylogeny was Jung's study *Wandlungen und Symbole der Libido* (1912), in which Jung pointed out numerous analogies between the phantasies and representations of psychotic patients and mythological, religious and philosophical cosmologies. On the debate between Freud and Jung on the issue of phylogeny, religion and culture, see Vandermeersch (1991).

16 According to Freud, this is notably the case for those cultural phenomena – art, religion and philosophy (Freud 1912–1913a: 73) – that cannot be defined in functional terms, that is, those that serve neither the function of self-preservation nor that of the preservation of the species. On this issue, see also Westerink (2020).

17 In our reading of the various versions of *Three Essays* and in several other publications in which we explored Freud's theories of sexuality, Philippe Van Haute and I have argued that the 1905 version of *Three Essays* clearly presents a non-oedipal theory of infantile sexuality (Van Haute & Westerink 2021). Contrary to the secondary literature that defines the abandonment of the seduction theory in 1897 as the point of Freud's turn to oedipal phantasies, the non-oedipal theory presented in Three Essays suggests that the oedipalization of Freudian theory only becomes possible after Freud discovers the objectal aspects of infantile sexual life in his studies of infantile sexual researches and his case study of Little Hans (Freud 1908c; 1909b).

18 For a detailed discussion of the Wolf Man case study as a contribution to trauma theory, see Fletcher (2013: 220–275) and Westerink and Van Haute (2025: 95–126).

19 On this issue, see also Silveira (2013).

20 See also the following quotation from "The Dissolution of the Oedipus Complex":

> Although the majority of human beings go through the Oedipus complex as an individual experience, it is nevertheless a phenomenon which is determined and laid down by heredity and which is bound to pass away according to programme when the next pre-ordained phase of development sets in.
>
> (Freud 1924d: 174)

21 Haeckel's recapitulation theory was widely accepted and integrated by other authors Freud knew and studied – his teacher Carl Claus, Gustav Fechner and August Weismann to name but the most important (Claus 1872: 96; Fechner 1873: 40–41; Weismann 1892: 58–60). It was Haeckel who coined the terms phylogeny and ontogeny (Willner 2023: 94).

22 The biogenetic law also makes it possible for Freud to understand man's cultural creations on the basis of the principles and functions that apply in nature (Geyskens 2005: 23–26). Cultural history is an extension of the evolution of organic life. It therefore progresses from "primitive" to advanced, more complex and

differentiated forms. The evolution of the human species and the individual includes cultural history and its recapitulation in sexual development and the formation of the self from a newborn to an adult (Freud 1916–1917a: 354). This affords Freud the opportunity to identify analogies between child, primitive man and neurotics. After all, if sexual development and ego-formation at the level of ontogeny are a repetition of phylogenetic developments, then the same is true of developmental disorders (fixations, regressions, inhibitions). The biogenetic law allows the developmental disorders of individuals to be seen as repetitions of inherited and imperishable fixations acquired by ancestors in the evolutionary lineage.

23 The biogenetic law as formulated and conceived by Haeckel was largely based on embryology. In fact, many nineteenth-century scholars were convinced that findings from embryology could compensate for the lack of paleontological evidence (Darwin's "missing link"), and that a continuous progressive evolution could be demonstrated (Bowler 2003: 191). Even though the law has older roots in nineteenth-century biology, it could be considered "Darwinian". In *On the Origin of Species*, Darwin suggests that findings from embryology would support his theory of evolution: "the embryo is the animal in its less modified state; and in so far it reveals the structure of its progenitor", this is, of "ancient forms of life" (1859: 330–331).

24 With the rejection of a drive towards perfection, Freud situates himself closer to Darwin and his idea that coincidental (accidental) factors produce advantages and disadvantages for individuals and species.

25 The haunting aspect of death comes to the fore in "The Uncanny". In a reference to Ernst Jentsch's *Die Psychologie des Unheimlichen* (1906), Freud argues that uncanny feelings are created when clear distinctions between animate and inanimate objects are no longer possible (Freud 1919h: 230, 233). What fascinates Freud here is the inanimate aspect of the animate: the rigid and mechanistic presence of forces and principles that oppose a conception of organic life as dynamic, progressive, coherent, creative and well adapted to the demands posed by the external world.

26 This reference to "spontaneous generation" analogous to traumatic shock sets Freud apart, to some extent, from his predecessors, such as Haeckel, who argues that the spontaneous generation of organic life (protoplasm) must be situated in an inorganic fluid environment with a specific composition of interacting (attracting and repelling) chemical elements (Haeckel 1866, vol. 1: 143–144).

27 Freud may have taken intuitions from Haeckel who referred to the most simplified living substance as "plasm without structure" (*strukturlose Plasmakörper*) or "organism without organs" (*Organismus ohne Organe*) or "vesicle" (*Bläschen*), to its plasmatic core as source of sensation (pleasure, pain) and active movement and development, and to its first "differentiations" (*Differenzierungen*) (Haeckel 1866, vol. 1: 112, 276, 279ff). Similar ideas concerning the first plasmatic organic life forms (*protoplasmatische Schleimkügelchen*) can also be found in Fechner's *Einige Ideen* (Fechner 1873: 12ff). In his *Grundzüge der Zoologie*, Carl Claus also mentions the protoplasm as first living substance, elaborating on its capacity to fuse (verschmelzen) and divide (teilen) (1872: 16–17).

28 This is, among others, evidenced in the 1895 "Project" in which there are several references to protoplasm and its "general irritability" (Freud 1950c: 296, 298).

29 Freud has a profoundly Darwinian perspective on evolution when highlighting the threat of extinction and the notion of survival. After all, in *On the Origins of Species* Darwin argues that "the greater number of species" have left "no descendants but have become utterly extinct" (1859: 359).

30 Such is the case with the radiolaria, described by Haeckel in the appendix to Lamarck's *Zoological Philosophy* (Lamarck 1910: 97–98), and the rhizopods

(Haeckel 1866, vol. 1: 186 ff). Descriptions of organic substances attracting inorganic matter can also be found in Fechner's *Einige Ideen*, notably in the chapter in which he discusses the elasticity (spontaneous production of forms) of protoplasms and the non-elasticity of *Rädertierchen* (Fechner 1873: 12–24), and other biological literature with which Freud was familiar. As early as 1895, in "Project", Freud mentions the "irritability of protoplasm" and the creation of a "non-irritable surface" (Freud 1950c: 296).

31 According to Haeckel, the formation of differentiations on the surface of the protoplasm can be seen as "products" of secretion (*Ausscheidung*) (Haeckel 1866, vol. 1: 279ff).

32 The reference to a spatial concept such as *Umweg*, which implies a notion of movement and change of place, can be seen as echoing a Helmholtzian perspective on the effects of *Bewegungskräfte*, namely the fact of spatial movement (from one place to another) in matter and the "direction" (*Richtung*) in which a material object is moved (Helmholtz 1847: 6).

33 Donna Haraway (1976) has convincingly shown that the crystal is often referred to in late nineteenth-century organicist biology as a model for exploring the formation of structure and architecture in organic life forms. In this context, the crystal is sometimes referred to in order to define the difference between inorganic and organic matter: the crystal is characterized by absolute material stability, whereas organic life is characterized by a dynamic approximative stability and the capacity to transform (what Helmholtz called) kinetic energy into functional energy (du Bois-Reymond 1891: 30–31).

34 In "Repression" from 1915, Freud writes that in order to explore the nature of repression one needs to learn more about the origins and differentiation between what is unconscious and what is conscious (Freud 1915d: 148). Freud's elaborations in *Beyond the Pleasure Principle* can thus also be seen as a contribution to the theory of repression.

35 Freud takes up this issue again in "A Note upon the 'Mystic Writing-Pad'" (Freud 1925a: 228, 230, 231).

36 The reference to projection and hence to the mechanism that defines psychosis and paranoia (in the Schreber case) is relevant in view of Deleuze's reading of Freud's theory of the drives in *Logique du sens*. Whereas the traumatic neurotic patient leads Freud to elaborate the undifferentiated vesicle and its first functional and intentional differentiations, Deleuze makes a similar claim with regards to schizophrenic experiences in which he detects a complete breakdown of the individual's organization. What remains after this elimination of functions and structures is what he calls "organism without parts" or "body without organs". In this context, Deleuze associates this body without organs with Freud's "protoplasmic vesicle". Here, Deleuze combines two different elements from Freud's reflections on the initial life forms: the undifferentiated nature of the vesicle (in Chapter 5) and the plasticity and self-creative potentiality of the protoplasm (in Chapter 6) (Deleuze 1990: 186–201, 203; see also Schuster 2016: 75–78).

37 Although it is beyond the scope of our study to provide a detailed account of the many parallels between the 1895 "Project" and *Beyond the Pleasure Principle*, we can note here that in both texts Freud theorizes the conditions and emergence of the basic structure of psychic life and eventually of consciousness and ego-formation from physiological and evolutionary processes – the irritability of the living substance and the gradual advancement in modes of responsiveness and capacities of processing.

38 In this tenet, Freud follows Richard Avenarius's *Kritik der reinen Erfahrung* and others writing on related topics. Avenarius had tried to theorize the emergence and

historical development of consciousness from psycho-physiological processes (notably the impact of stimuli – *Reize*) while criticizing those philosophies (such as Kant's) that start from the givenness of consciousness (*unmittelbaren Gegebensein des Bewusstseins*) and of capacities (categories) to organize perceptions (Avenarius 1888: xxii).

39 This becomes explicit in Freud's brief reference to "the Kantian theorem that time and space are 'necessary forms of thought'" (Freud 1920g: 28). We should note that Freud's reflection on this theorem is not un-Kantian when one considers that also for Kant without "synthesis" (binding) into a unity or sequence of representations, the manifold of "intuitions" would be chaotic and impossible to receive and grasp by understanding. Where Freud differs from Kant is that, for the latter, the synthesis is produced by imagination as an efficient psychic function that is able to organize haphazard impressions into stable representations (Kant 1788: A77–78, A120; also Ingala 2020: 185).

40 For example, in his "Entwicklungsstufen des Wirklichkeitssinnes" (1913), Ferenczi explores intuitions with which we have become familiar in the course of our reading of *Beyond the Pleasure Principle*: the return to a state of absence of stimuli, fixation and repetition, the tendency to persist and regress, the need for protection, the traumatizing influence of external catastrophes and modifications, and the references to biology including Haeckel's biogenetic law (Ferenczi 1913; also Willner 2024b: 196–197). In a footnote added in the 1920 edition of *Beyond the Pleasure Principle* (Freud 1920g: 41–42 n.), Freud refers to Ferenczi's (1913) text, crediting it with reaching "the same conclusion along different lines" on obligatory modifications and the conservative character of the drives. On the cooperation between Freud and Ferenczi on phylogeny and biology, see Grubrich-Simitis (1985) and May (2024: 143–151).

41 For an example, we can refer here to the hysterical reaction formations of disgust at the excremental and the anxiety of sexual longing. Perhaps the most important effect of the traumatic experiences of the prehistoric hominids concerns the fact that sexual development is interrupted after an initial flowering of infantile sexuality. That the urges enter into the service of reproduction is a delayed development that does not begin until puberty (Freud 1985a: 14–15; see also 1905d: 234; 1939a: 74–75).

42 On Lamarck and Lamarckism, see among others Gould (1977), Bowler (1983; 2003), Ritvo (1990: 31–59), Burkholz (1995) and Willner (2024b).

43 This already forms the core of Schopenhauer's critique of Lamarck in *Über den Willen in der Natur* of 1836. Against Lamarck's emphasis on perception and subsequent knowledge, Schopenhauer proposes to explain the physical modifications of organisms from a will for life preceding the individual organism (Schopenhauer 1854: 42–43).

44 On this issue, see Wagner (1909: 213–222), Gould (1977: 96–97) and Westerink and Van Haute (2025: 138–140).

45 In Freud's personal library there is a copy of Richard Semon's *Die Mneme als erhaltendes Prinzip im Wechsel des organischen Geschehens* from 1908. In this influential study, Semon defends a Lamarckian theory of organic memory-traces he referred to as "engrams" engraved in and the altering the "disposition" of the excitable (irritable) substance which as such largely depends on the morphological state of and physico-chemical processes in an organism. The inherited memory-traces will be revived in individuals when these encounter similar stimuli as previous generations did (Semon 1908).

46 Freud had been familiar with Hering and his work since his student days. His 1870 text on the inheritance of unconscious memories was included as a chapter in

Samuel Butler's *Unconscious Memory* (1880). In a 1926 translation of Israel Levine's *The Unconscious*, edited by Anna Freud, the paragraph on Butler was translated by Freud. In a footnote to that paragraph, Freud wrote that, instead of Butler, Hering should have been foregrounded in Levine's book, because of his contribution to the knowledge of "unconscious soul activities" (Freud 1926g; see also Burkholz 1995: 129ff). In *Beyond the Pleasure Principle*, Hering is mentioned, but for a different aspect of his work.

47 According to Hering, in animals, the unconscious memories inherited from previous generations express themselves in instinctual "knowledge" and habits. Freud implicitly adheres to this idea, given his views on the urge in organic life to return to a previous situation, as evidenced in the migratory flight of birds or the migration of certain species of fish. Such instinctual knowledge of a previous or original place presupposes some form of unconscious memory, since it is only in the mnemic systems that traces of earlier experiences and impressions can be preserved.

48 Despite Freud's reservations against (classical) Lamarckism because of its overvaluation of the capacity for need-motivated expedient self-modifications, he defends the notion of the inheritance of acquired characteristics – even in his late texts written at a time when Lamarckian thought was increasingly subjected to critique, especially in the biological sciences. "I cannot do without this factor", he writes in *Moses and Monotheism* (Freud 1939a: 100). In the Moses study, Freud argues that a theory of inheritance of acquired psychical characteristics and contents is crucial for understanding the gradual development of a people's character from inner motive forces. In this concrete case, moreover, trauma can only be effective when stored (as "archaic heritage") in the (collective) unconscious. In this text, Lamarckism is crucial for Freud's argument that past traumatic experiences produce transgenerational effects. On this issue, see also Kitcher (1992: 174–180).

49 This focus on the dialectics of law (symbolic order) and desire leans heavily on Lévi-Strauss's structuralist perspective on distinctions between nature and culture, biological beings and social individuals, and instinct and desire. These, however, are distinctions that find no support in *Beyond the Pleasure Principle* as a text in which Freud explores the fundamental forces and principles that define all organic life.

50 We note here that, for Haeckel, evolutionary theory (and parts of biology and geology such as palaeontology) were not natural sciences, but historical sciences, in which speculation and subjective theory would be guides in the search for factual evidence. In this view, evolutionary theory was close to archaeology (Richards 2008: 313).

51 The example Pauly gives is that of the difference between throwing a stone and throwing a bird. Whereas the stone will follow a direction according to mechanical laws, the bird will use the mechanical forces in order to redirect its flight in a chosen direction (Pauly 1905: 150).

52 In New Introductory Lectures, Freud situates psychoanalysis in the tradition of psycho-biology with the following statement: "Actually what we are talking now is biological psychology, we are studying the psychical accompaniments of biological processes" (Freud 1933a: 95–96).

53 Freud was familiar with the writings of Alfred Binet (an assistant of Charcot), notably his work on fetishism and animal magnetism (suggestion, hypnosis).

54 Notably in section 61 in his *Critique of Judgement*, Kant had argued that mechanistic theories allow for explanations of contingent causations and productions of a variety of life forms, but need to be supplemented with a notion of purpose, i.e., a teleological principle of design as a regulative principle or law in nature (Kant 1790; see also Van de Vijver, Van Speybroeck & Vandevyvere 2005). Indeed,

it was Johann Friedrich Blumenbach who in his 1781 *Über den Bildungstrieb* had introduced the term and defines it as a fundamental force that explains the self-organizing capacities in organisms beyond sheer mechanistic explanations of movement and change. Arguably, this can be seen as the starting point of discussions that continue throughout the nineteenth century. On this issue of drive in German Idealism, see Kisner and Noller (2021).

55 In the references to Schopenhauer's philosophy, Freud adopts arguments and ideas from students such as Alfred von Winterstein and Otto Juliusburger, who in various articles had explored Schopenhauer's relevance for psychoanalytic theory. They notably highlight Schopenhauer's ideas of the unconsciousness of the will, death as the purpose of life, and the sexual drive as the main expression of the will to live (Gödde 1999: 282–289).

56 In later texts, Freud will associate the "source" of the drives with chemical processes (Freud 1915c: 123).

57 In 1905, Freud argues that it is likely that the stimulation of erogenous zones, and the subsequent sexual excitation, trigger the thyroid gland to produce a substance that is disseminated throughout the whole body. The decomposition of this substance acts – in a manner comparable to a toxic substance – as a stimulus upon the reproductive organs.

58 For Freud, Steinach's biochemical research was important because of its insights in the "organic determinants of homo-eroticism and of sexual characters in general". What Freud expected from this line of research was that it would "produce a direct confirmation of this presupposition of bisexuality" which he had always regarded as a constitutional factor in homosexuality and in the aetiology of hysteria (Freud 1905d: 147 n., 215; 1905e: 114). These remarks are also echoed in "The Psychogenesis of a Case of Homosexuality in a Woman" – a text Freud wrote in January 1920 (Freud 1920a: 171).

59 In *The Ego and the Id*, Freud associates the life and death drives with chemical processes, more specifically, anabolism and catabolism, that is, metabolic processes of biosynthesis and decomposition of molecular and cell structures (Freud 1923b: 41). These processes occur "in every particle of living substance", but in "unequal proportions", such that in some particular substance, the life drives may be dominant while in others it might be the death drives.

60 Freud was familiar with Roux's work in experimental embryology. In two references to Roux's experiments on germ cells and early embryonic life, Freud views these experiments as contributions to trauma theory, that is to say, to the study of the physiological effects of creating breaches in the cell structure (Freud 1916–1917a: 361; 1940a: 185).

61 It is these internal processes that cause functional differentiations and neo-formations. Chemistry is the model here: the fusion of two different substances produces a new third substance with different properties (A+B=C/C≠AB). The expedient properties of a complex organism cannot be reduced to the properties of its components (cells), but emerge as new properties in the course of the formation of the unity (Haraway 1976: 33f).

62 The notion of cell state or "community of cells" (*Zellenstaat*) is mentioned by Freud in Chapter 6 (Freud 1920g: 50). The concept was introduced around 1850 by Rudolf Virchow, whose work Freud was familiar with. Freud's reference to cell states links his work to Virchow and others who argue that all higher organic life forms have to be seen as compositions of individual cells. According to Haeckel, referencing Virchow, "the organism as a whole is an organized community, a state of cells", and the life functions of the organism are "the sum of life functions of individual cells" (Haeckel 1866, vol. 1: 264). See also Richards (2008: 47).

63 Freud was also familiar with writings of Wilhelm Ostwald – Freud had a copy of his *Vorlesungen über Naturphilosophie* and several other publications in his library (Davies & Fichtner 2006). Ostwald had argued that "chemical affinity" should be explained in terms of transformations of chemical energy as the most elementary form of energy producing motion and action in matter. He had also suggested that "psychic energy" and the processes in organic life can be traced back to chemical energy, thus suggesting continuity between energetic processes in inorganic and organic matter (Ostwald 1902: vii, 233). From Freud's reference to "chemical affinity", we should, however, not conclude that he adopted Ostwald's pan-energetics (Assoun 1981: 168–194; Bergo 2025).

64 In the 1920 version of the text, Freud changes this to "in the highest degree significant" (Freud 1920g: 40; compare 2024: 59). This new phrasing can be understood from Freud's new drive theory in which Eros is the drive that binds cells (see Chapter 4).

65 Recently, Étienne Balibar has argued that the statement "to die in one's own fashion" can be read against the background of the First World War and the impossibility of so many people dying a natural death – and instead dying a violent death. The statement would then imply a kind of "recourse against the violence of life" and "a principle of anti-violence". What human beings (and animals) desire is to put an end to violent deaths (Balibar 2022). Our reading suggests that this idea can be integrated into the broader perspective Freud develops: "to die in one's own fashion" expresses the idea that organic life forms seek to avoid any potential life-threatening external influence.

66 Weismann discusses and rejects in particular Karl Wilhelm Nägeli's theory of "idioplasm", i.e., an inner formative and purposeful principle and innate tendency towards perfection. Nägeli strongly opposed the Darwinian notion of selection and adaptation (Wagner 1909: 76–78; Ritvo 1990: 38–39; Bowler 2003: 248). On Weismann, see also Churchill (2015).

67 In the 1920 version of *Beyond the Pleasure Principle*, Freud shifts the focus to the various forms of reproduction as these emerge in the course of evolution. Darwin had paved the way for Weismann's views on reproduction as a fundamental force in evolution with his notion of sexual selection and the idea that the creation of both physical and psychological differences between species and individuals largely depends on the evolution of sex (Darwin 1871, vol. I: 278; vol. II: 402). On Darwin and sexual selection, see also Grosz (2004; 2011). With regards to sexual selection Grosz notes that Darwin's references to attractiveness provides an explanation as to why sexual activities are pleasurable, that is, rewarding in itself but without any value in relation to survival (natural selection) (Grosz 2011: 130). With this suggestion, we can establish a link between the shift in Beyond the Pleasure Principle from natural selection to sexual selection, on the one hand, and Freud's formulations of the pleasure principle (from zero excitation to constancy) and the life drives' contribution to the increase of excitation, on the other.

68 The term "appearance of immortality" (*Schein der Unsterblichkeit*) is taken from Johannes Müller's well-known *Handbuch der Physiologie des Menschen*; it puts forward the idea that, although individual organic bodies are transient (vergänglich), on the level of the species, life continues through the organic force (organische Kraft) inherent in organic life, producing next generations (Müller 1834: 33). Freud owned and studied a copy of Müller's *Handbuch*, which was published in 1834–1840 (Davies & Fichtner 2006; May 2024: 151). It is quoted by Weismann in the opening paragraph of *Über die Dauer des Lebens* (Weismann 1882: 1).

69 On this point, Freud almost literally quotes Weismann (compare Weismann 1886: 44).

70 In a letter written in 1912 – thus long before the publication of *Beyond the Pleasure Principle* – Jones expresses his scepticism about Freud's interest in various biological theories and informs Freud that Lamarckism is irreconcilable with the theories of Weismann (Freud & Jones 1993: 150).
71 In addition, we cannot avoid the impression that Freud does his best to present the new formulations on the sexual drives as his own, that is, as derived from earlier metapsychological considerations, notably his theory of sexuality. The references to Ewald Hering on assimilation (Freud 1920g: 49) and Darwin on amphimixis and growth (Freud 1920g: 56) contribute to masking Weismann's views as the main inspiration for the new concept of the life drives.
72 This articulation of drive dualism leads Freud to make several minor but highly significant changes and additions to the 1919 text. Most relevant is the following passage in which Freud inserts an important remark in italics:

> Let us now hark back for a moment ourselves and consider whether there is any basis at all for these speculations. Is it really the case that, apart from the sexual instincts, there are no instincts that do not seek to restore an earlier state of things? that there are none that aim at a state of things which has never yet been attained?
> (Freud 1920g: 41)

73 Freud refers to three of Weismann's works in particular: *Über die Dauer des Lebens* (1882), *Über Leben und Tod* (1884) and *Das Keimplasma* (1892).
74 The fact of natural death and mortality does constitute a psychological problem, that is, a fact ("law of nature" and *Ανάγκη*) that is either believed or negated – both options can also be ways to find comfort (Freud 1920g: 44–45). Freud's remarks on losing in death "those who are dearest to us", have been taken to refer to the death of his daughter Sophie in January 1920. It gave rise to the idea that *Beyond the Pleasure Principle* could be seen as the result of a personal process of grief and mourning. Freud himself was among the first to deny this: the large part of the text was already finished in 1919. Nevertheless, this one passage can be seen as a more personal reflection, even though the content is in line with earlier elaborations on the topic, notably in *Totem and Taboo*. See also May (2024: 91–92) and Rose (2021: 44ff).
75 Freud clearly assumes here that the two drives – ego-drives (now also called death drives) and sexual drives – must have arisen at the same time.
76 To be clear, this is not the same as the question, "How is life possible?". For Freud, the answer to this question remains undisputed throughout the two versions of the text: an external force disturbing inorganic matter.
77 This may explain Freud's references to "living substance" (*lebende Substanz*) – a concept regularly used by Lipschütz (and others) as equivalent of unicellular organism.
78 Minor sources are Wilhelm Fliess's *Der Ablauf des Lebens* (1906) and Max Hartmann's *Tod und Fortpflanzung* (1906), of which Freud gives a short account. Other authors mentioned by Freud such as Woodruff are probably known to him through the studies of Lipschütz and Doflein. In her commentary on *Beyond the Pleasure Principle*, Ulrike May provides an overview of the referenced biological literature but also identifies several sentences and passages in which Freud merely paraphrases others, notably Lipschütz (May 2024: 154–155).
79 This connects to Max Hartmann's view of life and death in *Tod und Fortpflanzung* from 1906. Freud refers to Hartmann because of his definition of death as "the termination of individual development" and cell division as always producing the death of the individual cell (Hartmann 1906: 9, 29; Freud 1920g: 47).
80 Freud's reference to Schopenhauer in relation to the new drive dualism is problematic. Schopenhauer's concept of the "will" refers to the fundamental and original unity of

being; the negation of this will cannot be traced back to a death principle, but to the lived experiences of the effects of the will in individual lives (Gödde 1999: 401–402).

81 Whereas Freud traces the origins of the capacity to experience pleasure and unpleasure back to the first differentiations in the vesicle, Ferenczi, in Thalassa and other texts, argues that there is proto-psychic activity in organic life from its very beginning. Ferenczi's ideas on plasticity build on the idea that in all organic life forms psychic motives can prevail over existing anatomical structures (see also Soreanu 2023). Ferenczi thus radically thinks through Freud's early clinical finding that hysteria's manifestations behave "as though anatomy did not exist or as though it had no knowledge of it" (Freud 1893c: 169).

82 Haeckel's introduction of the term "protist" (and the scientific study of protists in Protistologie) in his *Generelle Morphologie* can be seen as part of the larger trend in the emerging field of cell biology in the late nineteenth century that Freud was already familiar with due to his zoological and neurological research.

We have already noted (see p. 78) that among others Fechner elaborated on the "elasticity" (that is, plasticity) of protoplasmatic amoebae in their interaction with their environment (Fechner 1873: 14ff).

83 In "On Narcissism", Freud draws parallels between the protoplasm's "putting out" (*ausgeschickt*) of pseudopodia and the ego's "sending out" (*ausgeschickt*) libido towards objects (object cathexes) as the fundamental principle in the formation of groups (group psychology) (Freud 1914c: 7576, 100–101).

84 In the writings of Nietzsche, we also find references to protoplasm and their pseudopodia as informative about the fundamental characteristics of life. According to Nietzsche, the activities of protoplasm show that not the instinct for self-preservation but the will to power is the fundamental force in life: the will to dominate and achieve mastery and that, as such, "can manifest itself only against resistances" and "therefore seeks that which resists it" (Nietzsche 1901: 346).

85 Compare also, for example, the following from "A Case of Homosexuality in a Woman": "From very early years, therefore, her libido had flowed in two currents [*lief in zwei Strömungen*], the one on the surface being one that we unhesitatingly designate as homosexual" (Freud 1920a: 168).

86 Their capacity to "stretch out" is continued in the development of organisms – notably in plants reaching into the air towards the light – that "live in and of their relations with the sun" (Freud 1920g: 38).

87 In *Thalassa*, Ferenczi connects to this train of thought on biogenesis in a fluid space, and the subsequent "traumatic" exile from the sea (that is, the development of life on land). The drives would then aim to restore an initial situation (see Freud 1920g: 36). For ontogeny, this means re-establishing the intra-uterine situation, the recapitulation of embryonic life (Ferenczi 1924: 52–59; see also Willner 2023; Soreanu 2023).

88 Lacan and Laplanche distance themselves from Freud's references to biology and physics. Lacan argues that the unconscious and its functioning should not be understood from an explanatory science such as biology, but from its structures, as determined by culture and language. The psychogenesis of each subject should not be understood from organic drive activity and natural needs, but from a desire to eliminate the subject's existential "lack", manifested in object relations and their cultural encoding. Laplanche will argue that psychoanalysis should limit itself to a psychological theory of sexual trauma that can do without reference to biology and to the "mythological" concepts of the life and death drives (Laplanche 2015b). In that case, sexuality would not primarily be a bundle of physiological processes; it would take shape only when the confrontation with an enigmatic sexual object calls for phantasmatic processing (Laplanche 1989; 2015b).

Chapter 4

Theories of the drives

So far, we have not explicitly addressed the question of what prompted Freud to put the first version of the text aside, only to publish it a year later after adding substantial new theoretical and clinical material. In this chapter, it will be argued that the "extreme line of thought" (Freud 1920g: 37 n.) developed in the first version of the text led to conclusions and implications that Freud could not accept. His discussion of the pleasure principle, the compulsion to repeat, the traumatic neuroses and the conservative character of all drives led to a theoretical impasse. The 1920 additions to the text can be seen as responses and answers to the main theoretical problems and questions that the first version of the text had generated. This implies that the inquiries into the traumatic neuroses, children's games, transference neuroses, and tragic theatrical figures were not intended to prepare the ground for the introduction of a theory of death drives and life drives. *Beyond the Pleasure Principle* cannot be taken as a text that intended to systematically introduce a new drive theory. It can more appropriately be said to comprise several drive theories. I will argue in this chapter that the different drive theories Freud presents in the text are at least partly contradictory. More precisely, it is with the introduction of the concept of the life drives that Freud undermines his views on the conservative character of all drives, the role of trauma and the nature of "progress" in evolution, and the interaction between organisms and their environment, as he set them out in the first version of the text. The investigation into Freud's drive theories ultimately leads to an alternative interpretation of the life and death drives and gives his theory a place in discussions about the fundamental principles and characteristics of life. Henri Bergson's *Évolution créatrice* will be an important discussion partner in the last section of the chapter.

Constant forces

In Chapter 4 of *Beyond the Pleasure Principle*, Freud describes the traumatic neuroses in terms of amounts of excitation flooding the psychic apparatus such that this apparatus is unable to bind these excitations to representations.

DOI: 10.4324/9781003680413-4

Subsequently, he turns his attention to the pulsional sources of these amounts of excitations. He writes:

> The most abundant sources of this internal excitation [*Erregung*] are what are described as the organism's 'instincts' [*Triebe*] – the representatives [*Repräsentanten*] of all the forces [*Kraftwirkungen*] originating in the interior of the body and transmitted to the mental apparatus – at once the most important and the most obscure element of psychological research.
>
> (Freud 1920g: 34)

The "obscure element" Freud mentions refers not only to the fact that he considers the study of the drives to be "beyond" the realm of empirically observable phenomena in clinical practice. Indeed, beyond the clinical-empirical, there is the domain of "constructions" that remain uncertain as long as there is no confirmation from the patient, and "speculations" that remain uncertain as long as scientific confirmation or falsification is not provided (Freud 1920g: 18, 60). The obscurity also refers to the different perspectives – the physiological and the biological – that Freud had explicitly distinguished in "Instincts and Their Vicissitudes". The physiological (or physicist) perspective comes to the fore in the reference to *Kraftwirkungen*. A drive is like a constant force (*Kraft*) that pressures the nervous or psychic apparatus. In "Repression", we find similar statements on the repressed exercising "continuous pressure in the direction of the conscious" and "an uninterrupted expenditure of force [*Kraftausgabe*]" that "must be balanced by an increasing counter-force" (Freud 1915d: 151). Here, we recognize the mechanistic paradigm we discussed earlier. From this perspective one can clearly distinguish between the drive as a constant force (*Kraft*), the effects of this force on higher systems, and the psychic efficiency and expediency of the processing of this force.

From a biological perspective, however, the drive appears to be a "concept on the frontier" (*Grenzbegriff*) between the somatic and the psychical (Freud 1915c: 121). It is "the psychical representative [*Repräsentant*] of the stimuli originating from within the organism and reaching the mind" (Freud 1915c: 122). Though firmly anchored in the somatic, the forces and stimuli are represented in psychic life by "concepts". He adds that such a representative of stimuli in psychic life implies that the psychic apparatus is fully operative and organized, and as such regulated by the pleasure principle (Freud 1915c: 120). From this perspective, the drives are part of the psychical that seeks to master stimuli. Hans Loewald has convincingly argued that in Freud's biological perspective, the drives are no longer external and opposed to the psychical but play an active part *within* psychic life. They participate in the organism's responses to incoming stimuli from somatic "sources". The drives are part of the totality of responses to modifying forces (Loewald 1980: 120–123; Fong 2016: 10).[1] In other words, Freud uses the concept of drive in two different ways: drive is the motor force from which to understand a multitude of physical movements and psychic responses; and drives are the concrete impulses that can be represented in psychic life that can be satisfied through concrete actions. He can use the concept of drive metaphysically in order to define the elementary characteristics of life, i.e., of all living substances, while simultaneously he uses the term in reference to the variety of individual psychic representations.

In *Beyond the Pleasure Principle*, the study of traumatic neuroses leads to the conclusion that one can no longer presuppose the automatic regulatory principles of psychic life. This implies that one cannot take for granted that the drives are psychical representatives of somatic forces. More precisely, it is the compulsion to repeat traumatic situations that undermines not only the assumption of automatic regulation of psychic life by the pleasure principle, but also the idea of correspondence between drive and representation. In so far as the drives are pure somatic forces, they are "beyond" representation, beyond the "frontier" of conceptualization. What we find in the traumatic neuroses are amounts of unbound drive energy flooding the psychic apparatus, without this apparatus being able to bind and assimilate these stimuli. In these cases, in which the influx of the drives is unhindered and does not meet any resistance or inhibition, the drives reveal their "daemonic" character – their "essence", namely the amount of force exercising pressure (*Drang*) on the psychic apparatus (compare Freud 1915c: 122). The drives are like constant forces without any intention and aim. They are inexpedient and non-functional forces that manifest themselves in continuous "activities" and repetitions for the sake of repetition. The drives manifesting themselves in the compulsion to repeat are autonomously operating forces. They are not concerned with their effects. They are indifferent to whether they result in pleasure or unpleasure or contribute to progress or not. The drives are aimless forces which persist in pressuring everything they encounter, producing tension and excitation in every cell, tissue, organ or system susceptible to stimuli. The character of the drives is Mephistophelean: it "[*drängt*] *ungebändigt immer vorwärts*" without concern for the tragic consequences (Freud 1920g: 42). The drives are "the driving factor which will permit no halting at any position attained" (Freud 1920g: 42). The drive is the inner propelling "remorseless law of nature", the inner purposeless and restless "necessity" (*Ανάγκη*) to which every individual is submitted (Freud 1920g: 45). If and for as long as a drive does not encounter an obstacle or counter-force, it will persist in its movement and direction. Concretely, in the case of traumatic neurotic patients, this is manifested in the compulsory repetition of an accidental life-threatening situation.

This physiological perspective of the drive as an indifferent, non-functional and aimless force can be found throughout Freud's writings.[2] In the 1905 edition of *Three Essays*, the first definition of drive is phrased as follows:

> In addition to an 'instinct' [*Trieb*], which is not itself sexual and which has its source in motor impulses, we can discern in the partial drives a contribution from an organ receiving stimuli (e.g., the skin, the mucous

> membrane, or a sense organ). An organ of this kind will be described in this connection as an 'erotogenic zone' – as being the organ whose excitation lends the instinct a sexual character.
>
> (Freud 1905d: 168 n.)

Here, the drive is defined in purely physiological terms without any reference to representations or ideas. It is merely a stimulus producing excitation in sensitive organs and zones. One of the reasons for deleting this definition of the drive and replacing it with a definition in line with "Instincts and Their Vicissitudes"[3] was the following. The sentence can be read – as, for example, Jung did[4] – as a definition in which one primal drive is assumed. In such a reading, the drive is a certain quantity of undifferentiated force or energy that only comes to be further differentiated into domains and functions through the various organs receiving the drive stimuli and producing excitation. This will lend the drive either a sexual or a self-preservative character (Van Haute & Westerink 2021: 20–21). As Jung had already pointed out, beyond Freud's drive dualism, one finds a latent drive monism, as evidenced in references to the drive as a quantity in flow (*Q*), a constant force (*konstanter Kraft*) or an urge (*Drang*) (compare Freud 1920g: 36).[5] One occasionally finds Freud hinting at such monistic conception, for example, when he writes that one may have to consider "an indifferent psychic energy" which only later becomes differentiated into ego-libido and object-libido (Freud 1914c: 78). A comparable remark on "displaceable and neutral energy" nourishing the life drives and death drives can be found in *The Ego and the Id* (Freud 1923b: 44; also Bernet 2020: 204).[6]

From this physiological perspective, drives produce excitation, tension and disturbance, and thus a workload for psychic apparatus. Psychic life is therefore first and foremost the totality of responses to these drives. This includes the creation of stable contact barriers, permanent traces, side-cathexes, neural pathways and facilitations which the excitations will have to follow before being discharged (Freud 1950c). The drives evoke psychic reactions of anxiety, attention, anticipation, wishes, etc., and higher psychic functions such as memory, phantasy, thought and judgement (Freud 1911c). Freud concludes "that instincts, not external stimuli, are the true motive forces behind the advances that have led the nervous system, with its unlimited capacities, to its present high level of development" (1915c: 120). But this does not mean that the drives aim at advancement. Freud is quick to deny the idea of a drive towards higher development (*Trieb zur Höherentwicklung*) or a drive towards perfection (*Trieb zur Vervollkommnung*) (Freud 1920g: 41–42). In so far as drives contribute to progress, they do so unintentionally. As the drives persist in producing tension, they pressure the psychic systems to bind impulses to representations, to seek satisfaction of demands and needs. Drives unintentionally generate a variety of psychic activities and differentiations. They constantly push life towards activity. From this perspective, progress is the effect of the reactions to blind repetitive forces. Or in dynamic-mechanistic terms: a body will only move when moved by forces that act on it; action is reaction.

Sexual drives and self-preservative drives

The introduction of the concept of "drive" in the 1905 *Three Essays* went hand in hand with the introduction of a drive dualism. Drawing upon Darwinian thought, Freud distinguishes self-preservative functional drives – notably, drives producing excitation as signalling the need for food intake – and non-functional sexual drives that seek to experience pleasure at autoerotic excitations. It is only in puberty that the latter drives find a new aim in the discharge of sexual products (Freud 1905d: 135, 207). This new aim paves the way for a more functional and heteronormative – and oedipal – perspective on the sexual drives.[7] A reading of the various editions of *Three Essays on the Theory of Sexuality* thus shows that the first drive theory is the nucleus of a non-oedipal sexual theory in which infantile sexuality is defined in terms of organic processes and repeated polymorphous perverse, autoerotic pleasurable activities (see also pp. 66–67). These repetitions and stimulations produce new (non-self-preservative) functions of, and associations between, different organs and body parts. Different body parts can become susceptible to stimulation and thus acquire qualities previously characteristic of the lips or genitals (Freud 1905d: 180–184). From his observations of the repetitions of pleasurable activities and the associations and interactions between different organs, tissues and body parts, Freud concludes that the body is not so much a functional unity of parts but rather consists of "connecting pathways" (*Verbindungswege*) between erogenous zones. Freud pursues and broadens this line of reasoning in the studies of Little Hans and Schreber in which one or more erotogenic zones become the organizing element in a philosophy of life and a delusional conception of reality. Hans's "widdler-centric" *Weltanschauung* results from sexual researches solely informed by his own autoerotic activities, and his subsequent interest in the genital organs of others (Van Haute & Westerink 2021: 57). Central in Schreber's delusions is his wish to be transformed into a woman – a wish Freud traces back to infantile genital fixations (Freud 1911c: 55–56, 77).

In the period of these case studies, we can witness the beginning of a progressive oedipalization of the sexual theory and a growing focus on the significance of infantile object relations. The formative aspects of autoerotism are gradually eclipsed by a focus on the normalizing and repressive effects of the Oedipus complex.[8] In this context, notably in the 1915 edition of *Three Essays*, Freud introduces new theoretical material in sections on the libido theory and narcissism, the phases of development of the sexual organization, the sexual researches of children, and the diphasic object choice (Freud 1905d: 194–200, 217–219). These new sections undermine the radical sexual theory of the 1905 edition and progressively introduce a theory of sexuality in which infantile sexuality is seen as organized in developmental phases relative to object-finding, through early object-finding. The infantile period is now seen as preparing the normal and functional sexual organization (Van Haute & Westerink 2021).[9] And yet, all these reconsiderations of the role of sexuality do not lead Freud to fundamentally question his drive theory. He maintains the distinction between "the *ego*, or *self-preservative*, instincts and the *sexual* instincts" as "a working hypothesis, to be retained only as long as it proves useful" (Freud 1915c: 124; Freud's italics).

In the 1919 version of *Beyond the Pleasure Principle*, there is no indication that Freud sets out to fundamentally reconsider the drive dualism he had introduced in 1905 and reaffirmed in 1915. In discussing occasions for the release of unpleasure in the first chapter, for example, Freud points towards psychic conflicts and the repression of sexual drives by the ego (Freud 1920g: 11). This reference to psychic conflict implicitly confirms the theory of sexual drives and ego-drives. A similar train of thought can be found in Chapter 3 in which Freud discusses unpleasure for one system as satisfaction for another (Freud 1920g: 19–20). His brief elaborations of "the early efflorescence of infantile sexuality" and its "extinction" due to its inadequate state of development, are in line with the theory of sexuality that he had articulated in 1915. This includes references to the child's first defining object choices, the experiences of loss of love from these objects, and the early effects of socialization (Freud 1920g: 20–21).

But most significant are the references to the sexual drives and self-preservative drives in Chapter 5 after Freud has introduced the idea of a first drive that came into being as the immediate reaction to the first attributes of life (inner disturbance, tension). This first drive is a drive that seeks to cancel out the – unpleasurable – tension and return to an inanimate state (Freud 1920g: 38) while at the same time, forced through modifications of the living organism, embarking on "ever more complicated *détours*" before reaching its aim (Freud 1920g: 39). The insistence on the conservative character of *all* drives – again – does not lead Freud to fundamentally reconsider his former drive theory. Instead, he fleshes out the implications "in regard to the great groups of drives which, as we believe, lie behind the phenomena of life in organisms": the self-preservative drives and the sexual drives (Freud 1920g: 39).

For Freud, the question is how to consider drives of self-preservation when the aim of all life is the inanimate. If the aim of life is death, what explains the further development of organic life into forms that no longer "die easily" and generate self-protective measures? In the 1919 version of *Beyond the Pleasure Principle*, Freud argues the following: the fact that there are ever more complicated life forms with lengthened life-spans is not determined by self-preservative drives, but by organic life being subjected to modifications in changing circumstances. We have already seen that these modifications force living organisms to diverge ever more widely from their original course of life (Freud 1920g: 38–39). The evolution of the species from the undifferentiated vesicle to increasingly complex organisms such as human beings thus makes the journey back to the inanimate longer and more laborious. Every species has developed its own unique detour, seeks to "follow its own path to death" and "wishes to die only in its own fashion" (Freud 1920g: 39). This means that every organism seeks to preserve itself up until it unavoidably dies a natural death. Under normal circumstances, it will resist all possible short-circuits. It will flee from life-threatening danger and will avoid situations in which it could "die easily". Every organism wishes to die from internal causes and therefore tries to avoid every external event that would cause its death. What "natural death" in this context means can be understood from Freud's references to Haeckel's biogenetic law: organisms are directed towards the inorganic only through the repetition of the history of the species – including the repetition of the life-span of the same species. According to Freud, the self-preservative drives can thus be said to be "myrmidons of death" as they urge the living organism to live until it dies from internal causes (through metabolic processes, exhaustion and ageing). The self-preservative drives aim stubbornly at the repetition of the same detour through life taken by previous generations. They resist further evolution and development; instead, they seek to repeat the same death as that of previous generations. They seek to repeat the same life-span of previous generations, faithfully maintaining and securing (*getreulich festhalten*) a certain fashion of dying (see also Freud 1933a: 106).

Freud also attributes the conservative character of all drives to the sexual drives. In this case, likewise, Freud calls upon the biogenetic law. With the appearance of multicellular organisms (and the subsequent more complicated organic life forms), a form of reproduction was introduced in which two similar (belonging to the same species) and yet different (belonging to two sexes) germ cells would coalesce and generate offspring. The sexual drives safeguard the emergence of more of the same new individuals who will repeat the same detour towards death as the previous generation. According to Freud, these drives are conservative "in the same sense as the other drives in that they bring back earlier states of living substance". In a way, Freud writes, the sexual drives are even more conservative "in that they are peculiarly resistant to external influences" and "preserve life itself for a comparative long period" (Freud 1920g: 40).

The self-preservative and sexual drives are profoundly conservative and answer to the principle of repetition. The group of self-preservative drives "rushes forward to reach the final aim of death", that is, the natural death that, depending on the species, comes either very swift (*möglichst bald*) or takes a bit longer. The group of sexual drives "jerks back to a certain point to make a fresh start and so prolong the journey", that is, repeats the journey of the previous generations (Freud 1920g: 40). Freud thus suggests that the two drive groups are formally analogous. Echoing Spielrein, Freud argues that in multicellular organisms the sexual drives are conservative because of the implied death of a portion of the germ cells in coalescence which, as such, is the initial "state" from which a new individual develops. The self-preservative drives are conservative in the sense that they spur life on for as long as possible, that is, until the organism dies a natural death. Freud thus suggests that the aim of all life equals the aim of all living beings. But can this be maintained? One could argue to the contrary: the very fact that life emerged from inanimate matter (and would seek to return to the inanimate) has no analogy on the level of living beings who are, after all, always born from other living beings (Bernet 2020: 206).

To the mention of the vacillating rhythm (*Zauderrhythmus*) of groups of drives rushing forward and jerking backward, Freud adds a few sentences in the 1919 text that will be reformulated in the published version. The original passage reads as follows:

> But sexuality and the distinction between the sexes did not exist at the start of life, and the sequence just depicted appears to us to be a later complication of an originally simpler one. In fact it appears to repeat a moment (one unknown to us, but for certain a very important one in the history of living substance) which is the point from which, in order to prolong its life, it learned to develop a second goal, one that stood opposed to the first goal.
>
> (Freud 2024: 60)

In the reformulation of this passage in the 1920 version of *Beyond the Pleasure Principle* Freud argues that "the possibility remains that the instincts which were later to be described as sexual may have been in operation from the very first". He adds: "it may not be true that it was only at a later time that they started their work of opposing the activities of the ego-instincts" (Freud 1920g: 41).

This reformulation clearly results from the introduction of the new drive theory in the 1920 version of *Beyond the Pleasure Principle.* In the 1919 version of the text, Freud argues that immediately after the emergence of life "the first drive came into being: the instinct to return to the inanimate state" (Freud 1920g: 38). It is only later in evolution – with the emergence of more differentiated organisms – that the self-preservative drives were the first to come into being, followed at a later stage by the sexual drives aiming at coalescence of germ cells. As we will see below, in the new drive theory, Freud argues that the death drives and life drives spontaneously originate with the first living substance. In this new version of the emergence of life from inanimate matter, the sexual drives – as drives aimed at reproduction – are a specific manifestation of the life drives (Eros) that seek to "reunite" what "was torn apart into small particles" (Freud 1920g: 58). In other words, the life drives do not aim at reproduction; they are nor reproductive drives (*Fortpflanzungstriebe* – see also Van Haute & Westerink 2021). But they do become manifest in the reproductive activities of multicellular organisms. Freud thus argues, contrary to his 1919 statements, that the sexual drives are not a later acquisition, but are in fact the expression of the life drives in multicellular organisms.[10]

While it seems at first sight that Freud continues the trains of thought articulated in the first version of the text contrasting the sexual drives and self-preservative drives, he fundamentally changes his argumentation in the 1920 version of the text:

> The upshot of our inquiry so far has been *the drawing of a sharp distinction between the 'ego-instincts' and the sexual instincts*, and the view that the former exercise pressure towards death and the latter towards a prolongation of life. But this conclusion is bound to be unsatisfactory in many respects even to ourselves. Moreover, *it is actually only of the former group of instincts that we can predicate a conservative*, or rather retrograde, character corresponding to a compulsion to repeat. For on our hypothesis the ego-instincts arise from the coming to life of inanimate matter and seek to restore the inanimate state; whereas as regards the sexual instincts, though it is true that they reproduce primitive states of the organism, what they are clearly aiming at by every possible means is the coalescence of two germ cells which are differentiated in a particular way.
>
> (Freud 1920g: 44; my italics)

Contrary to what Freud had been arguing in the 1919 version of the text, the sexual drives are now said to be profoundly non-conservative. In order to underscore this, Freud adds an interjection towards the end of the fifth chapter. In the first version of *Beyond the Pleasure Principle*, the question was raised as to whether there are indeed any instincts that do not seek to restore an earlier state of things. In the subsequent version, however, Freud adds "apart from the sexual instincts" (Freud 1920g: 41). In the second published version from 1921, Freud italicizes this short addition, thus further emphasizing its importance.[11] This insertion of 1920 clearly contradicts the 1919 paragraph in which Freud had described sexual drives as conservative "to a higher degree" in comparison to the self-preservative drives.

In the opening section of Chapter 6 of *Beyond the Pleasure Principle*, Freud argues that the sexual drives do not aim at a return to the inanimate or to an earlier state of things, but in fact seek to prolong life in order to "lend it the appearance of immortality" (*Schein der Unsterblichkeit*) (Freud 1920g: 44).[12] It is undeniably true, he argues, that the coalescence (*Verschmelzung*) of germ cells can be said to be a reproduction of the most primitive state of the organism. The question is then, what "important event" provoked this tendency towards coalescence? Freud's speculations in Chapter 5 on the origin of life, the appearance of the first conservative drive, and the first functional organization in the undifferentiated vesicle provide no clue as to what circumstances were decisive for the appearance of coalescence as an aim of a group of drives. This will lead Freud to review his reconstruction of the emergence of life, as is discussed below.

From these first reformulations of the drive theory in the 1920 version of the text, Freud draws the conclusion that his argumentation developed a year earlier may have been mistaken. He ends the paragraph by spelling out the implication – namely that "the compulsion to repeat would no longer possess the importance we have ascribed to it" (Freud 1920g: 44). If, indeed, the sexual drives are no longer conservative, they are also no longer primarily characterized by the return to a previous state and an implied (partial) death, or the recapitulation of the life trajectories of previous generations. On the contrary, they would be characterized by a progressive tendency to create and prolong new life forms. They "push life forward". This means that the sexual drives and the life drives would tend to connect to and maintain aspects of what Freud had, in 1919, termed the "daemonic" character of the drives. The sexual drives and the life drives are "troublemakers", continuously producing new tension and excitation in processes of coalescence. In this new conceptualization, however, the non-conservative drives are no longer aimlessly insisting on repetition for the sake of repetition. The sexual drives and the life drives do have an aim: the creation of ever larger unities.

And there is more. Freud now also suggests that the opposition between the self-preservative drives and the sexual drives ceases to hold, since this opposition had been articulated in terms of vacillating forces rushing forward and jerking backward. The idea that the sexual drives aim at prolongation of life – even lending the cell's life "appearance of immortality" – implies that the aim of the sexual drives coincides with the aim of the self-preservative drives which seek to prolong each individual life until it ends in natural death. If the sexual drives can be placed in the service of self-preservation, there is no opposition between these drives. For the first time Freud is explicitly questioning the "working hypothesis" of the distinction between self-preservative and sexual drives.

In this context, Freud mentions "ego or death instincts and sexual or life instincts" (Freud 1920g: 44). In Chapter 5, he had once referred in passing to the sexual drives as "the true life instincts" (Freud 1920g: 40), yet without adding any specific significance to this statement. He now also introduces the term "death drives". In the context of the 1920 version of *Beyond the Pleasure Principle*, the new concepts are first introduced as synonyms for the self-preservative drives and sexual drives. Having said this, Freud prepares his readers for a new conceptuality that will define a new drive theory. And yet, in the first part of Chapter 6 (i.e., in the transition from the definition of all drives in Chapter 5 to the new drive theory), he keeps referring to the death drives and life drives as equivalents of the self-preservative and sexual drives, respectively (Freud 1920g: 44–50). This is still the case in the reference to Schopenhauer in which Freud associates the sexual drives with the "will to live", while death drives or self-preservative drives are said to be conservative, aiming at death (Freud 1920g: 50).[13] Only from this point in the text onwards does Freud introduce his new drive theory in which the self-preservative and sexual drives are both seen as aspects of the life drives. We should note, however, that in his discussion of the concept of life drives, Freud clearly gives priority to the sexual drives over the self-preservative drives. In this context, he does not mention the self-preservative drives further, but appears to include them in the general "life-preserving" (*lebenserhaltende*) character of the sexual drives (Freud 1920g: 55).

The urge to restore a previous state

We have seen that Freud's starting point for a new definition of the concept of drive in the 1919 version of the text is the phenomenon of the compulsion to repeat highly disturbing life-threatening traumatic situations. Since the compulsion to repeat concerns the reliving of traumatic situations over and over again, and since this compulsion cannot be considered as a function or tendency in the service of secondary processes, this compulsion must be seen as expressing an aspect of the drives. Repetition must reflect the character of the drives. For this reason, Freud reasons that the drives are to be seen as urges seeking to restore a previous situation; they are the motive forces behind concrete compulsions to repeat:

> At this point we cannot escape a suspicion that we may have come upon the track of a universal attribute [*Charakter*] of instincts and perhaps of organic life in general which has not hitherto been clearly recognized or at least not explicitly stressed.[14] *It seems, then, that an instinct is an urge* [*Drang*] *inherent in organic life to restore* [*Wiederherstellung*] *an earlier state of things* [*früheren Zustand*] which the living entity has been obliged to abandon under the pressure of external disturbing forces; that is, it is a kind of organic elasticity, or, to put it another way, the expression of the inertia inherent in organic life.
>
> (Freud 1920g: 36; Freud's italics)[15]

At first sight, this definition seems to be in line with Freud's elaborations of the traumatic neuroses and their daemonic repetitions. Yet, instead of defining the drives relative to the repeated return to trauma, Freud associates the drives with the restoration of a situation that precedes any disturbing impact of external forces. This step is not self-evident. It allows Freud to move from trauma as a life-threatening interruption of psychic life, and more generally, of life, towards a conception of life as "awakening" (*erwecken*) (Freud 1920g: 38) from the inanimate into the animated. The choice of the verb *erwecken* indeed suggests that Freud associates the evocation of life with an "awakening" to life, or more concretely, with the awakening from a fright-dream in which the traumatic situation was relived.[16]

And, yet, it is telling that the manifestations of the compulsion to repeat on which he comments in this context do not include the fright-dreams he had discussed at length in a previous chapter. Instead, Freud once again mentions children's play and their repetitions of unpleasurable experiences in attempts at mastery, the pleasure experienced at repetitions of identical activities such as rereading a book or listening again to a nice story or a joke being told more than once. And he refers to the repetition evinced in transference and in negative therapeutic reactions (Freud 1920g: 35–36). According to Freud, these are all illustrations of a pulsional tendency to repeat "identical" impressions and sensations (*Identität des Eindrucks*) – independently of whether these generate pleasure or unpleasure (Freud 1920g: 35).[17] What he takes from his analyses of the fright-dreams in the traumatic neuroses is not the repetition of highly disturbing situations of influx of amounts of drive energy, but merely the insistence on the repetition of the same impression. Drives insist on the repetition of "the same course of life" and of identical situations and impressions (Freud 1920g: 38). They thus resist enforced modifications that not only bring change and development, but also novelty as "the condition of enjoyment" (*Bedingung des Genusses*) (Freud 1920g: 35). Such modifications, change and new possibilities of enjoyment give meaning to life. The drive as an urge to restore an earlier state of things, in contrast, persists in the inexpedient and meaningless repetition of the same. The daemonic character of the drives is seen here as manifesting itself in an urge to restore situations in which there is no psychic activity and creativity. The drives pressure towards a meaningless life devoid of any impetus to act, move and enjoy. Seen from this perspective, Freud can maintain a defining aspect of the traumatic neurotic's tragic repetitions: the uncanniness of paralyzed psychic life, and the deadly way in which a person can be subjected to drives that do not produce liveliness and enjoyment in new activities. The drives empty life out in such a way that ultimately it no longer has to respond to stimuli. The urge to restore a previous situation thus results in a form of death that can best be described in terms of lethargy and monotony. The drives turn an organism into lethargic matter, into a monotonous automaton with no interest in and excitement about anything new. The drives pressure not towards enjoyment at novelty, but towards desensitized and dull machinal repetitions.[18] Even pleasant stories and jokes may fall prey to this tendency of the drives.

Freud describes these drives as "conservative" (*konservativ*) (Freud 1920g: 36). The drives are conservative in the sense that they are "restorative", always pressuring the organism to return to a situation before some external force provoked disturbance and change. But the drives are also conservative in the sense that they are "historically determined":

> Every modification which is thus imposed upon the course of the organism's life is accepted by the conservative organic drives and stored up for further repetition. Those instincts are therefore bound to give a deceptive appearance of being forces tending towards change and progress, whilst in fact they are merely seeking to reach an ancient goal by paths alike old and new.
>
> (Freud 1920g: 38)

The drives and their characteristics are acquired by previous generations and thus inherited and repeated by all later generations. They "conserve" (preserve) the acquired characteristics of ancestry, that is, the characteristics of their distorted and diverted – traumatized – lives. Seen from this perspective, another aspect of the daemonic character of the drives comes to the fore. The daemonic is what binds us to previous generations and makes us repeat their detours (*Umwege*) as our own inevitable course of life (Freud 1920g: 39).[19] The daemonic is the compulsion to recapitulate the inherited, persistent and "imperishable" (Freud 1915b: 286) – to repeat what is hence, strictly speaking, not ours and yet defines our lives. The biogenetic law turns out to define the uncanny character of inheritance.

The aim of all life

From his exploration of the drive as an urge to restore an earlier state of things, Freud turns his attention to the question of the "final goal [*Endziel*] of all organic striving" and "the aim [*Ziel*] of all life" (Freud 1920g: 38). We should note that up to this point, Freud's statements on the restoration and repetition of previous situations and impressions have not addressed the question of the aim of the drives beyond the mere insistence on repetition. In fact, it appears that such repetitive movements would likely never come to an end unless they encounter an obstacle or counter-force. The fact that the urge to restore results in lethargic life and repetitions of the same does not necessarily imply that the drives aim at a life devoid of any disturbance, excitation, tension, conflict or unpleasurable sensations. In fact, the urge to restore does not consider the implications and results, pleasurable or unpleasurable, of its insistence. In the case of children listening to a nice story over and over again, there clearly is pleasure experienced at the repetition. The reference to transference points in the same direction. There is the re-enactment of the repressed and of past experiences, including feelings of pleasure at excitation. The fright-dreams of traumatic-neurotic patients, in contrast, attest to the repetition of highly unpleasurable and life-threatening situations. In other words, the fact that the urge to restore an earlier state of things goes hand in hand with repetitions of the same does not inform us about the final aim of all drives beyond the mere insistence on the repetition of the same (see also Bernet 2020: 207).

Freud's arguments for the next step in the drive theory derive mainly from evolutionary biology – and not from clinical observations. If indeed evolution can be described in terms of recapitulations, if the characteristics of organic life forms are acquired through external modifying forces, and if we can assume that the drives are fundamental and original characteristics of the living substance, the ultimate state of things that the drives seek to restore would have to be the very first state of things. This is the inorganic state which the first living substance was forced to abandon because of the incomprehensible force that created the first modification:

> It would be in contradiction to the conservative nature of the drives if the goal [*Ziel*] of life were a state of things which had never yet been attained. On the contrary, it must be an *old* state of things, an initial state [*Ausgangszustand*] from which the living entity has at one time or other departed and to which it is striving to return by the circuitous paths [*Umwege*] along which its development leads. If we are to take it as a truth that knows no exception that everything living dies for internal reasons – becomes inorganic once again [*ins Anorganische zurückkehrt*] – then we shall be compelled to say that '*the aim of all life is death*' and, looking backwards, that '*inanimate things* [*das Leblose*] *existed before living ones*'.
>
> (Freud 1920g: 38; Freud's italics)

The drives are now said to aim at the restoration of the initial state of inertia that precedes life – inanimate matter. The compulsion to repeat is rephrased here in terms of a single tendency towards the final aim of death. Death is the only finality of all drives. The first spontaneous reaction formation resulting from the transformation of the inorganic into the organic is that of the drives seeking to restore the inanimate. The drives are urges seeking to return to dead matter. They aim at the elimination of life and thus also the elimination of themselves. Life seeks to leave itself behind, to make itself into a past state.

According to Freud, the inanimate is a pleasurable state in which, after all, there is no tension or excitation. Or in other words, death is absence of unpleasure; and therefore death is pleasure. This means that the aim of all drives coincides with the pleasure principle – the reduction and ultimately the removal of all unpleasurable tension. Indeed, in the final paragraphs of the 1919 edition of *Beyond the Pleasure Principle*, Freud draws a conclusion along these lines:

> The pleasure principle, then, is a tendency operating in the service of a function whose business it is to free the mental apparatus entirely from excitation or to keep the amount of excitation in it constant or to keep it as low as possible. We cannot yet decide with certainty in favour of any of these ways of putting it; but it is clear that the function thus described would be concerned with the most universal endeavour of all living substance – namely to return to the quiescence of the inorganic world.
>
> (Freud 1920g: 62)

The pleasure principle is a tendency operating in the service of the drives – all drives – that endeavour to return to the inanimate.[20] The pleasure principle is the representative in psychic life of the drives that aim at inertia from the outset.

How does this universal endeavour relate to the daemonic character of constant forces and repetitions? It appears that the drives can be seen as urges that aim at the discharge of excitation produced by themselves. It appears that the drives are in conflict with themselves, seeking to master themselves. In his reading of *Beyond the Pleasure Principle* (and notably the section on the *fort-da* play and the final chapter), Derrida has developed this idea, arguing that the drives can be defined in terms of drives for mastery (*Bemächtigungstriebe*). The drives themselves aim at the dominance of the pleasure principle. The drives seek to bind themselves to representations through repetitive activities in which tension and excitation can be drained off. In the process of mastering themselves, they produce differentiated psychic life (Derrida 1987: 403; 2020: 347 ff). The drives would thus aim to bring their daemonic character to an end.

Such a reading can find support in Freud's writings, especially in "Instincts and Their Vicissitudes". In that text, Freud had not only argued that the drives can be "constant forces" comparable to external stimuli operating as an internal-outside upon the higher psychic functions. He had also argued that the aim of a drive is satisfaction which can only be obtained by removing the state of stimulation (Freud 1915c: 122).[21] The aim of the drives is thus to remove any disturbance or excitation originating from somatic stimuli, that is, the constant forces that pressure the psychic system. One could thus argue that the drives aim not only at self-mastery, but even at self-elimination.

But is this what Freud is telling us in Chapter 5 of *Beyond the Pleasure Principle*? Freud's reconstruction of the origin and emergence of life leads him to describe the drives solely in terms of reactive forces. Drives are not considered here as producing pleasurable (polymorphous-perverse) excitations or pushing life forward through the creation of new forms, but, on the contrary, as forces seeking the return to the inanimate. If this is true, if all drives are conservative, there are no forces "beyond" the pleasure principle that push organisms forward. Drives do not create forms; they are not plastic tendencies. Deleuze recognized this problem of what he called "the triumph of reactive forces" over the repeated disturbances generated by internal and external creative forces (Deleuze 2006: 135).[22] He criticizes the fact that Freud, in the course of his analyses of repetition, loses sight of the productive differentiating character of repetition, and that he favours the repetition of the same instead. This is despite the fact that in Freud's writings, one does find the idea of repetition producing not the same but something different (Deleuze 2004: 19). Deleuze here points to the notion of "displaceable energy" and the notion of the life drives producing new "vital differences" (Deleuze 2004: 19ff, 128ff; 2018: 99ff).[23] He thus contests the association in *Beyond the Pleasure Principle* of repetition with a compulsion to repeat the same. He reads this text as a metaphysical exercise in which the creative potential of the life drives is eclipsed by the introduction of a transcendental principle expressed in the compulsion to repeat the same: the drives towards death, that is, the conservative, regressive and entropic forces aimed at the inanimate. What Deleuze may not have fully realized is the fact that the theory of the life drives is Freud's solution to the problems that emerge with the introduction of the "conservative" character of all drives. We will return to this issue below.

This short reference to Deleuze indicates the main problems and questions arising in the first version of *Beyond the Pleasure Principle.* The different conceptualizations of the drives ranging from constant daemonic forces to conservative urges are difficult and probably impossible to reconcile (see also Johnston 2005: 183). Deleuze highlights the fact that displaceable drive energy or force manifesting itself in the compulsion to repeat cannot be identified with the conservative character that would define all drives. He thus points at a fundamental problem in Freud's reasoning. If all drives are conservative and restorative, there appear to be no drives that can push life forward, creating new modes and forms of life. This conservative character is confirmed and underscored by Freud's Lamarckism: all change and progress are said to be due to external modifying forces and reactive processes of adaptation.[24] What started as exploration of the "beyond" of the pleasure principle becomes a theory of a living monad seeking the elimination of inner tension vis-à-vis modifying external stimuli. All psychic organization in the secondary processes would be merely derivative of tendencies characteristic of living substances from the very beginning of life.

Freud's train of thought on the concept of the drive in Chapter 5 thus leads to an unforeseen and problematic conclusion: there is no "beyond" the pleasure principle. The drives and the pleasure principle that regulates psychic life both aim at the discharge of all tension – a conclusion also Derrida has drawn in his reading of Chapter 5 (Derrida 1987: 338–386). The pleasure principle is not only operating in the service of the drives, genetically speaking, it is the heir of the drives. From this perspective, all repetitions – whether succeeding or tragically failing – would be reparative and restorative. In addition, it seems that the question as to what produces tension and disturbance can therefore only be answered with reference to external modifying influences that repeatedly produce fresh inner tensions. At the end of Chapter 5, it becomes clear that the prioritization of the "economic point of view" has resulted in a conflation of the dynamical and the economic: change and movement (returns, restorations) through internal forces only serve the reduction of tension. The primacy of the economic perspective on psychic life threatens to lead to a methodological monism in which the dynamic processes become subjected to economic principles.

And there is more. At the end of Chapter 5, Freud stares drive monism in the face: all drives are conservative; the self-preservative and sexual drives are merely two expressions of the same drive character and aim. The problem here is not so much that any form of monism would be a genuflection to Jung. A more serious problem lies in the fact that this drive theory undermines the notion of psychic conflict, such as the conflict between sexual drives and ego-drives, primary and secondary processes. If all inner urges, tendencies, principles and systems aim at pleasure and the elimination of tension, what remains is only one major conflict, namely that between an organism and its hostile environment.[25]

The conclusion that the pleasure principle operates in the service of drives aimed at inertia, and that there is therefore no "beyond" the pleasure principle, is likely the main reason why Freud did not to publish the 1919 manuscript. He will likely have realized that he needed to find an answer to the question as to how to consider psychic conflict and the productivity of drives. And yet, when writing the text additions for the 1920 edition, Freud does not decide to completely rewrite Chapter 5. Apparently, he wants to maintain the key intuitions and insert these into the theory of life drives and death drives.[26] What then does he want to preserve from his 1919 drive concept? There is, above all, the idea that life is characterized not only by drives that ceaselessly push life forward and upward; life is also characterized by internal forces that pressure against life and that seek to avoid (further) interactions with the external world and (new) relations with objects. This is at the heart of the notion of the conservative character of drives seeking to restore the inanimate, the initial state of inertia in which matter was not yet disturbed and subjected to the principles of evolution and the enforced prolongation of living substances. There are drives that resist change and interaction; this resistance can be defined as "inertia inherent in organic life" and as "a kind of organic elasticity".[27]

Libidinal binding in groups

A month after finishing the first version of *Beyond the Pleasure Principle*, Freud started working on what a year later, in August 1920, would be a first draft of *Group Psychology and the Analysis of the Ego*. In the "Editor's Note" to the English translation of this text, James Strachey writes that "there is little direct connection between the present work and its close predecessor, *Beyond the Pleasure Principle*" (Freud 1921c: 67). Strachey most likely came to this conclusion because the concept of the death drive is not mentioned in the text on group psychology. However, from correspondence we know that Freud was in fact associating the two projects with each other. In a letter to Eitingon, dated 8 March 1920, he mentions working on "group psychology and death drives". This letter, written almost a year after completing the first version of *Beyond the Pleasure Principle*, contains the first written mention of the term "death drives" (May 2024: 90).[28]

A closer look reveals a direct connection between *Group Psychology* and the second version of *Beyond the Pleasure Principle*. In the text on group psychology, Freud explores the principles and mechanisms that organize interactions between individuals and "bind" people together in larger units. This study can be read as preparing the introduction of the concept of the life drives that seek the binding of parts (cells, organs) into larger unities (Ffytche 2022: 175; May 2024). Even in the first paragraphs of the text Freud introduces a quote from Gustav Le Bon's *Psychologie des foules*, which inspires him to associate the binding between individuals in groups with the binding of cells into larger unities: "The psychological group is a provisional being formed of heterogeneous elements, which for a moment are combined, exactly as the cells which constitute a living body form by their reunion a new being" (Freud 1921c: 73). This association is based on the argument that whatever binds people together in a group must be a principle or mechanism of binding that has a "libidinous and selfish" character (Freud & Jones 1993: 373). In other words, binding is what characterizes both libidinal and self-preservative drives. If we can assume that binding is not a late acquisition in evolution, this phenomenon must be characteristic of (a certain group of) drives from the outset.[29]

Referring to Wilfred Trotter's (1916) *Instincts of the Herd in Peace and War*, Freud writes "that the tendency towards the formation of groups is biologically a continuation of the multicellular character of all the higher organisms" (Freud 1921c: 87). He pursues this idea in discussing Trotter's work in some detail:

> Trotter derives the mental phenomena that are described as occurring in groups from a herd instinct ('gregariousness'), which is innate in human beings just as in other species of animals. Biologically, he says, this gregariousness is in analogy to multicellularity and as it were a continuation of it. (In terms of the libido theory, it is a further manifestation of the tendency which proceeds from the libido and which is felt by all living beings of the same kind, to combine [*vereinigen*] in more and more comprehensive units [*umfassender Einheiten*].)
>
> (Freud 1921c: 118)[30]

Despite his criticisms of both Le Bon and Trotter, what Freud takes from their studies is the notion of the continuation of processes of binding throughout evolution. This involves, in Trotter's words, the "aggregation of units" as evidenced in the two major "advances" in the evolution of species – "the passage from the unicellular to the multicellular, and from the solitary to the social" (Trotter 1916: 7). We may have expected Freud to expand on the nature of continuations and analogies by hinting at the biogenetic law in *Group Psychology*. But this is not the case. And, yet, Freud does adduce the notions of recapitulation and repetition in arguing that individuals and groups repeat the same "emotional ties" (*Gefühlsbindingen*) that operate in the primal horde. Group formation is a "revival" (*Wiederaufleben*) and the "reconstitution" (*wieder herstellen*) of the primal horde. It is not only the individual who repeats or "reanimates" (*Wiederbelebung*) the Oedipal object relations that characterize the primal horde – so does the group (Freud 1921c: 123, 127).[31] In other words, the focus here – as in *Totem and Taboo* – is on recapitulations and repetitions within the domain of social organizations, and, hence, within the domain of culture.

In *Group Psychology*, Freud also expands on binding as expression of "libido" which he further defines in terms of a "quantity of energy".[32] This libido is said to express itself in love. The nucleus (*Kern*) of love, according to Freud, is "sexual love with sexual union as its aim" (*Geschlechtsliebe mit dem Ziel der geschlechtlichen Vereiniging*) (Freud 1921c: 90). But the libido does not only aim at union between the sexes. In fact, the word "libido" is used to describe every libidinal investment in an object – the self, parents, children, friends, and also artefacts and abstract ideas. In this "wider" sense, Freud writes, the libido and its manifestations in love can also be named Eros. Because of its orientation towards objects, Eros does not only bind people together; it also "holds together everything in the world" (Freud 1921c: 92). Eros is a concept that defines all formative interactions between heterogeneous elements.

In *Group Psychology* and in the 1920 Preface to the fourth edition of *Three Essays*, the mentioning of Plato's Eros as a synonym for libido includes a reference to an article by Max Nachmansohn on a comparison between Freud's concept of libido and Plato's Eros (Freud 1905d: 134; 1921c: 91). The reference reveals the likely source of the concept of "life drives". Nachmansohn's text from 1915, which largely consists of a reconstruction of the difference between Freud's and Jung's libido theory, is relevant because of several aspects. First, Nachmansohn argues Freud cannot maintain that libido and the sexual drives are synonyms as he had suggested in the 1905 *Three Essays*, but in fact uses the term libido in a "wider" sense, such that reproduction and human sexuality are merely "manifestations" of the libido. Second, he suggests that the concept of libido includes all progressive, productive and creative strivings, and that for this reason the libido can be named "the life drive of nature" (*Lebenstrieb der Natur*), expressing itself in the variety of ways and forms of preservation of the species, notably in processes where there is unifying (*vereinigen*) (Nachmansohn 1915: 76). Nachmansohn's text appears to be one of the main sources not only for Freud's references to Plato's concept of Eros in *Beyond the Pleasure Principle* (Freud 1920g: 50ff), but also for rethinking the concept of libido in the "wider" sense of "life drives" characterized by creative strivings for binding, growth and even progress.

Why would Freud want to introduce such a concept of libido that – as I argue – leads to him abandoning the drive dichotomy introduced in *Three Essays* and continued in the first version of *Beyond the Pleasure Principle*? What clinical and theoretical problem does Eros help to explain or understand? *Group Psychology* gives us an idea of what is at stake. For, in this text, Freud argues that identification is the "earliest expression of an emotional tie" (Freud 1921c: 105). This idea is largely based on the study of melancholia and its key characteristics: the identification with a lost object. This identification is the regressive way through which the object-tie can be substituted and hence maintained (Freud 1917e: 249, 251; 1921c: 107–109). This identification then leads to destructive self-reproaches that further characterize melancholia. This begs the question why the sexual drives are so reluctant to give up their objects, or, which amounts to the same, what motivates identification, such that the emotional tie is continued despite increasing unpleasure? If indeed identification is the earliest expression of an emotional tie, identification must reflect characteristics of the drives. But how to situate identification in the theory of sexual and self-preservative drives (Van Haute & Westerink 2021: 90ff)? The problem Freud is confronted with is that identification in melancholia describes a process of desexualization. The ego is the substitute for a lost love object, but it is not a sexual object.[33] Identification thus transcends the drive dichotomy introduced first in *Three Essays*. It is not sexual (reducible to sexual object relations) and it is not self-preservative because of its mimetic character and the subsequent internal division between ego and ego-ideal (or superego) and the accompanying aggressive self-reproaches. Freud's elaborations of the concept of identification thus call into question the first drive theory and pave the way for the concept of Eros defined in terms of binding.

Freud's inquiries into *Gefühlsbindungen* between individuals and in groups are crucial for understanding the introduction of the new drive theory.[34] His "bold attempt at another step forward" in *Beyond the Pleasure Principle* consists of applying "the libido theory which has been arrived at in psychoanalysis to the mutual relationship of cells" (Freud 1920g: 50). From his study on group psychology, Freud also takes the idea that binding always has a provisional and temporary character. What is bound can be dissolved. There is no binding without the possibility of its opposite.

It is relevant to note here (in view of Freud's references to aggression in *Beyond the Pleasure Principle* – see below) that in *Group Psychology*, aggression or destruction is not the opposite of binding. On the contrary, Freud argues that aggression accompanies binding and supports internal unity. A group bound through love – such as Christian communities or socialist movements – can be extremely intolerant and aggressive towards those outside of the emotional ties of the group (Freud 1921c: 98–99). According to Freud, groups are not violent to outsiders because these would pose a real threat to the existence of the group. Neither is coherence of the group an effect of aggression to outsiders. The violence towards outsiders is the equivalent of the love for insiders; it results from the processes of binding. Aggression is an epiphenomenon of binding. To maintain the inner cohesion of the group, and prevent the group from dissolving, aggression needs to be projected outwards. That is the reason why the weakening of libidinal ties goes hand in hand with the decline of aggression towards others. This idea finds its way into *Beyond the Pleasure Principle*: narcissistic self-love seeks to redirect the disintegrating effects of the death drives towards external objects.

The force driving the dissolution of groups is not aggression but panic, Freud writes. What is panic? Panic involves the disintegration of what was bound. According to Freud, it is not because of an external danger that panic will break out. Panic emerges from within the group when the *Gefühlsbindungen* weaken and individuals begin to be solicitous on their own account (Freud 1921c: 96). This weakening of ties is a trigger that activates the actual cause of panic: unbound drive energy overwhelming the psychic apparatus, resulting in anxiety.[35] The phenomenon of panic thus resonates with clinical findings revealing the inner causes of modes of disintegration. Panic is a phenomenon that echoes Freud's views of psychosis as experience of "world-catastrophe" (*Weltuntergangserlebnis*), and the withdrawal (*entziehen, loslösen, ablösen*) of libidinal investment in people in one's environment (compare Freud 1911c: 69–70). His views on panic resonate with his ideas on the traumatic neuroses as the result of the sudden increase of amounts of excitation – unbound libido – due to "a breach in an otherwise efficacious barrier against stimuli" (Freud 1920g: 29). In panic, the psychic apparatus is suddenly overwhelmed by an influx of excitation.[36]

Through the inquiries into Eros, binding and unbinding in *Group Psychology*, Freud could find an answer to the fundamental problems and questions arising in the first version of *Beyond the Pleasure Principle.* While working on *Group Psychology*, he realizes that the libido theory can be applied to cells and organic substances. This insight impels him to rearticulate the productive non-conservative aspect of the drives in terms of binding. Also, it allows him to integrate the conservative character of the drives into a new drive theory that also takes into account an innate tendency towards disintegration and aggression. It is through reflection on binding and unbinding in groups that Freud is able to conceptualize the life drives (Eros) as productive and creative forces, and the death drives as forces that lead to decomposition of units. In addition, taking the libido theory as a model for understanding the interactions between cells and organs allows a different conception of the bodies of complex multicellular organisms, such as human beings. The human body is no longer conceived after the model of the differentiated crusted vesicle vis-à-vis a hostile environment, reacting against which it develops increasingly complex systems to reduce tension. Like groups, bodies are considered the provisional results of assimilatory and dissimilatory interactions between heterogeneous elements. Bodies are in states of flux in so far as they are continuously reshaped – within the realm of physiological and biological possibilities.

The next step in drive theory

What follows Freud's statement on the "attempt at another step forward" (Freud 1920g: 50) is a brief overview of the theory of the drives, starting from its first conceptualization in *Three Essays.* In this sketch, he wants to clarify the relation between ego-drives and sexual drives.[37] In *Three Essays*, the focus had been the sexual drives, so as to introduce a theory of sexuality and the drives covering "many things which could not be classed under the reproductive function" (Freud 1920g: 51). He is obviously referring here to his innovative theory of the partial drives, erotogenic zones and the polymorphous-perverse character of infantile autoerotics. Turning his attention to the formation and organization of the ego, Freud could take the step towards a second drive theory. In the course of studying the psychoneuroses, Freud had come to take it for granted that the ego was a "repressive, censoring agency, capable of erecting protective structures and reaction formations" (Freud 1920g: 51). However, the study of the psychoses had shown him that efficient ego functions were not self-evident. In the Schreber case, Freud had investigated narcissism as the stage in which a person takes his own body as love-object; this had afforded him insight into the process of ego formation (Freud 1911c: 60, 72). From his exploration of narcissism and the libidinal investment in the body, Freud concludes the following: first, the ego is the first actual object of libidinal investment. Second, the ego should be thought of as a libidinal construct. And, third, this libidinal construct is the condition for any subsequent object relations (Freud 1912–1913a: 88–89; 1914c). In conclusion, Freud writes:

> Thus the original opposition between the ego-instincts and the sexual instincts proved to be inadequate. A portion of the ego-instincts was seen to be libidinal; sexual instincts – probably alongside others – operated in the ego. Nevertheless we are justified in saying that the old formula which lays it down that psychoneuroses are based on a conflict between ego-instincts and sexual instincts contains nothing that we need reject today.
>
> (Freud 1920g: 52)

The next step in the drive theory starts with underscoring the libidinal character of the self-preservative drives. What does Freud mean with this? The answer can be found at the very beginning of his "bold attempt": the binding and capacity to attach (*aneinanderhaften*) of cells into multicellular organisms is "a means to prolong their life" through interactive cooperation. Such bindings continue the primal form in which two single cells (germ cells) preserve their lives when taking each other as objects and form a union. If, as Freud argues, the sexual drives can be defined in terms of establishing libidinal relations between cells, cell states, organs, bodies and individuals, the sexual drives can be said to aim at preserving and prolonging the lives of all elements involved. In other words, the sexual drives serve self-preservation. There is only prolongation – and hence preservation – of life through libidinal processes. This leads Freud to conclude that what he called self-preservative drives "are of a libidinal nature" (Freud 1920g: 52). From this point onwards, he will therefore regard both the sexual and self-preservative drives as expressions of the life drives or Eros, "the preserver of all things" (*den alles erhaltenden*). Eros is that "which holds all living things together" (*der alles Lebende zusammenhält*) (Freud 1920g: 50, 52). In this context of the introduction of the Eros, Freud again seems to distance himself from a Spielreinian perspective of the coalescence of germ cells. The germ cells behave narcissistically, Freud writes, and seek to maintain themselves in order to be able to perform the "momentous constructive activity" for which they are meant. Freud does not refer to self-sacrificial death through coalescence, but mentions "other cells" that "sacrifice" their lives for the prolongation of the community of cells.

If indeed the self-preservative drives are of a libidinal nature, are there perhaps no drives other than libidinal ones? Are there perhaps only life drives? This question not only follows from his earlier ideas on the narcissistic libido, but also echoes the problems with which Freud was confronted at the end of Chapter 5. If all drives are conservative, how would it be possible to maintain the distinction or opposition between conflicting drive impulses? The 1920 and 1921 references to Jung's genetic theory of the libido show that Freud is aware of coming close – again – to a monistic drive theory (Freud 1920g: 52–53). Although Chapter 6 departs from a "distinction between ego-drives, which we equated with death drives, and sexual drives, which we equated with life drives" (Freud 1920g: 52–53), Freud's argumentation leads to the unintended result of Eros coming close to what Jung had referred to as "pulsional force" (*Triebkraft*) or "primal libido" (*Urlibido*) (Jung 1912: 137–142). From this point onwards, Freud attempts to rethink the drive dualism. He does this from the intuition "that instincts other than those of self-preservation operate in the ego" (Freud 1920g: 53).[38]

These "other drives" are what Freud will now call "death drives". These drives can be said to maintain the conservative character of the self-preservative drives in the way Freud had sketched in the 1919 version of the text. They are the "myrmidons of death" that "ward off any possible ways of returning to inorganic existence other than those which are immanent in the organism itself" (Freud 1920g: 39). These drives seek immunity from any modifying external stimuli or internal drive energy. They protect life by smothering it, by reducing and eliminating tension and excitation, and by resisting any possible disturbing complication. Instead of energetic and creative forces binding cells to cells, organic substances to other organic substances, and individuals to objects, these drives manifest themselves in tendencies in another direction, namely the withdrawal from what is bound and has attained increasing complexity (Freud 1920g: 55, 63). Freud explains this by pointing out that binding goes hand in hand with the increase of tension and excitation, and hence with unpleasure. Referring to Barbara Low's "Nirvana principle", Freud recalls that "one of our strongest reasons for believing in the existence of the death drives" is the fact that these drives seek "to reduce, to keep constant, or remove internal tension due to stimuli" as a "tendency which finds expression in the pleasure principle" (Freud 1920g: 55–56).[39] The death drives aim at the reduction of tension inherent in the life drives' pursuit of larger unities. In their "unobtrusive" (*unauffällig*) pursuit of pleasure and the elimination of "vital differences", the death drives must be the motive forces behind the decomposition of whatever the life drives unite.[40]

Regarding the death drives, Freud argues that, like the life drives, these drives are pressuring forces. How can we understand this? After all, does not the idea that death drives aim at the reduction of tension contradict the idea that these drives are forces? Is it not paradoxical to say that there is constant insistence on the reduction and removal of tension? Freud appears to argue that the life drives produce new tensions and excitations in the process of binding. The death drives seek to reduce tension, and this reduction can only be accomplished by dissolving unities, unbinding what was bound. In this sense, the death drives must be considered forces that can dissolve and decompose. By virtue of their capacity to redirect and redistribute investments (e.g., in the withdrawal of libido), the death drives are to be seen as proper forces.[41] This is in line with the physiological perspective we have already discussed: Freud maintains that the death drives are energetic forces, and that forces such as life drives can only be inhibited or obstructed by other forces. In other words, the death drives cannot merely be the privation or spontaneous weakening of life drives.[42] They are not the "lack" of life drives.[43]

The puzzling question regarding the life drives and notably the sexual drives that Freud now needs to answer is analogous to the question of whether death is a later acquisition in the course of evolution (Freud 1920g: 55–57). If the death drives are operative in the very first living substances as urges that aim to reduce or remove internal tension by decomposing what has been unified, then we must assume that the life drives are also present in the first living substance. The problem is, Freud reasons, that we can only know its later concrete manifestations in the conjugation of protists and in the reproduction of multicellular organisms. "In other words", Freud writes, "we need more information on the origin of sexual reproduction and of the sexual drives in general" (1920g: 56). Since science "has so little to tell us about the origin of sexuality", Freud turns his attention to a source that, at first sight, seems unlikely: Plato's *Symposium*. More precisely, he takes up Aristophanes' "theory" of the original human nature, the three sexes – man, woman, and the union of the two. In Aristophanes' fable, Zeus cut the primeval human being into two separate parts, whereupon each of these parts desired the other half, longing to restore union of the parts (Freud 1920g: 57–58). We should note here that Freud had referred to this myth in *Three Essays*; there he had called it a "poetic fable" reflecting the popular opinion in contemporary psychiatry and sexology that sexuality must be defined in terms of reproductive activities between heterosexual partners (Freud 1905d: 136). It may appear, as Laplanche has argued, that the two references to this myth are opposing each other – with *Three Essays* dismissing it and *Beyond the Pleasure Principle* approving it, for its heteronormativity and it focus on reproduction (Laplanche 2015a: 162–163, 167). However, Freud does not deny this myth's accurate description of adult sexuality in either text. What is also noteworthy in both of Freud's texts is the fact that the myth falls short in defining the sexual processes and activities that precede it. The myth merely articulates the question of the origins of sexuality, and thus paves the way for a systematic inquiry, while failing to deliver an accurate answer. In *Three Essays*, the poetic fable is merely the starting point for exploring polymorphous-perverse autoerotic infantile sexuality. In *Beyond the Pleasure Principle*, it initiates speculations on the origin of the life drives and the processes of binding.

Freud continues introducing a new speculative account of the origins of life and its first characteristics. The incomprehensible force that produced life to emerge in inanimate matter caused the first living substance to internally explode and to be "torn apart [*zerrissen*] into small particles" (Freud 1920g: 58). In response to this initial fragmentation, the life drives arise seeking to reunite the particles within the cell in order to re-establish the cell's unity. These life drives thus arise spontaneously in response to an original fragmentation. Or rather, they continue processes already present in inorganic matter, namely "chemical affinity" (Freud 1920g: 58). It becomes clear that the development of organic life into increasingly complex forms is no longer considered exclusively as the result of acquired modifications or protective measures against external stimuli. Instead, change and progress in evolution result primarily from the life drives seeking reunion of particles and parts.

The life drives thus originate as reactive forces and appear to be conservative in character. Freud takes up an aspect of the lines of thought he had developed in 1919. The reference to Aristophanes confirms this: "it traces the origin of an instinct to a *need to restore an earlier state of things*" (Freud 1920g: 57; Freud's italics). It is not only the death drives that seek to reduce or remove internal tension and to return to the inanimate; the life drives, too, have a conservative character in the sense that they initially are drives striving for "reunification" (*Wiedervereiniging*).[44] This argument is clearly meant to indicate that the new drive theory pursues the lines of thought articulated in Chapter 5.

But is Freud's argument for the conservative-restorative character of the life drives convincing? Several aspects of Freud's reasoning undermine and even contradict this. First, the reference to chemical affinity introduces what will be the dominant character of the life drives: the capacity to form new fusions, amalgamations and intermixtures.[45] The life drives proceed with chemical processes when aiming at binding particles into cells, cells into cell states, cell states into organs, organs into bodies, and eventually individuals into groups. None of these formations can be said to restore an initial unity that was lost. Second, Freud's reference to restoration and the reunification of fragments is undermined by his own speculative account of the emergence of life. If the emergence of life coincides with the moment of fragmentation, there is, strictly speaking, no unity before fragmentation. There is no original model for the unity of the living substance. Third, the life drives do not aim at preserving an established state of stability and relative tranquillity. They preserve and prolong life by including components, adding energy through continuous assimilation of material (metabolism) and increasing energy levels (through eating, drinking, breathing).[46] They preserve life through growth and development into ever more complex substances. There is thus an irreducible difference between what the life drives supposedly seek to refind and what they actually establish.[47] And last but not least, Freud explicitly states in the 1920 version of the text that the sexual drives are not conservative. This implies that the life drives are not characterized by an urge to restore an earlier state of things.

Beyond the pleasure principle: Eros

Freud conceptualizes the life drives as dynamic and creative, that is, as producing change and movement. The integration into larger units goes hand in hand with increase of internal tension. The life drives are constantly producing "the influx of fresh amounts of stimulus". Processes of binding – we can think, for example, of sexual activities that produce fore-pleasure – go hand in hand with the increase of excitation and imply the introduction of new "vital differences" (Freud 1920g: 55).[48] For this reason, the question as to why the death drives aim at the reduction or removal of tension is no longer answered by reference to external forces pressuring to modifications and adaptations, but by a reference to an internal source of tension and excitation – the life drives.

From this we can conclude the following. Whereas Freud's "economic" reasoning on the characteristics of the drives in the 1919 version of *Beyond the Pleasure Principle* ultimately implied that there was no "beyond" of the pleasure principle, there is a "beyond" in the 1920 edition. It is Eros, the life drives – the "breakers of the peace" that are "constantly producing tensions" (Freud 1920g: 63). Eros is a "troublemaker" and "the force that introduces disturbances into the process of life" (Freud 1923b: 46–47). The life drives produce tension and excitation without concern about whether this generates pleasure or unpleasure, and hence without concern for the well-being of the parties involved in the process of binding. By virtue of continuously pushing the living substance forward towards new unities and forms, these drives can be said to maintain a Mephistophelean character. In this way, Freud reinstalls what he had been arguing in previous texts: in order to understand ontogeny and psychic life, one needs to distinguish between dynamic factors (the interaction between forces producing movement in certain directions) and economic factors (the management of these quantities towards stability) (see Freud 1916–1917a: 374–375).

In *Beyond the Pleasure Principle*, and in later texts, the life drives are first and foremost presented as drives that bind components into unities. They are not aimless constant forces that keep pressuring everything they encounter. Their aim is not to merely continue and repeat their movement and direction, but to form unities and to prolong life by taking a variety of detours (Freud 1920g: 56). In the following years, Freud will confirm and develop this idea. The aim of the life drives, he writes in an encyclopaedia article from 1923, is "to form living substance into ever greater unities, so that life may be prolonged and brought to higher development [*Höherentwicklung*]" (Freud 1923a: 258). He inserts a similar formulation in the 1923 edition of *Beyond the Pleasure Principle*; two years later, he adds that the life drives are an internal impulse towards "progress" (*eine innere Tendenz zum 'Fortschritt'*) (Freud 1920g: 40 n.). Here Freud presents the life drives as the true modifying forces in phylogeny and ontogeny.[49] In the 1923 edition of the text, he also adds a passage at the end of Chapter 5, arguing that Eros provides a "substitute" for the drive towards perfection that he had previously so vehemently rejected and still rejects (Freud 1920g: 43). Although Freud maintains rejecting any notion of progress in terms of a tendency towards perfection, the life drives are increasingly regarded as the motive forces of change and of the development of living beings into more complicated forms. This means that the theory of the life drives is at odds with the arguments in Chapter 5 on progress and change being the effects of external modifying forces only (see Bernet 2020: 205).

In Chapter 5 of the 1925 edition of *Beyond the Pleasure Principle*, Freud adds a footnote to his thoughts on the conservative character of all drives, stating that "the reader should not overlook the fact that what follows is the development of an extreme line of thought" that will be corrected in the course of the text (Freud 1920g: 37 n.). This is significant: Freud self-critically observes that the assumed restorative and repetitive tendencies in the life drives no longer rest upon material from clinical practice presented earlier, that is, on the compulsion to repeat in transference and traumatic neuroses. He concludes that he may have "over-estimated" the significance of the compulsion to repeat (Freud 1920g: 59). But what Freud affirms in the 1925 footnote above all is this: if the life drives are the motive forces that "push forward towards progress and the production of new forms" (Freud 1920g: 37), it is impossible to maintain that all drives are conservative and restorative.

Aggression, sadism and destruction

In Chapter 6 of *Beyond the Pleasure Principle*, Freud writes that the various speculations "demand that we should produce an example of a death instinct" (Freud 1920g: 54). The example he adduces is one that had not been mentioned in the first version of the text at all: aggression. His starting point is the idea that the "polarity" of love (affection) and hate (aggression) is "similar" to the polarity between life drives and death drives (Freud 1920g: 53). This similarity prompts him to find out whether the polarity of love and hate can be traced back to these drives. To give this inquiry some plausibility, he assumes that not all aggression is functional. Not all aggression is a response to actual life-threatening circumstances or actual provocations; nor is it a matter of the ambitious pursuit of goals involving some sort of struggle against obstacles. Aggression, in short, cannot be reduced to an indispensable capacity in the service of self-preservation, pursuit of power, growth and advancement. This does not mean that hatred cannot be motivated by self-preservative drives. In "Instincts and Their Vicissitudes", Freud had argued that the relation of the ego to the external world is always already from the onset a relation of hatred – indifference only being "a special case of hate or dislike" (Freud 1915c: 136). After all, the external world is always and in principle a source of stimuli that threaten the individual's life and prevent the satisfaction of needs.

In *Beyond the Pleasure Principle*, Freud turns his attention to sadism and masochism as clinical phenomena that can shed light on the polarity of the life drives and death drives. The argument is this: an urge to injure an object cannot be an expression of the life drives and must therefore be the manifestation of other drives. This implies that Freud first of all needs to make plausible that love and hate are related to sadism and masochism. He does not present any new argument for this; instead, he uses the opportunity to reconsider his previous views on this matter. With regard to the question of the relation between sadism and hate, Freud had maintained, from the *Three Essays* onwards, that the various forms of aggression (including anger, hostility, etc.) should all be traced back to a sadistic component of the sexual drives (Freud 1905d: 158–159; 1909d: 240).[50] In "Instincts and Their Vicissitudes", he had argued that sadism must be defined in terms of "the exercise of violence and power upon some other person as object" and "the infliction of pain" (Freud 1915c: 127, 128). This new formulation seems to suggest that sadism is not the expression of the sexual drives, and in fact may not be sexual in character. This is confirmed by Freud's observation that it is only in masochism – as transformed sadism – that the infliction of pain (self-injury) "trench[es] upon sexual excitation and produce[s] a pleasurable condition" (Freud 1915c: 128). In other words, here the question arises (again) whether and how sadism and masochism are related to the sexual drives, or whether sadism is the result of an as-yet-unknown factor that cannot evidently be traced back to self-preservative drives.

But there are additional reasons why Freud considers sadism a better "example" of the death drives than hatred. In "Instincts and Their Vicissitudes", Freud had argued that hate can be understood as originating from a "primal psychical situation" of narcissism in which the ego is cathected with drive energy and preoccupied with autoerotic pleasure, while the external world is not cathected with any interest. In this situation, the world is not yet perceived as a relevant source of pleasure or unpleasure, nor is it even perceived as external, that is, as something different from the ego (Freud 1915c: 134–135). This changes when under the dominance of the pleasure principle a further development takes place: the ego finds itself capable of experiencing mastery over external stimuli in such a way that this is felt as pleasure. It will therefore no longer treat its outside with disinterest. It will seek to "introject" objects from the external world that are sources of pleasure, and vice versa, it will try to expel – "project" – whatever causes internal unpleasure into the external world. The part of oneself which was felt as source of unpleasure, and which has been projected into the external world, is then perceived as a hostile object and thus will be hated. It is only through projection and with the appearance objects that hate becomes the first form of investment in objects (Freud 1915c: 135–136; De Vleminck 2013: 92ff).

This suggests that it is far from self-evident that hatred stems from the death drives. Whether one regards hate as originating in narcissistic self-love or as self-preservative reaction against external objects in a hostile environment, hate would have to be seen as an expression of the life drives seeking to prolong the unity of the ego. In terms of the life drives, hate can in fact be regarded either as operating in the service of (preparing for) processes of binding to external objects, or as being itself a form of persisting and enduring form of binding to objects. After all, what characterizes hate is not the insistence on the (immediate) destruction of the object, but the continuous investment in an object in order to efficiently project internal tension and unpleasure onto it. This would also be in line with Freud's argument in *Group Psychology*: aggression to outsiders is instrumental for the cohesion of the group.

Sadism therefore seems to be a more promising clinical example of the death drives. Freud asks, "how can the sadistic instinct [*sadistischer Trieb*], whose aim it is to injure the object, be derived from Eros?" (Freud 1920g: 54). How could (a component of) the life drives produce an object's annihilation (*Vernichtung*) when these drives are said to aim at binding and forming larger unities? Sadism involves destruction that cannot be traced back to Eros, that is, it cannot be related to binding, and therefore must stem from drives resulting in decomposition:[51]

> Is it not plausible to suppose that this sadism is in fact a death instinct which, under the influence of the narcissistic libido, has been forced away from the ego [*vom Ich abgedrängt wurde*] and has consequently only emerged in relation to the object [*erst am Object zum Vorschein kommt*]?
> (Freud 1920g: 54)

After the ego has been established as union of parts established through binding, the life drives seek to maintain, prolong and expand this union. This inevitably creates new tensions and excitations. The death drives that seek the reduction of tension, for their part, threaten to dissolve any union of parts. The "narcissistic libido" (as more concrete manifestation of the life drives) reacts in defence of the unity of the ego; it will "force away" the death drives from the ego towards substitute objects which are subsequently cast as potential threats to the ego. In this way, the death drives can no longer harm the unity of the ego. This "forcing away" of the death drives implies that these drives which are originally indifferent to external objects now lead to a first interest in such objects – i.e., as objects of aggression.[52] This will prepare the ground for other "interests" in objects – more precisely, for the transformation of narcissistic libido into object-libido. (The "forcing away" of the death drives is thus the condition for the Oedipus complex.)

This implies that every libidinal investment in objects will inevitably and from the outset be contaminated by the death drives. Freud refers to this contamination as "mitigation" (*Ermäßigung*) and – in chemical terms – "intermixture" (*Verschmelzung*) (Freud 1920g: 54). According to Freud, the polarity of love and hate, which usually takes the form of "ambivalence" of feelings in relation to specific objects, results from this intermixture of life and death drives in the investment in objects.[53] Aggression and destruction are always involved in processes of binding to objects. Freud thus presents a tragic view of object relations which are inevitably characterized by ambivalence. There is no love relation without hate intermingling with it in the process of binding. This means that love and hate are not opposites; they are related to each other in the form of a "polarity" present in all object-relations.

Freud goes a step further. There is no binding without unbinding. There is no love-hate relation, no investment and interest in objects, without the tendency towards undoing of that relation. Such unbinding usually consists of withdrawal of libidinal investment in objects so as to reduce tension. The death drives thus never show themselves in a pure unmediated form. The death drives become manifest in a variety of object-related phenomena that result from attempts to defend the ego from the death drives.

This train of thought leads Freud to reconsider his former views of sadism and masochism and to show that if the ego was forced to expel the death drives, masochism need no longer be seen as sadism turned against oneself, but may in fact be primary (rather than secondary).[54] For this reason Freud focuses on the "turning from an object to the ego" (Freud 1920g: 54).[55] In such cases, the ego becomes the object of cruelty and destructiveness.[56] Since this "turning" is a regressive movement, Freud concludes that "there might be such a thing as primary masochism" (1920g: 55). This idea cannot be inferred from the simple fact that libidinal investments can be withdrawn. One must assume, Freud avers, that the narcissistic libido is not capable of leading all of the death drives away from the ego to external objects. Some of the death drives remain, threatening to dissolve the unity of the ego and to restore a previous situation of less internal complexity, instability and vital differences.

Must this "previous situation" necessarily be associated with the reduction of tension? Laplanche has argued in his critique of the concept of the death drives that the more productive insight one can take from *Beyond the Pleasure Principle* concerns the distinction between binding and unbinding tendencies. The life drives, he writes, are aimed at integration and synthesis through narcissism and object relations; unbinding does not point towards the existence of a (speculative or biologistic notion of) death drive, but to "another kind of sexuality", namely the anarchic, untamed, autoerotic polymorphous-perverse infantile sexuality that threatens the unity of the ego and stability of object relations. Binding and unbinding then are a new way to formulate a conflict within sexuality that Freud already elaborated in the 1905 *Three Essays* with the introduction of two regimes of sexuality, of which the first one is repressed by the second (Laplanche 1985: 123; 1999: 197–199; 2015a). Laplanche can thus argue that the life drives and death drives are both "sexual". The question should be raised here whether this interpretation of the new drive theory in terms of two conflicting regimes of sexuality finds support in Freud's *Three Essays*. What Laplanche loses from sight is that, first, infantile sexuality is merely (the repetition of) pleasurable excitation derived from autoerotic sensations, and, second, adult sexuality is largely characterized by continuation of pleasurable sensations and polymorphous-perverse elements in and through object relations. The two regimes of sexuality are thus not opposed regimes. Also, infantile sexuality, according to Freud, is relatively unproblematic as it does not include negativity, that is, it is not aimed at any form of annihilation, elimination or destruction.

Freud's tentative views of masochism and sadism in *Beyond the Pleasure Principle* will be further elaborated in "The Economic Problem of Masochism" (1924). In that text, various forms of masochism will be traced back to the death drive (here in the singular) that seeks "to disintegrate the cellular organism and to conduct each separate unicellular organism into a state of inorganic stability" (Freud 1924c: 163). It is only after the libido has been able to divert the death drive towards external objects, that this drive can be properly named "destructive instinct, the instinct for mastery, or the will to power".[57] The portion of the death drive that does not share in this transposition outwards will retain "the self as its object". What needs to be explained, Freud argues, is the pleasure in pain that defines masochism (Freud 1924c: 159, 161). To answer this question, Freud turns his attention to the most elementary form of masochism, erotogenic (primary) masochism. The portion of the death drive that is not directed towards external objects "becomes libidinally bound" (Freud 1924c: 164; also De Vleminck 2013: 167–171). As to why, how and to what extent such binding of the death drive takes place, Freud gives no clear answer. The main argument appears to be that the life drives pushing life forward prefer the sensation of pain over the radical aim of the death drive, namely the annihilation of any excitation. In their effort to maintain and prolong life at all costs, the life drives seek the "taming" (*Bändigung*) of the death drive by integrating it in all libidinal self-preservative and object-related processes. With the concept of the life drives, Freud takes up elements of his earlier views of the drive as "the driving factor which will permit no halting at any position attained" (Freud 1920g: 42). Drives push life forward in an "unrestrained" (*ungebändigt*) manner, without concern for whether the accompanying internal tension and excitation is pleasurable or not. They restrain ("tame") the death drives by integrating them in their own unrestrained movement.[58]

The life drives are "beyond" the pleasure principle. It is these drives that produce tension and excitation. And it is through their taming of the death drive that pleasure can be experienced as pain. This is what gives the death drives the appearance of a self-destructive force.[59] On the question as to whether the death drive can be seen as essentially self-destructive, Freud will answer in the negative. Self-destruction is either the effect of the taming of the death drive by the life drives, or of the introjection of the destructiveness towards external objects, turning the ego into an object of aggression. The former shows itself in primary erotogenic masochism. The latter is evidenced in moral masochism (need for punishment) and melancholia (self-reproaches) (Freud 1924c: 164).

Freud will also explore these self-destructive manifestations of the death drives in *The Ego and the Id*. Here Freud turns his attention to melancholia in which he recognizes the effects of the defusion (*Entmischung*) of drives that had previously been fused.[60] The study of melancholia shows that the "destructive component" of sadism has "entrenched itself [*sich abgelagert*] in the super-ego and turned against the ego" (Freud 1923b: 53). In melancholia, the super-ego "rages" with merciless violence against the ego, making use of the available amounts of "displaceable energy". Melancholia results from two displacements. First, there is the displacement from sadistic tendencies against an external object towards aggression against the ego (through identification with an object that is lost but cannot be given up). And, second, there is the entrenchment of energy in the super-ego which results from the extraction of energy cathected to other invested objects, including the ego. As a result, the psychic organization disintegrates into opposing parts, with one part raging against another.[61]

Considering the examples of primary erotogenic masochism and melancholia, we can understand why Freud defines the death drive in terms of "destructive drive" (*Destruktionstrieb*) from *The Ego and the Id* onwards (Freud 1923b: 41, 1940a: 148). In his study on Freudian thought, Paul Ricoeur registers two shifts in Freud's *Beyond* essay: "one notices a twofold shift of emphasis: first, from the tendency to *repeat* to the tendency to *destroy*; next, from more *biological* to more *cultural* expressions" (Ricoeur 1970: 294; original italics). Although it is not evident that the cultural expressions of destructive tendencies dominate the last part of *Beyond the Pleasure Principle*, what can be said is that the paragraphs on aggression and sadism pave the way for Freud's later articulations of the death drive in terms of a *Destruktionstrieb* and its cultural manifestations. Considering studies such as *Civilization and Its Discontents* and *Why War?*, one can argue for a definition of the death drive in terms of the violent dissolution of social bonds (compare Butler 2020: 152). This, however, is not what is at issue in *Beyond the Pleasure Principle*.

The later conceptualization of the death drive in terms of a destructive drive has an important advantage for Freud: it underscores a dualistic conception of the drives in which the drives are opposing forces in conflict with each other. However, in an attempt to be less speculative – less metaphysical – Freud opts for a definition of the death drive for which there are more plausible clinical examples (notably melancholia) and cultural expressions (notably violence).[62]

The drive theory contested

When Freud introduces the notion of primary masochism in *Beyond the Pleasure Principle*, he adds a footnote in which he credits Sabina Spielrein and August Stärcke in particular with having anticipated the idea of sadistic components of the libido as self-destructive impetus towards death (Freud 1920g: 55 n.). This reference is rather ambiguous, since the new drive theory which Freud introduces in this text cannot simply be seen as an extension of Spielrein's and Stärcke's ideas. We have already briefly referred to Spielrein's book entitled *Destruktion als Ursache des Werdens* (1912), in which she raised the question of how to understand the aspects of sexual life (such as disgust), which obstruct the final aim of the sexual drive – reproduction. In search for an answer, she turned to Jung's genetic theory of the libido and his suggestion that the primal libido can be both creative and destructive. According to Spielrein, inherent in the sexual drive, there is a destructive component that disregards the aim of the self-preservative drives to safeguard and continue the life of the individual. This destructive factor becomes manifest in every object-love and eventually in the sexual act in which two germ cells merge. Such assimilation of individual cells implies the discontinuation of the individual cells as distinct units (Spielrein 1912).

In a short text from 1914, Stärcke had voiced ideas quite similar to those of Spielrein. According to Stärcke, there is an ego-drive that seeks to accumulate energy for self-aggrandisement and prolongation of life, and there is "libido" that seeks to sublate individuality, displace energy towards objects, and strives for immortality through reproduction and the death of the individual (Stärcke 1914). He repeats this position in several letters to Freud written from September 1922 onwards (May 2017). Stärcke argues that since the libido is a "centrifugal" force aiming at assimilation (coalescence), it is inherently self-destructive and self-sublative. The libido ultimately is death drive ("*Libido = Todestrieb*"), in opposition to which the self-preservative drives (ego-drives) seek to maintain and isolate the ego. In response, Freud berates Stärcke for coming close to the "Jungian heresy" (May 2017: 100).

The correspondence with Stärcke shows that Freud considered a Spielreinian interpretation of the life drives as problematic.[63] Whereas, as we have seen, Freud's remarks on the sexual drives and the coalescence of cells in Chapter 5 can be read as echoing Spielrein's views on the annihilation of the germ cells as the condition for the development of a new individual, in Chapter 6 the life drives primarily aim at binding parts in ever greater unities, thus prolonging the life of living substances. It is no coincidence that the most significant additions to the text editions of 1923 and 1925 are meant to prevent further misunderstandings on this point. In a footnote added in 1925, Freud writes that the reference to "ego-drives" must be understood as a provisional description deriving from his earlier drive theory (Freud 1920g: 41 n.). This clearly indicates that one can no longer uncritically refer to or defend the notion of ego-drives versus libido, as

Stärcke does. Also, Freud further highlights the creative character of the life drives (Freud 1920g: 42–43). More importantly, he maintains that his new drive theory is a dualistic theory in which the drives are forces working in "opposition" to each other:

> Our views have from the very first been *dualistic* and today they are even more definitely dualistic than before – now that we describe the opposition as being, not between ego-drives and sexual drives but between life drives and death drives.
>
> (Freud 1920g: 53)[64]

The question can be raised as to whether this drive dualism of opposing forces, and parallel to that, the tendency to associate the death drives with aggression (destruction) and the life drives with sexuality, are the best answer that Freud could have offered in response to the readings of others, and against the alleged threat of Jungian monism (see Bernet 2020: 222).[65] One could in fact argue that Freud in his response to his trains of thought on the conservative character of all drives, in the 1920 version of the text does not put forward a new "sharp distinction" between opposing drive forces (Freud 1920g: 44), but instead introduces a new drive theory based on a notion of drive energy (as "displaceable energy"), "ambivalence" and "polarity". In this new drive theory, the death drives are conceived as "unobtrusive" and "associated from the very first with the life drives". They manifest when mitigated by and intermixed with the life drives (Freud 1920g: 57). Thus, the new drive theory does not so much describe opposing forces, but the interaction of two different aims at different levels – the energetic binding of components into unities and the reduction of tension. In short, there is good reason to critically question Freud's added references to monism and dualism, and to conceive of the relation and interaction between the drives in different terms.[66]

The discussions following the publication of *Beyond the Pleasure Principle* concern not only the libido and the drive theory. Another controversial topic is that of trauma. In previous chapters, we have seen that Ferenczi was Freud's closest companion in working on the bioanalytical project. Notably the first version of *Beyond the Pleasure Principle* can be read as Freud's contribution to this project. However, in the 1920 additions, Freud nuances the significance of the compulsion to repeat. Moreover, he abstains from any further discussions of trauma and traumatic neuroses, and from further references to Lamarckism. What is significant in this context is the fact that Freud does not associate somatic and psychic fragmentation with trauma. The introduction of Eros and sexuality in the second version of *Beyond the Pleasure Principle* goes hand in hand with the disappearance – once again – of traumatic neurosis.

Although Ferenczi will follow Freud in regarding the life and death drives as the pulsional motivational forces in organic life (Ferenczi 1929: 251), he is among the first to recognize that the new drive theory no longer depends on a theory of trauma and on a clinical engagement with traumatic neuroses. Trauma seems no longer fundamental for understanding phylogeny and ontogeny. In *Thalassa*, however, Ferenczi strongly emphasizes the significance of trauma in evolution. From this point onwards, he will continue to further develop his own trauma theory. In several publications from the late 1920s and early 1930s, he will argue for a general theory of trauma in which psychic fragmentation results from the child's inevitable confrontation with the enigmatic character of adult sexuality (Ferenczi 1929; 1933).[67] This leads to a "slight modification" of the theory of life and death drives (Ferenczi 1995: 41). According to Ferenczi, the death drives do not react against the life drives, nor are they opposed to the life drives. Both drives are the spontaneous response to fragmentation and atomization of psychic life, which result from trauma. The life drives seek to establish protective psychosomatic cooperations in the interactions with external objects and conciliations between fragmented parts. The death drive's response consists of an urge to restore an earlier, pre-traumatic state which Ferenczi associates with relaxation, absence of irritability (homeostasis), and the return to the moist environment of the mother's womb. From this perspective, he can insist on the importance of restorative repetitions. If the death drives are reparative responses to traumatic fragmentation, as Ferenczi argues, these drives must be seen as self-preservative, aiming at mastery.[68] It is from fragmentation and disintegration of the "former self" that the death drives seek the "neoformation of the self" (Ferenczi 1995: 181).[69] The death drives become manifest in the egoistic and parasitical tendencies of organs and body parts which – like embryos in the mother's womb – seek to prevail at all costs and as such become the "foundation stones for a further development" (Ferenczi 1924: 90).

Although Ferenczi could find support for his ideas in various trains of thought in *Beyond the Pleasure Principle*, Freud could not accept his insistence on the importance of trauma and the attempts at mastery for the conceptualization of the drives. It was not the mere fact that Ferenczi returned to the seduction theory and its premise of accurate accounts (as opposed to mere phantasies) of childhood traumata that Freud found difficult to accept.[70] Ferenczi's conceptualizations in this regard implied a return to a theory in which extraordinary traumatic events would be decisive in phylogeny and the aetiology of neuroses. Ferenczi's rethinking of the life drives and death drives takes trauma as starting point: the drives are reactive and reparative forces. For Freud, however, the drives are forces that do not originate in response to repeated and new traumatic fragmentations, but, on the contrary, can be seen as motive forces in processes of fragmentation and self-destruction without the interference of external stimuli.

Having said this, Ferenczi's interpretation of *Beyond the Pleasure Principle* does raise the question whether the death drives can be conceptualized in terms different from destruction or aggression. This question has more recently been raised again by Catharine Malabou. She argues that when Freud associated the death drives with elasticity and entropy, he overlooked the plasticity inherent in processes of decomposition fomented by the death drives (Malabou 2012: 177–178; 2022: 281). As an example, she mentions war traumata resulting in psychic change and transformation of identity (Malabou 2012: 15, 179). The death drives are here seen as a kind of psychic compliance with destructive impacts (see Malabou 2012: 70, 166). These drives are understood to mark the endogenous process towards "death in life". They are characterized by the tendency to return to earlier states of mental functioning, the capacity of letting oneself perish or of being indifferent towards the outside world, and of creating protective shields against suffering. These characteristics point towards a certain plasticity of the death drives, a capacity to neo-formations.

Indeed, Freud, in associating the death drives with unbinding, fragmentation and aggression, seems not to be able to conceive of the death drives as forces producing new forms and figures. And yet, as we will further discuss below, there is a train of thought in *Beyond the Pleasure Principle* that leads in another direction: in their attempts to "neutralize" the life drives, the death drives can be said to produce fixity and stability of forms. This would not be a destructive plasticity, but could be named "adhesive" plasticity.

The libido of cells and organs

In Chapter 2, we have seen that the traumatic-neurotic compulsion to repeat leads Freud to speculate "beyond" sexual trauma on the devastating effects of war trauma. Thinking beyond the pleasure principle implies thinking beyond the sexual. The traumatic neuroses confront Freud with the limits of his theories to the extent that these are anchored in clinical observations of neurotic conflicts. The 1920 third step in the drive theory can be seen as redefining these limits through "enlarging" and "stretching" the concept of sexuality, and "extending" the concepts of libido and life drives to individual cells (Freud 1905d: 134; 1920g: 60 n.). More specifically, this "extension" implies that the sexual drive manifesting itself in adult sexuality becomes a historically acquired form of the life drives aiming "by every possible means" at binding.

This step entails a fundamental reconsideration of the original drive dualism which Freud had introduced in *Three Essays*. It is for this reason that Freud makes no attempt to integrate his new drive theory into the later editions of *Three Essays* (Van Haute & Westerink 2021). There is no place for an enlarged concept of libido within the framework of the existing theory of sexuality. The life drives are "beyond" human sexuality. There are manifestations of the life drives earlier and other than the sexual reproduction one finds in humans. And yet, the relation between the new drive theory and theory of sexuality in *Three Essays* is more complicated than this. At first sight, it may appear that Freud brings to the fore a heteronormative perspective on sexuality in the 1920 edition of *Beyond the Pleasure Principle*, particularly when it comes to his ideas on reproduction through the coalescence of germ cells. But, in actual fact, the concept of the life drives prompts Freud to rethink the continuity between autoeroticism, narcissism and object choice.

Although the new drive theory is not integrated in the 1920 and 1924 editions of *Three Essays*, the concept of the life drives can be said to shed light on problems in the theory of sexuality that Freud found difficult to resolve. This mainly concerns the transformation of autoeroticism into functional adult sexuality (Davidson 2001: 66–92; Van Haute & Westerink 2021). How to consider the transition from non-objectal autoerotic pleasurable activities such as sensual sucking to the primacy of the genitals, and the subjection of fore-pleasure to the ultimate aim of end-pleasure? Are the object and the functional organization of sexuality introduced from the outside, that is, through adults (parents) and cultural norms? Does the introduction of the object depend on specific attractive or enigmatic qualities of the object? This is not what comes into consideration for Freud in *Three Essays*. Through the introduction of a developmental approach and the concept of narcissism (in the 1915 edition), he can reason that the transformation of infantile into adult sexuality depends solely on psychic aspects of sexual life and physiological processes such as the maturation of the sexual organs and the production of chemical substances. In *Beyond the Pleasure Principle*, Freud radicalizes this train of thought on the inner motive forces and processes that generate transformations in the various regimes of sexuality. The life drives – and hence the sexual drives – aim at binding with objects from the outset. Hence, all possible varieties of sexuality can be considered objectal. More specifically, particles seek assimilation with particles, cells with cells, organs with organs, bodies with bodies. What Freud had called non-objectal autoerotic sexuality now appears to be inherently objectal. Is this not a contradiction? It would be if "object" was to be taken to mean "person" – as Freud had specified in *Three Essays* (Freud 1905d: 135–136). The application of the libido theory in *Beyond the Pleasure Principle*, however, implies that cells and organs can also be objects.[71]

In the years preceding the writing of the sixth chapter we can already find statements that pave the way for a perspective on autoeroticism as inherently objectal. In a letter to Oskar Pfister, dated the 9th of October 1918, Freud writes:

> Do you not see that the multiplicity of these components [*Triebe*] derives from the multiplicity of the organs, all of which are erotogenic, i.e., fundamentally all aspire to reproduce themselves in the future organism? And has the fact that all the organs combine to form a living unit [*lebende Einheit*], all influencing [*beeinflussen*], aiding [*unterstützen*] or checking [*hemmen*] one another and remaining dependent [*abhängig bleiben*] on one another even in the process of their development, prevented the anatomists from studying and describing them separately?
>
> (Freud & Pfister 1963: 62)

Thus, even in 1918, Freud was conceptualizing the drives as a multiplicity of (partial) forces active in each cell, each organ and body part, forging organic components together into a unity.[72] This may be taken to suggest that cells and organs can behave narcissistically in directing all libidinal investment towards themselves, in order to prolong and reproduce their lives. For example, germ cells but also cancer cells ("malignant neoplasms")[73] can behave narcissistically and independently of other cells in their search for the prolongation and reproduction of their own lives at all costs. They do not consider the well-being of other cells (Freud 1920g: 50). Having said this, Freud also suggests that the life drives never stop insisting on further formation and prolongation of unities:

> We might suppose that the life instincts or sexual instincts which are active in each cell take the other cells as their object, that they partly neutralize the death instincts (that is, the processes set up by them) in those cells and thus preserve their life [*am Leben erhalten*]; while the other cells do the same for *them*, and still others sacrifice [*aufopfern*] themselves in the performance of this libidinal function.
>
> (Freud 1920g: 50; Freud's italics)[74]

Cells interact and communicate, can level out and inhibit each other's drive impulses, keep each other alive, prolong each other's lives, and even sacrifice themselves for other cells.[75] Cells can attract other cells, or be attracted to other cells; they can behave passively or actively. In Darwinian terms, one could perhaps say that the application of the libido theory to the relations between cells implies rethinking sexual selection as an internal organizing principle enhancing individual differences.[76]

According to Freud, the libido theory can similarly be applied to organs and body parts. The quote from the 1918 letter to Pfister already points in this direction. Here Freud associates the erotogenic character of all – and not merely some – organs with partial drives seeking the "reproduction" of the organ through the cooperation with other organs in one living unit capable of reproduction in conjunction with another unit (of another sex). Freud further seems to suggest that the organs assembled in this unit will influence, aid and inhibit each other while at the same time remaining an identifiable unit, such as the lungs, the stomach, the bowels or the skin. This seems to imply that organs, too, can behave narcissistically, withdrawing their libidinal investment in other organs and body parts, and redirecting (withdrawing) the libido towards themselves.

This would be in line some of the arguments in *Three Essays*. In infantile sexuality, the sexual activities are "derived from a number of separate instincts and erotogenic zones which, independently of one another, have pursued a certain sort of pleasure as their sole sexual aim" (Freud 1905d: 207). From "Instincts and Their Vicissitudes" in 1925 onwards, Freud adduces the term "organ pleasure" to designate the pleasure that organs experience at their own irritability and excitability through rhythmically repeated stimuli (*Organlust*)

(Freud 1915c: 125–126; 1916–1917a: 323). The main examples are those he had previously explored in *Three Essays*: sensual sucking, holding back the excreta, and infantile masturbation. Each one of the sexual partial drives emanating from a variety of organic sources strives "independently of one another" for the attainment of organ pleasure. And only when the synthesis of these sources, drives and organs is achieved do these drives "enter the service of the reproductive function and thereupon become generally recognizable as sexual instincts" (Freud 1915c: 125–126). Without the various organs striving for pleasure, there can be no synthesis in the service of reproduction. In other words, there can be no release of tension in end-pleasure without a prior accumulation of excitation in fore-pleasure. This idea is taken up again in the 1920 version of *Beyond the Pleasure Principle.* The body with its reproductive organs is not presumed to be given as a unity at the outset; rather, it is a composition of heterogeneous interacting components – the multiplicity of erotogenic organs made up of cells and cell states. All these organs are susceptible to stimulation from within and from without and can thus sense pleasure and unpleasure from their own internal processes or from external sources in other organs and body parts.

The application of the libido theory to the mutual relationship of cells and *mutatis mutandis*, of organs, does not tend towards a new drive dualism of two opposing forces, but towards a pluralistic conception of the drives. We could say that in 1920 edition of *Beyond the Pleasure Principle*, Freud deploys the libido theory in such a way that it allows for further reflection on the partial drives and the polymorphous-perverse character of all organs and tissues. Just as organs and tissues can be thought of as a composite network of interacting cells and cell states, so too can the entire body be thought of as a composition of interacting parts – bones, muscles, organs and tissues. These interactions are further defined and differentiated by a number of factors Freud mentions in the text. There is, first, the ratio of life drives to death drives depending on the amount of "unbound" energy and the appropriation of that energy by this or that drive for displacement and condensation. Second, there is the factor of the degree of mutual fusion, neutralization and uncoupling of the drives. What comes into consideration, third, is the nature of the object of libidinal investment (the "ego" or an external object). And, finally, what has to be taken account of is the change in magnitude of the excitation generated in the interaction between components within a given time as a determinant of whether this excitation is perceived as pleasurable or unpleasurable. These factors form a matrix to think of the (human but also animal) constitution as a differentiated and fundamentally unstable entity. This instability explains various pathological or perverse phenomena – at least partly. But, if we follow Freud, we should not infer that this instability ideally gives way to the kind of stability sought by the pleasure principle. Rather, Freud's references to Fechner's constancy principle and the "tendency towards stability" seem to suggest that differentiated interactions between drives are characteristic of the complexity of being human. This is particularly evident in Freud's observation that sadistic aspects are also present in sexual development and in "normal" sexual life. This is in line with earlier suggestions in *Three Essays* in which he argues that the normal *vita sexualis* is not conceivable without perverse components (such as kissing, watching, grasping): "No healthy person, it appears, can fail to make some addition that might be called perverse to the normal sexual aim" (Freud 1905d: 160).[77] "Normal" in the constitution of complex organisms are the variations in the integrative interplay between life drives and death drives.[78] It is precisely the – purely theoretical – possibility of a distinction into pure drives that would destroy any organism. The organism would be either threatened in its existence because of the unlimited polymorphic plasticity of the life drives or because of the solidifying effects of the death drives.[79]

We can now also understand why Freud uses the plural – life drives and death drives – in *Beyond the Pleasure Principle*. This can be seen to correspond to the use of the plural in the theory of self-preservative (ego-) drives and sexual drives. Notably in *Three Essays* Freud had used the plural in his analyses of the partial drives and polymorphous character of sexuality. But this is not the only reason. The application of the libido theory to the mutual relationship of cells implies that life drives and death drives are operative in each cell. In each cell there are intermixtures, and unequal proportions and strength of the drives (see Freud 1923b: 41). The same goes for cell states, organs, tissues and body parts, and their interaction with other cell states, organs, etc. The references to Eros and the death drive in the singular in later writings including *The Ego and the Id* or *Civilization and Its Discontents* indicate a shift of attention from the interactions between cells, organs and tissues towards the opposition of drives as forces associated with internal conflicts between ego and super-ego, and in relation to external (or internalized) objects.

Creative forces

In a short article published in 1922, Ferenczi remarks that Freud's conceptualization of the life drives comes close to Bergson's *Évolution créatrice* and its central concept of *élan de la vie.* Both concepts suggest that all development and change is largely endogenously produced and immanent to all organic life. But Ferenczi realizes that Freud does not become a representative of a contemporary "mystical" vitalism. What sets him apart from this school of thought is the fact that he argues for an exogenous, and hence natural and reactive origin of the drives – trauma, to be precise. Freud denies the drives any spiritual essence or unity that precedes material formations (Ferenczi 1922: 120–121). This reference to Bergson may seem surprising when we consider what we have argued in previous chapters in particular: Freud aligns himself with biological theories that take their starting point in mechanistic – and hence non-vitalist – principles. What then could be the arguments for the suggestion that Freud's notion of the life drives resembles Bergson's concept of *élan de la vie* (*élan vital*)?[80]

We have already discussed Freud's rejection of a formative drive towards growth and perfection, stated in the 1919 version of *Beyond the Pleasure Principle*. This rejection implies the dismissal of any reference to an organicist conception in the tradition of Kant's formative drive as a purposive impetus or supra-organismic force directing life and organisms towards a predisposed set of ends.[81] The same goes for the vitalist theories of Hans Driesch – a student of Haeckel and Roux, and the most important representative of vitalism in German biology at the time. Notably from his research on urchin embryos Driesch concluded that the mechanistic theories of his time could not account for the specific formation of organic forms and for individual variations and characteristics. He therefore assumed a formative immaterial and non-mechanical (non-physical-chemical) principle which he named *Entelechie* (Driesch 1905: 208–209; also Bennett 2010: 69–76). According to Driesch, the potentialities of living beings were directed and organized by an innate self-directing force that operated as an agent deciding and arranging which possibilities inherent in cells and organs would be actualized.[82] This "autonomous" organizing force or "judging principle" did not aim at the realization of the perfect individual form from a plurality of potentials, but at maintaining and regulating the unity and harmony of organic development by continuously checking the expediency of actualizations and their implications (Driesch 1905: 4, 174ff).[83] Freud remains aloof from any references to organizing principles making for a putative purposiveness and harmony of organic life forms. And he is certainly not the only one. In a context of a variety of theoretical positions seeking to complement mechanistic approaches with psychological principles, Pauly and Wagner, among numerous other biological theorists, criticized Driesch for introducing the (Aristotelean and Leibnizian) concept of *Entelechie* (Pauly 1905: 181ff; Wagner 1909: 182–183).

And yet, we have seen that the introduction of the concept of the life drives necessarily implies a revision of ideas developed in the 1919 version of *Beyond the Pleasure Principle*. These revisions eventually lead Freud to admit that "the efforts of Eros to combine organic substances in ever larger unities" may be seen as a "substitute" for the "drive towards perfection" (Freud 1920g: 43). The fact that Freud does not admit of such a drive indicates that he does not want to associate the productivity of the life drives with finality and (pre-given) harmony. Instead, he highlights the binding of parts in larger unities as the aim of the life drives, while maintaining the idea that these drives are "the driving factor which will permit no halting at any position attained". In other words, there are drives that constantly "impel towards change and development". In Chapter 6, Freud affirms that the "phenomena of repetition" in embryonic developmental processes are "no doubt extremely rich" (Freud 1920g: 56); yet the concept of the life drives implicitly undermines the status of Haeckel's recapitulation theory (and Weismann's theory of the repetition of the properties of germ cells). This is for two reasons. First, in Haeckel's view, progress is always based on the repetition of previous forms. Freud, however, does not assume that the creation of new forms necessarily implies or includes the repetition of previous formations. Second, to explain the emergence of new variations and forms, the recapitulation theory referred to the acquisition of characteristics in processes of adaptation to challenging circumstances. In Chapter 6, Freud does not deny the significance of external influences "especially in the plant world", where sunlight, temperature, climate, etc. determine the features of species and individuals (Freud 1920g: 45). But when raising the question about "the origin of sexual reproduction and of the sexual drives in general", he argues, we should understand these phenomena foremost on the basis of the life drives. Every variety is one possible "manifestation of growth" (*Teilerscheinung des Wachstums*) among others, such as "multiplication by fission, sprouting or gemmation" (*Teilung, Sprossung, Knospung*) (Freud 1920g: 56). Referring to Darwin, Freud then adds that if such manifestations by chance prove advantageous in a certain environment, these manifestations will be retained, that is, they will be acquired and inherited by future generations. In other words, acquisition and inheritance follow the inner impetus to growth. The life drives are the motor force for the "increase in the variability of the organic life forms" (*Variabilität der Lebewesen*) (Freud 1920g: 56 n.). These drives are endogenous forces that continuously seek to produce transformations and neo-formations.

Freud thus distances himself from the biological theories that had been the main arguments for his views on the conservative character of all drives in the 1919 version of the text. At the same time, in the 1920 version of the text, he distances himself from Weismann's anti-Lamarckism through a critique of the potential immortality and immutability of germ plasm. He sides with Weismann, however, in prioritizing reproduction as the key factor in evolution and the emergence of variations of species and individuals. In this way, Freud responds in a way similar to Bergson to the dominant paradigms in the contemporary biology. Bergson also sides with Weismann against Lamarck when arguing that "the essential causes of variation are the differences inherent in the germ borne by the individual, and not the experience or behaviour of the individual in the course of his career" (Bergson 1907: 85). But he rejects Weismann's theory of inheritance and germ plasm as the sole explanation for the variety of species and individuals. According to Bergson, the germ cells set in motion embryonic life and thus secure continuity between generations, but in each new individual this is just a "bud" from which a new individual will develop in which new germ cells will be generated. Continuity does not depend on immutable germ plasm, but on "genetic energy", i.e., an impetus towards ceaseless variation manifesting itself in the unpredictable development of each individual (Bergson 1907: 27–28; also Posteraro 2022: 179–185).

It is from a reflection on the variability of the organic life forms that we can find analogies between the problems with which Freud was confronted in *Beyond the Pleasure Principle* and the kind of problems Bergson in *Creative Evolution* identifies in the contemporary biology. The fundamental problem is how to explain the enormous variety of organic life forms – species and individuals – and how to explain change, transformation and differentiation. The introduction of the concept of *élan de la vie* in Bergson's *Creative Evolution* is meant to answer these questions. Bergson defines it as an original "tendency" or "impetus" of life that, while being passed on from generation to generation, is the energetic fundamental cause of the creation of new species and variations in evolution (Bergson 1907: 87)?[84] Unlike Driesch's *Entelechie*, this vital impetus is not an expedient organizing principle in individual life forms directing them to a harmonious actualization of potentials.[85] It is a tendency that manifests itself in the whole of creation, that is, in the evolution of and differentiations within the multiplicity of organic life. Life unfolds in a continuous, undetermined and increasingly complex and unstable movement of becoming. The *élan* is a permanent "push" towards new forms, new "directions" and "deviations" (including regressions and "setbacks") emanating from organic matter's compository organization of relatively independent yet interacting cells, tissues and organs (Bergson 1907: 16, 42–44, 83, 104).

The undetermined character of continual creation does not only imply a critique of the contemporary organicist and vitalist theories maintaining purposiveness, finality and goal-orientation in concrete individual life forms. It also implies a critique of theories prioritizing use-inheritance and adaptation. Life cannot be explained by approaches in which development and change are reduced to a series of accidental effects of advantageous external influences (Bergson 1907: 54, 70). This critique of theories that explain the variations of species and individuals on the basis of enforced acquisitions is part of a larger critique of mechanistic theories organized around notions of phylogenetic repetition – as, for example, represented by Haeckel's biogenetic law – and ontogenetic physico-chemical processes – as, for example, in Roux's developmental mechanics.[86] Of course, Bergson does not deny the significance of metabolic and chemical processes for understanding the assimilatory and dissimilatory processes in protoplasms or organic tissues (Bergson 1907: 31–37, 86, 98–99). But these physico-chemical processes can only cause ontogenetic cyclical repetitions of syntheses and disintegrations, and vacillations of rising and falling quantities of energy. These tendencies do not produce new creations and evolutionary trajectories; they are indicative of the fact that organic matter organized according to mechanistic principles tends towards permanency and stability through phylogenetic and ontogenetic repetition.[87] Organic matter tends towards the reproduction and maintenance of stable morphological forms. It tends to repeat previous states and anticipates predictable trajectories to come – as evidenced in reproduction and the prolonging of advantageous directions

(Bergson 1907: 63, 77, 86, 102). Seen from this perspective, organic life, according to Bergson, has the tendency to return to inert matter, to develop into automatisms and fixities regulated by physical and chemical forces, to refuse further evolution, and to continue in a habitual "slumbering" fashion "with the least possible trouble" (Bergson 1907: 98, 109, 129). In *Creative Evolution*, we thus do not so much find an opposition between a spiritual life force and inert matter, but the unfolding of interactions and conflicts between two tendencies in organic matter. On the one hand, there is the "tendency" towards inertia, i.e., towards the stability and fixity of forms and a resistance to modifications. On the other hand, there is the *élan vital*, the tendency that defines "life", explosively expressing itself in the whole of creation as an impetus towards the generation of new directions, new forms, new variations (Bergson 1907: 254).[88] This impetus cannot be reduced to physico-chemical processes, but instead is characterized by the fact that each organism is a "historical being", a being whose structure, activities and trajectory can only be understood in terms of *durée*, that is, in terms of the way the past is prolonged into the present (Bergson 1907: 15, 36).

If indeed Bergson can be seen as a thinker exploring the conflict between the creative impetus and tendencies towards fixity and repetition in organic matter, and as a philosopher critical of the contemporary broad variety of mechanistic and vitalist theories,[89] Freud's tentative thoughts on the life drives in Chapter 6 of *Beyond the Pleasure Principle* can indeed be said to come close to his philosophy of life.[90] Both Bergson and Freud can be said to be following in the tradition of Darwin when arguing that the creation of new forms is inherent in the nature of organic life, and that this creativity is not predetermined – for example, in a notion of archetypes such as Jung proposes – but irregular and open-ended. And like Bergson, Freud's life (and death) drives are not so much reducible to physico-chemical processes, but need to be understood from the way in which they continue history and carry an evolutionary past into the present and beyond.

We should be careful, however, not to assert similarities too uncritically. In fact, Bergson's philosophy of life includes a conceptualization of tendencies towards fixity and repetition that appears to come close to Freud's elaborations of the conservative character of all drives in Chapter 5 of *Beyond the Pleasure Principle*. Organic life forms seek not to be modified, not to change, not to transform into something new, but rather to repeat and to re-produce the same detours and directions. But whereas Freud puts forward a theory in which conservative drive tendencies oppose modifications caused by external stimuli in processes of adaptation to changing circumstances, Bergson associates the "refusal to evolve" with a resistance to the *élan de la vie* (and hence to life as such) and with a tendency towards a dormant and convenient way of living in an advantageous environment that does not cause much trouble (Bergson 1907: 109, 129). It is through adaptation that such refusal and resistance are facilitated. Freud, on the contrary, in Chapter 5 (1919), reasons that the refusal to evolve, motivated by urges towards inertia, is a matter of resistance against further modifications and adaptations in a hostile environment. This is why Freud in Chapter 6 in 1920 will not conceptualize the death drives in terms of urges or tendencies to maintain a certain fashion or form in an advantageous environment. In the new drive theory, references to external stimuli, modifications and the necessity of adaptation are largely absent. The death drives are not primarily associated with wrinkle-free and undisturbed living in advantageous circumstances. Having said this, there are good arguments to further consider another aspect of familiarity between Bergson's and Freud's ideas: the association of the refusal to change with tendencies towards fixity, stability and continuity.

Adhesiveness, resistance and stability

With the introduction of the concept of the life drives, Freud decisively moves beyond his argumentations in Chapter 5 in which he introduced a theory of all drives urging the return to the inanimate. With the application of the libido theory to the mutual relationship of cells, it is clear that organic life forms can no longer be solely defined in terms of their resistance to further modifications. And yet, Freud maintains and continues his main intuitions on the conservative character of all drives in the new concept of the death drives. The concept of the death drives preserves the main aspects of what the 1919 version of *Beyond the Pleasure Principle* had made out to be the characteristics of all drives: the reduction (*Ermäßigung, Abgleichung, Aufhebung, Herabsetzung*) of excitation, the aim of inertia and "death", the resistance to new modifications, the elasticity and the need to restore an earlier state of things. How to consider these conservative tendencies in relation to the life drives? In Chapter 6 of *Beyond the Pleasure Principle*, we find relatively few clues to answer this question. One would expect Freud to devote ample attention to processes by which the intensity of excitation generated by the life drives can be slowed down or dissipated, but this does not seem to be the case. The problem Freud might be facing here is that such examples cannot easily be provided without lengthy discussions of other forms of intermixture of life and death drives than the ones briefly sketched in the discussion of sadism and masochism. After all, the clinical examples of libido withdrawal or incapacity towards new bindings (object-relations), detachment or regression – in paranoia, melancholia or hypochondria – show the displacement of the libido but not the diminution of excitation. In melancholia, for example, Freud argues, the detachment from an object does not lead to the displacement of libido towards a substitute object, but to the withdrawal of the libido into the ego. Here the libidinal relation with the lost object is maintained such that the ambivalent feelings of love and hate for the object are reinforced and intensified. As a result, one finds in melancholia an extraordinary and even catastrophic self-abasement (Freud 1917e).

If the 1920 version of the text conceptualizes the death drives in response to the life drives, we need to answer the question, how and in what sense do these drives react to the vitality and plasticity of the libido? We could take our starting point here in reflections on an aspect of drive theory that Freud had already explored in earlier texts: the "adhesiveness" (*Haftbarkeit*), "pertinacity" (*Zähigkeit*) or viscosity (*Klebrigkeit*) of the libidinal drives (see also Laplanche & Pontalis 1973: 12–13). The very idea of "viscosity of the libido" shows that Freud does not consider viscosity to be a counter-force operating from without. It is thought of as characteristic of the libido. In systematizing his views on the human sexual constitution through the introduction of the concept of drive in *Three Essays*, he had noticed that the sexual life of a person can become fixated, tending towards compulsory repetition of the same sexual aims and object relations (Freud 1905d: 242). While Freud attributes this phenomenon to a psychical factor "of unknown origin" in *Three Essays,* the problematics of fixation and adhesiveness of the drives are repeatedly addressed in the years preceding the publication of *Beyond the Pleasure Principle.* Freud is more and more convinced that the fixations one finds in the neuroses and perversions cannot be explained by reference to accidental factors only but must be understood as an expression of a constitutional factor, that is, as characteristic of the drives. In the case of the Wolf Man, for example, Freud argues that his patient's inclination to fend off all novelties and defend any position of the libido once taken, that is, his fixations, should be seen as manifestations of the "sluggishness" (*Schwerflüssigkeit*) of libidinal cathexes, the lack of "mobility" (*Leichtbeweglichkeit*) and "plasticity" of psychical energy (Freud 1918b: 115–116).[91] Fixation puts an end to the mobility of the drives (Freud 1915c: 123). In such a case, Freud argues, the drives remain attached to a certain representation persisting unaltered in psychic life. This adhesiveness of the libido is a general human phenomenon found where a subject's libido clings to (types of) an object while stubbornly resisting renouncement even when the object is lost (Freud 1916a: 306–307; 1916–1917a: 348).[92]

It seems evident that the adhesiveness or pertinacity of the libido as a tendency in conflict with progress, change and recovery (Freud 1915f: 272), cannot be associated with the aim of the life drives. These are mobile and plastic; their objects are variable; there is no tendency in the life drives towards persisting in attachment and fixation. According to Freud, it is not external frustration or contentment with the environment that hinders or inhibits the life drives in their mobility towards new objects or growing complexity, but an internal factor that is now assigned to the death drives. Just as the life drives seek new attachments in order to "neutralize" the death drives (Freud 1920g: 50), the death drives seek to neutralize the life drives from within. They work against the life drives by insisting on the continuation of existing attachments and libidinal investments. They seek to slow down and smother psychic and somatic mobility and plasticity. They strengthen the aspect of *-haften* in cells that are attached to one another (*aneinanderhaften*) (Freud 1920g: 52). It is thus the adhesiveness of the drives as evidenced in fixations that determines the death drives' apparent resistance to change and insistence on more-of-the-same.[93] Whereas the life drives continuously push forward, creating new investments, the death drives insist on repetition of compulsory actions thus unobtrusively undermining and inhibiting the life drives' mobility by clinging and sticking to positions and activities, objects and aims, that cannot be renounced. Seen from this perspective, the death drives should not be seen as forces aiming to unbind what the life drives bind into greater unities. It is more accurate to say that the death drives insist on remaining bound to an object and to persist in an activity or attitude. In fact, the capacity to unbind is in line with the life drives and their capacity to divert and displace drive energy from one investment to another. This is why Freud can write that melancholia is a "disorder in the distribution of libido" (Freud 1920g: 33). The problem here is not the fact of displacement of libido through withdrawal or regression, but the "hypercathexis" in the attachment to the object. In melancholia, the libido is insufficiently distributed. This is a new way to understand Freud's remark that melancholia is the "pure culture of the death drive" (Freud 1923b: 53).

The way Freud conceptualizes the death drives comes close to how Alexander Götte (in *Über den Ursprung des Todes* from 1883) and Max Hartmann – whose *Tod und Fortpflanzung* from 1906 Freud briefly refers to in his text (Freud 1920g: 47) – conceptualize death. It is the "standstill" or "termination" of individual development (Hartmann 1906: 9, 29). The death drives are insisting on repetition of more-of-the-same and a deadening stasis as a way towards the reduction of tension and abolition of vital differences. How to make sense of this repetition? Freud's discussion of transference in Chapter 3 of the *Beyond*-essay can be helpful here. In this context, he argues that the first step in analytic treatment consists in uncovering the resistances so as to oblige the patient to repeat the repressed material in the form of a contemporary experience. This resistance during treatment, Freud argues, "arises from the same higher strata and systems of the mind which originally carried out repression", that is, from the ego (Freud 1920g: 19). Resistance means that the ego is defending a certain psychic homeostasis and tranquillity against any possible intrusion of excitation, either in the form of repetitions of unpleasurable experiences or memories thereof. The ego stubbornly defends its stability. The ego is the obstacle to repetition of the repressed. And since the repressed insists on entering consciousness, the ego can do nothing but continuously resist. Or, what amounts to the same thing, to repeatedly resist.

The Wolf Man case offers a good example of this phenomenon. His treatment proved difficult because he remained entrenched "behind an attitude of obliging apathy" (*einer Einstellung von gefügiger Teilnahmslosigkeit*) and "unapproachable" over a long period of time. The first year of his treatment "produced scarcely any change". And when the patient finally developed a more active attitude, resulting in a first feeling of "relief" (of allowing excitation to enter consciousness and be discharged), the patient "immediately gave up working in order to avoid any further changes" and preferred "to remain comfortably in the situation which had thus been established" – that is, a situation of attachment to his current state of illness and resisting the "binding". This situation, Freud writes, is the same as "when today an enemy army needs weeks and months to make its way across a stretch of country which … only a short time before had been passed over by the defending army in a few days" (Freud 1918b: 11–12). It is, Freud will later write, like "having written on water" – whatever the analyst does (or does not do), makes no impression apart from some insignificant ripples on the surface that leave no trace underneath (Freud 1937c: 241).

In his reflections on this phenomenon of resistance, Freud refers to Jung's "psychical inertia" (*psychische Trägheit*) as a concept describing the sluggishness of the libido (Freud 1918b: 115–116).[94] In "Analysis Terminable and Interminable", Freud returns to this concept of psychical inertia or "psychical entropy". In a discussion of the resistances of the ego in analytic treatment and the adhesiveness of the libido, he notes that in some people, the processes set in motion by the treatment are "so much slower" than in other people.[95] Apparently, these patients "cannot make up their minds to detach libidinal cathexes from one object and displace them on to another". Instead, there is a depletion (*Erschöpfung*) of plasticity and the capacity to change; there are "unchangeable, fixed and rigid" (*unabänderlich, fixiert und erstarrt*) psychic processes, relationships and distributions of drive forces; and there is a certain "force of habit" and exhaustion (*Erschöpfung*) of receptivity (Freud 1937c: 241–242).[96] Freud suggests that this "psychic entropy" – the tendency of the psychic apparatus towards stability and decrease of tension (dissipation of energy) analogous to laws of physics (second law of thermodynamics) – can be seen as an expression of the death drives governed by the striving for pleasure (Freud 1937c: 242–243).

The references to aggression, masochism and destructive drives in *Beyond the Pleasure Principle* and other texts need not distract us from an important idea: the death drives are entropic forces that seek to run down energy, tension and excitation while isolating psychic life and seeking immunity to internal and external forces that pressure towards change. The death drives produce depletion and exhaustion, rigid habits and apathy. Seen from this perspective, the death drives do not oppose the life drives as counter-forces, but effectively work in fusions, agglomerations and intermixtures, depleting the life drives from within, that is, slowing down,[97] coagulating and clogging up their fluidity, wearing them out and solidifying their plasticity, and exhausting their vitality.[98] At first sight, Freud writes, these entropic processes seem to be typical only of old people who are close to their natural deaths. However, as expression of the death drives, this tendency towards entropy can be assumed to be inherent in all psychical and physical processes. This should not lead to the conclusion that the death drives can prevent severe unpleasure. But it does explain why the cathexis of an injured organ or a painful organic illness might be psychically preferable to the mobility of unbound drive energy flowing through the psychic apparatus (Freud 1920g: 33).

We have said that the life drives with their aim of binding have no concern for the well-being of the parties involved; they are not concerned with the well-being of an organism. From what we have said about the adhesiveness, pertinacity and fixation of drives, we can say that the reverse is also true. The death drives conceptualize the organism's lack of concern with the aims of the life drives. In this sense, the notion of the death drives maintains the aspects Freud introduced through the biological and evolutionary theories of Chapter 5. Every organism repeats (recapitulates) the acquired and fixated characteristics of its ancestors. An organism's acquired and inherited material composition and characteristics are the disposition for the kind of detour towards death an organism seeks to repeat. Seen from this perspective, all organic life gives evidence of adhesiveness and inertia, of resistance to morphological and psychical change. In the concept of the death drives, Freud continues an idea that was articulated in the 1919 version of *Beyond the Pleasure Principle*: the drives are "historically determined" and "conservative". They rather repeat what is fixated and resist change. They thus contribute to a relative stability in organic life forms and prevent an uncoordinated proliferation of forms. It is because of this aspect of the death drives that one could make a case for a certain formative tendency in the death drives (like Ferenczi and Malabou have suggested). The death drives would neutralize the most excessive consequence of the life drives – an outburst of proliferations of cells in organs, tissues and body parts such that no form can be maintained – and thus generate stability and duration. If indeed it can be said that the interacting life drives and death drives are at work in assimilations and fixations, movements and coagulations, plasticity and elasticity, vitality and exhaustion in organic life, Freud offers a theory in which organic matter is not merely the passive material suitable for the conversion of psychic conflicts. The "creation and transformation of organs" are not only the result of "the power of unconscious ideas over one's own body" (compare Freud & Abraham 2002: 361–362). In the living substances there are materializing forces at work, processes of organic transformation and stabilization, vitalization and crystallization, movement and congestion. Freud presents a theory of the dynamic character of organic processes and, as such, a theory of organic constitution and physiological "compliances" to psychic life.

From here, we can go a step further. We mentioned that in melancholia libido is insufficiently distributed. We know that Freud in *The Ego and the Id* refers to melancholia as "a pure culture of the death instinct" (Freud 1923b: 53). Could we then perhaps say that mania (the "counterpart" of melancholia) is the pure culture of the life drives, i.e., the clinical manifestation of uninhibited and excessive drive energy? For Freud, mania is a direct and uninhibited expression "in action" of the primary process with its unbound drive energy (Freud 1917e: 254, 258; 1921c: 132). In mania, there is excessive distribution of energy as evidenced in general excitement ("triumph") and impulsive behaviour. If so, the life drives when not inhibited by death drives do not only disregard well-being, but also undermine self-preservative urges. The life drives can be deadly, not because the process of binding implies coalescence and hence the death of the individual, as Spielrein and Stärcke argued, but because the freely mobile life drives aiming at binding in greater unities express themselves in unhinged and triumphant activities without consideration of reality. If so, the death drives could be said to be the forces that prevent the life drives from being deadly, i.e., from the deadly consequences of drives without "halting at any position attained".[99] It is at this point that Freud offers a possible critique of Bergson's optimism with regards to the "explosive" character of the *élan de la vie*: There is – materialized – fixity, adhesiveness and viscosity, and it is motivated by an inner urge to reduce tension and vital differences in order to establish what Freud refers to as "one or more optima".

Based on what we have said about the interaction between the life drives and the death drives, we can understand why Freud, after having prioritized the "diminution of the quantity of excitation" and the "lowering of excitation" in the 1919 version of *Beyond the Pleasure Principle*, inserts references to Fechner's ideas on "conditions of stability and instability". The introduction of the concept of the life drives makes it impossible to consider life only in conservative terms and as aiming at death or at static equilibrium. The notion of the "tendency towards stability" is introduced in order to relate the pleasure principle to the death drives. Given the continuous pressure from the life drives towards change and new forms, it is the death drives that work towards an aim "attainable only by approximation" (Freud 1920g: 8–10). For Freud, the approximate stability with its compromises and conflicts is the best way to describe a "normal" and "healthy" psychic life caught between the polarities of the plasticity and vitality of the life drives and the pertinacity and rigidity of the death drives. The consequences of this line of thought will be drawn in a few years later, in "The Economic Problem of Masochism" (Freud 1924c). Here Freud argues that we should not equate stability with "the inorganic state" and the "Nirvana principle". "Beyond a certain limit", deviations from stability – either in the form of a surplus of tensions or extreme "relaxations of tension" – are perceived as unpleasure (Freud 1924c: 160). Tensions are not necessarily unpleasurable; and complete absence of tension is not pleasurable (see Freud 1920g: 63).[100]

Final remarks

The new drive theory as introduced in the second version of *Beyond the Pleasure Principle* can be seen in response to "the development of an extreme line of thought" in Chapter 5 that needed to be "limited" and "corrected" (Freud 1920g: 37 n.). Freud presents this correction in terms of a reformulation of drive dualism, i.e., the opposition of two distinct drives. His brief overview of the development of his drive theory in Chapter 6 is meant to underscore this point (Freud 1920g: 50–53). Not all drives are conservative;

the sexual and self-preservative drives are not two expressions of the same tendency towards death. In fact, the introduction of the concept of the life drives leads to another, structurally similar, question: "If the self-preservative drives too are of a libidinal nature, are there perhaps no other drives whatever but the libidinal ones?" Are there perhaps only libidinal drives? If so, Freud writes, how to distinguish the concept of the life drives from what Jung had named "drive force" (Freud 1920g: 52)? The answer follows immediately: "We started out from the great opposition between the life and death instincts" (Freud 1920g: 53).

We should again raise the question whether Freud's explicit references to drive dualism added in 1921 and whether the rejection of Jung's monism are the most adequate way to frame the new drive theory. Freud's later affirmations of drive dualism in which the death drives are defined in terms of a destructive or aggressive drive and the life drives (Eros) are forces that bind people together, should not obscure the fact that in *Beyond the Pleasure Principle* all formulations of the drives are linked to the bioanalytical perspective. The application of the libido theory to the mutual relationship of cells means that Freud considers living substances as the "vital association" (*Lebensverband*) between cells that seek to prolong their lives by constructing ever larger unities (Freud 1920g: 50). He does not conceive this vital association in terms of a stable union, but, to the contrary, as a continuous growing and expanding substance in which there is "no halting at any position attained". In its most excessive manifestation, this is manic proliferation, which, as evidenced in the case of malignant cancer cells, can be deadly since they devour the vital association from within. It is in the excessive "manic" manifestations that the "vital differences" (tensions and excitations) increase such that the change in magnitude in a limited period of time produces sensations of unpleasure the death drives will seek to eliminate. Despite Freud's references to dualism, the new drive theory is not a theory of oppositional forces – as also Derrida has noticed in his seminar *La vie la mort* from 1975–1976 (Derrida 2020: 334ff). Both drives can – in different ways – be deadly as well as life-sustaining; both drives are inherent to "life" and the detour of every living organism; every change ("progress") or fixation implies death and maintenance of life.

In terms of trauma, Freud no longer assumes the primacy of external trauma he articulated in 1919, but returns to his first psychoanalytical intuition when he associated trauma with memory and *Nachträglichkeit*: trauma comes from within (Westerink & Van Haute 2025). The death drives seek to protect the organism from the traumatizing effects of unrestrained life drives that pressure the organism from within. The death drives do so not through facilitating immediate discharge, but, to the contrary, by "slowing down" and exhausting the libidinal energy, by pressuring towards fixations and repetitions. They operate against the life drives only after mitigation with the life drives. That is, they only work against the life drives from within, from being intermixed with the plasticity, mobility and fluidity of the life drives. In this way the death drives seek to protect the organism from the proliferating and disturbing – and hence potentially traumatizing – surplus of the life drives. But the reverse is also true. The life drives insist on "growth" against the deadly repetitions and fixations that – as, for example, evidenced in melancholia – do not necessarily imply pleasure. In answer to the sedimenting effects of the death drives, the life drives produce fresh vital differences that provide the opportunity for feelings of pleasure in the way Freud had already described in *Three Essays* and other texts: autoerotic pleasure experienced at rhythmic repetitions and organ pleasure. Repetitions can be vitalized such that pleasure is no longer felt as absence but presence of excitation.

If we consider again that Freud's starting point is the application of the libido theory to cells, we can further move beyond drive dualism. The "vital association" or "union" cannot simply be thought of as the momentary outcome of two contrasting (and interacting) forces but as a composition of individual elements (cells, organs, body parts) in which drives express themselves in different ways (including mitigations, intermixtures, ambivalences) at the same time. Freud's idea of "displacement" or "condensation" of unbound energy (and hence also symptom formation) hints at this possibility of shifting investments in different parts of the body. There is local plasticity and elasticity, processes of fusion and defusion, coalescence and fission, assimilation and dissimilation, rises and falls in the quantity and quality of libido, binding and unbinding, anabolic and catabolic processes. The body is a composition of these processes such that there is a multiplicity of effects, flows and inhibitions, displacements and fixations. It was notably Ferenczi who pursued this line of thought in *Thalassa* and later writings, while questioning Freud's drive dualism of contrasting negative and positive forces. He was not the only one who sought to overcome Freud's obsession with dualism (vs. Jung's monism).[101] Lacan famously argued that "every drive is virtually a death drive" (Lacan 2006: 848). In every drive there is an unstrained and repetitive insistence to move either beyond the pleasure principle towards excessive and painful-destructive excitation in *jouissance* or to insist on homeostasis and equilibrium such that the subject turns into an automaton, a living machine. These ideas find support in a reading of *Beyond the Pleasure Principle* but also highlight Lacan's focus on destructive tendencies in and beyond the symbolic order of culture. In my reading, however, the example of the death drives Freud provides – sadism and masochism – is not necessarily the paradigmatic clinical example, and certainly not the only way to consider the variety of possible vicissitudes and intermixtures of the life and death drives. Lacan's views on the destructive insistence on jouissance may be just one possible manifestation of intermixture of drives, repetition and fixation, excitation and pleasure-unpleasure-series.

In a footnote in *Three Essays*, added in 1924, Freud writes that the theory of the drives "is the most important but at the same time the least complete portion of psychanalytical theory" – *Beyond the Pleasure Principle* being the latest contribution to such theory (Freud 1905d: 168 n.). This statement parallels remarks in his autobiographical study on the general and fundamental concepts in psychoanalytic theory, such as "libido" and "drive", lacking precision. According to Freud, precision is impossible in any science, notably also in biology and physics, which lack adequate definitions of their fundamental concepts such as life, matter, force, energy, gravitation, et cetera. It is only through "progressive analysis of the material under observation" that psychoanalysis, like the other sciences, may reach a certain consistency in the its fundamental concepts (Freud 1925d: 57–58). Being trained in these sciences, Freud realizes that the fundamental postulates of physics and biology can only be known from their observed effects. In *Beyond the Pleasure Principle*, he also realizes that speculations on the fundamental concept may "diverge widely" from empirical observation, and that therefore one "must be ready, too, to abandon a path that we have followed for a time, if it seems to be leading to no good end". The development of science depends on the capacity to doubt, to give up a certain conviction, and to transform one's views (Freud 1920g: 59, 64). And this is exactly what characterizes the text: "limping" instead of taking a straight path (Freud 1920g: 64).

Limping in order to come closer to what? *Beyond the Pleasure Principle* was not written in order to speculate on the drives as such, but to gain insight into constitutional and hereditary factors that condition certain pathological phenomena. From the study of the traumatic neuroses and the bioanalytical perspective on evolution in the 1919 version of *Beyond the Pleasure Principle*, Freud maps the human constitution as the result of traumata, repetition and the resistance to enforced modifications. From this inquiry Freud provides insight in the "somatic compliance", i.e., the physiological-material and psychic structures and dynamics, in the aetiology of the traumatic neuroses. In the 1920 version of text, Freud articulates a theory of life and death drives as the fundamental plastic-creative and adhesive tendencies from which to understand the human constitution. Both theories are meant to provide insight into clinical phenomena such as the "motor symptoms" and materialization processes in traumatic neuroses, hysteria, melancholia and hypochondria (Freud 1920g: 12). They allow for different, yet not necessarily mutual exclusive, perspectives on the creation and transformation of organs (compare Freud & Abraham 2002: 361–362), the materialization in symptoms, the functions and disfunctions of organs, the processes of circulation and fixation in body parts, muscles or the digestive system, and the continuities between somatic processes and psychic organization. That Freud in the final chapter of *Beyond the Pleasure Principle* does not refer or return to clinical practice should not prevent us from raising the question of the clinical potential of considering the human body and the psychosomatic from the perspective of trauma and reaction formations, or from the proliferating and adhesive tendencies in the drives. The answers to this question are beyond the scope of this book.

Notes

1 The biological perspective of drives mentioned briefly in "Instincts and Their Vicissitudes" is clearly present in other texts from that period. In "The Unconscious", for example, he writes that "an instinct cannot be represented otherwise than by an idea [*Vorstellung*]". And when he speaks of "repressed drive impulses", he notes that this can only mean that the ideational representative is repressed and unconscious (Freud 1915e: 177). In the paper "Repression" from the same year, he describes the relation between the drive and its psychic representation in terms of an idea or group of ideas "cathected with a definite quota of psychical energy (libido or interest) coming from a drive", i.e., cathected with a "quota of affects" that "correspond" to the quantity of drive stimuli (Freud 1915d: 152).

2 In his writings before 1905, that is, before the introduction of the drive concept in *Three Essays*, Freud mentions "psychic energy" or "endogenous excitation" as "constant force" (1895b: 112) or "quantity in a state of flow" (Freud 1950c: 296).

3 This definition was replaced in the 1915 edition of the text by the description in line with "Instincts and Their Vicissitudes": "By an 'instinct' is provisionally to be understood the psychical representative of an endosomatic, continuously flowing source of stimulation" (Freud 1905d: 168).

4 In *Wandlungen und Symbole der Libido* (1912), Jung argues that Freud introduced the notion of a single primal drive (*Urlibido*) which, in the course of development, differentiates into various psychic functions and, in connection with certain bodily functions, zones, and objects, becomes cathected with sexuality. Through a process of differentiation of bodily functions, the primal drive will partly develop into a sexual drive connected to the sexual – reproductive – function of specific body parts (Jung 1912: 133ff; Van Haute & Westerink 2021: 60–61). According to Freud, however, Jung is wrong when attributing a voluntaristic and purposeful character to the drive. According to Freud, Jung's concept of the primal libido should therefore be distinguished from "the energy which must be supposed to underlie mental processes in general" (Freud 1905d: 217).

5 Laplanche writes that although Freud "does postulate the existence of two kinds of drive, Freud never accepts that there might be two kinds of instinctual energy" (Laplanche 1989: 146). He therefore proposes an "energetic monism" as a starting point for differentiations in sexual drives and ego-drives, life drives and death drives (Laplanche 1985: 124; also Hock 2000: 210–215).

6 Here we find an important starting point for a critique of the theory of life drives and, in particular, death drives. Otto Fenichel will argue that Freud's suggestion of an originally "neutral energy" should be a reason not to link the neurotic conflict to a speculative drive dualism, but to a conflict between the individual and a repressive culture that demands drive renunciation (Fenichel 1935). This idea can also be found in the writings of Wilhelm Reich and will have a strong influence on later post-Freudian theory formation, including Herbert Marcuse's *Eros and Civilization*. Marcuse, however, gives the death drives a place in his theory – they are destructive drives: the motive forces in man's striving for domination of nature, and in civilization's oppressive organization (Marcuse 1955).

7 In the 1915 edition of *Three Essays*, he states:

> The final outcome of the sexual development lies in what is known as the normal sexual life of the adult, in which the pursuit of pleasure comes under the sway of the reproductive function and in which the component instincts,

under the primacy of a single erotogenic zone, form an organization directed towards a sexual aim attached to some extraneous object.

(Freud 1905d: 197)

8 In *Anti-Oedipe*, Deleuze and Guattari vehemently criticize the oedipalizing moves in Freudian thought, and oedipal readings of Freud's work, while presenting a radical non-oedipal reading of the Schreber case, focusing on the creative internal forces that generate and organize his organs and body parts (Deleuze & Guattari 1997: 11ff). And in *Mille plateaux*, the authors present a non-oedipal reading of the case of Little Hans, drawing attention to Hans's "becoming-horse" as an affectively motivated rearrangement of the relations between one's own body and other bodies (Deleuze & Guattari 2021: 300ff). Given Freud's non-oedipal 1905 theory of sexuality, there are good arguments for these non-oedipal readings of these case studies.

9 We note here that Freud must have realized the undermining effect of his views of the Oedipus complex for his 1905 theory of infantile sexuality. For, there are no inserted sections or excursions on the complex and some associated issues (identification, superego formation, desexualization) in the later editions of *Three Essays*. The complex is only briefly mentioned in a few footnotes (Van Haute & Westerink 2021).

10 One can want to argue with Lynn Margulis and Dorion Sagan that sex/sexuality should not be defined in terms of copulation and reproduction, but in terms of the fusion of cells. The origin of such fusions can be traced back to a primal genetic repair system restoring damaged DNA through symbiosis. The damage would be caused by exposure to a hostile environment. Margulis thus defines sex in terms of symbiosis between various elementary organic life forms (Margulis & Sagan 1986). Freud's notion of the life drives as urges towards coalescence in and between cells appears to prelude a notion of symbiogenesis.

11 There are several short additions in the passages on the conservative character of the drives later inserted in 1920 and 1925, in which Freud nuances his "extreme line of thought" on the sexual drives, announcing "a correction of this extreme view of the self-preservative instincts" in what follows (that is to say, in Chapter 6) (Freud 1920g: 37, 39, nn.).

12 A similar statement can be found in "On Narcissism". Here Freud argues that reproduction provides the individual with the comforting illusion of immortality (Freud 1914c: 91).

13 In a letter to Lou Andreas-Salomé, dated 1 August 1919, Freud writes that he is exploring literature in order to substantiate his latest ideas on the drives, including the writings of Schopenhauer – though not with great pleasure (Freud & Andreas-Salomé 1972).

14 The final part of this sentence (six words) was added in 1921.

15 Italics were added from the 1923 edition onwards.

16 On this movement in *Beyond the Pleasure Principle* from trauma as interruption of psychic life (and life as such) towards the conceptualization of the "awakening" of life from death as the foundation of the drives and psychic life, see Cathy Caruth's reading of Lacan's Seminar 11, Chapter 5 (Caruth 1996: 94–115). Caruth suggests that this movement is based on Freud associating the life-threatening situation with (the inevitability of) actual death, and the awakening with survival. Just like the shell-shocked patient is the one who survived the horrors of the trenches, and relives this survival in his dreams and awakenings from the dreams, life is what survived the primordial catastrophic event of the incomprehensible force.

17 The translation of *Identität* in "identical" is accurate. The term *Identität* is used here in a classical sense, that is, as deriving from *identitas*, sameness.
18 Lacan critically concludes on this that, according to Freud, "all that life is seeking repose as much as possible while awaiting death … dozing off is the most natural of all vital states" (Lacan 1991: 233).
19 Is it possible to actively affirm this "daemonic" character of the inherited? In *Totem and Taboo*, Freud suggests in a famous reference to Goethe that indeed this is the case: "What thou hast inherited from thy fathers, acquire it to make it thine" (Freud 1912–1913a: 158). If the inherited is not opposed or inhibited by other forces, Freud suggests, it will continue its course (as constant force). To say that one can consider what is inherited as "mine", is to say that the inherited can be recognized as such and be critically opposed by the ego and by the capacity of conscious thought. In *The Ego and the Id*, Freud articulates this in terms of the ego's "conquest" of the Id as the realm of "the experiences of past ages" (Freud 1923b: 55–56).
20 See also Zupančič (2017: 98–99) and Allen (2021: 40).
21 Hans Loewald, and more recently Benjamin Fong, have convincingly argued that Freud's claim that the drives aim of discharge of tension is situated in a shift towards a biological model for understanding psychic life. This biological model must be distinguished from a physiological model in which drives are seen as constant forces and in which the psyche is defined as an apparatus regulated by the pleasure principle aiming at discharge of stimuli. In the biological model, the drives are no longer seen as "external" to the psychic apparatus, but as an integral part of the psychic organization (Loewald 1980: 116–124; Fong 2016: 8–12).
22 Deleuze is not the first and only one to recognize the problem we are discussing here. Lacan had taken this problem as starting point for rearticulating the "beyond" of the pleasure principle in terms of a desire for enjoyment (*jouissance*) that cannot be reduced to the pleasurable discharge of tension but, on the contrary, is to be described as a self-destructive tendency of repetition and excess. In a different way, Deleuze appreciates Freud's insight in describing compulsive repetition as an original pulsional force. What is unthinkable for Deleuze is the idea that all drives are reactive, conservative and regressive.
23 On Deleuze's reading of Freud on drive and repetition, see also Ansell-Pearson (1999: 104ff), Somers-Hall (2017), Ingala (2020) and Moyaert (2022).
24 Freud's remark that the development of organisms is ultimately to be seen as resulting from the relation between the earth and the sun (Freud 1920g: 38), is likely informed by Jacques Loeb's experimental research on heliotropic (mechanistic) reactions of plants and animals in several publications, copies of which Freud had in his library – such as *Die Bedeutung der Tropismen für die Psychologie* from 1909 (Haraway 1976: 21–22; Davies & Fichtner 2006).
25 One can argue that precisely this would reflect a clinical insight from the analyses of traumatic neuroses. Are these neuroses not manifestations of the conflict between external forces causing breaches and paralysis to the psychic systems, on the one hand, and an internal joining of forces to defend and restore, on the other? Such a conclusion would point towards a failure on Freud's part to integrate the traumatic neuroses into an existing theory of the aetiology and characteristics of the psychoneuroses, that is, a theory that implies inner conflicts between opposing drive tendencies.
26 Indeed, this intent is confirmed in later texts in which Freud discusses the death drives. In later texts, he will maintain that the conservative nature of the drives, the urge to restore an earlier state and to return to inanimate matter, are characteristic of the death drive (see e.g., Freud 1923b: 40; 1933a: 106–107). In fact,

Freud argues that the death drive deserves to be called such by virtue of these characteristics (Freud 1923a: 258; 1940a: 148).

27 The reference to Newtonian ideas of inertia and elasticity are telling in this context: A body remains at rest unless a force acts upon it; a body resists a distorting force and returns to rest once that force is removed. Freud applies these principles to the drives and hence to life as such.

28 This also means that Freud's first mention of the death drives in writing is dated after the death of his daughter Sophie. We know that Freud denied what, among others, Fritz Wittels in his 1924 Freud-biography suspected, namely that *Beyond the Pleasure Principle*, including the idea that "the aim of all life is death", could be read as a personal reflection on Sophie's death. However, the introduction of the death drives and the elaboration on death and immortality in Chapter 6 were written after her passing away. See on this issue, May (2024: 91–92) and Rose (2021: 44ff).

29 This is why Freud suggests that the study of the binding of individuals cannot do without palaeobiological research (Freud & Jones 1993: 373).

30 In the German texts there are no brackets in this passage.

31 In this context, Freud repeats his Lamarckian arguments from *Totem and Taboo*: primal emotional ties were acquired, fixated and inherited in every new generation as "archaic heritage", that is, as "predispositions that survived in the unconscious from the early history of the human family" (Freud 1921c: 127–128).

32 In "A Short Account of Psycho-Analysis", Freud defines the libido as "the force (thought of as quantitatively variable and measurable) of the sexual instincts directed towards an object – 'sexual' in the extended sense required by analytic theory" (Freud 1924f: 203).

33 Also, according to Freud, identification with the father cannot be reduced to sexual object relations. This is crucial when we consider the gradual oedipalization of Freudian theory. The fully-fledged Oedipus complex as defined in *The Ego and the Id* is based on a notion of identification as presented in "Mourning and Melancholia" and *Group Psychology*. Since it is through the new drive theory in *Beyond the Pleasure Principle* that identification and self-aggression can be accounted for that Freud is able to fully develop the concept of the Oedipus complex.

34 Borch-Jacobsen has correctly drawn attention to the significance of the concept of *Bindung* in both the theory of the life and death drives and in *Group Psychology*. However, we cannot agree with his reconstruction in which the concept of Eros as presented in the 1920 version of *Beyond the Pleasure Principle* was applied in Group Psychology (Borch-Jacobsen 1988: 154ff). The hypothesis brought forward in this study argues the opposite: Freud applies his views on Eros/binding in groups to processes of binding between cells and in organic life.

35 This anxiety is *sinnlos* as it results from the cessation of emotional ties, that is, from the cessation of libidinal cathexes, and not as a response to or expectation of concrete danger. Panic anxiety is anxiety in which decathected amounts of unemployed libido are discharged in the form of anxiety which only in a second moment will be bound to an external danger (compare Freud 1916–1917a: 407, 410). Panic anxiety is thus similar to fright, as it consists of amounts of drive stimuli (libido) flooding the psychic systems that seek to bind the impulses to representations. Freud had explored this phenomenon in an 1895 article in which he analyzed what he had called anxiety neuroses as a form of actual neuroses. The main idea is this: anxiety –one could also call it panic – results not from external factors, but from an internal "attack" of accumulated excitation pressuring and overwhelming the psychic apparatus and expressing itself in bodily

symptoms (disturbances in heart action, tremors, etc.) and other phenomena such as fright-dreams. Freud describes this endogenous excitation as being "in a freely floating state", that is, not bound to representations (Freud 1895b).

36 In mentioning the analogy between panic as "disappearance of the emotional ties" and "neurotic anxiety", Freud refers to an "interesting though somewhat over-imaginative" paper presented by Bela von Felszeghy in 1919 and published in *Imago* in 1920. The mention of this paper is significant: in von Felszeghy's text we find several elements that pave the way for various ideas we find in Freud and also in Ferenczi – namely, the analogy between panic and fright (in traumatic neuroses), the decomposition of group binding and the regression to narcissism, the idea of trauma of birth (primal catastrophe) and the tendency to return to the mother womb (Ferenczi), the drive as an urge to return to "the pre-existential Nirvana" as a tendency that implies self-annihilation, the application of psychoanalytic insights on cells, and the idea of progression through binding in variable unities (Von Felszeghy 1920).

37 In the 1920 proofs of the manuscript, Freud adds a footnote in which the terminology and development of the drive theory – or better, various drive theories – are further clarified. The various theoretical modifications lead Freud to extend the libido concept and eventually to introduce the concept of Eros and the death drive. (Here he uses the concept of "death drive" in the singular for the first time.) In the 1921 edition of *Beyond the Pleasure Principle*, Freud adds a passage to this footnote in which he describes how the concept of the ego-drives has been transformed – from one in which the drives stand in opposition to the sexual drives, to a theory in which the libido and ego-drives are cast as aspects of the life drives (Freud 1920g: 60–61 n.).

38 From the 1921 edition of the text onwards, this sentence reads as follows: "that instincts other than the libidinal ones of self-preservation [*die libidinösen Selbsterhaltungstriebe*] operate in the ego" (Freud 2024: 71). The 1920 formulation can be read to suggest that there are libidinal drives that do not aim at the self-preservation and the prolongation of life. In the second formulation, Freud clarifies his statement, arguing that besides libidinal self-preservative drives, there are other non-libidinal self-preservative drives operating. This is in line with an earlier remark in which he states that only "a portion of the ego-instincts was seen to be libidinal" (Freud 1920g: 52). The second formulation is thus merely elucidating the first so as to avoid possible misunderstandings. However, Freud immediately adds that in clinical practice, such non-libidinal ego-drives have thus far not been proven to exist (Freud 1920g: 53).

39 Freud read Low's *Psycho-Analysis* (1920) after Ernest Jones had sent him a copy. We should note here that Low's concept of the Nirvana principle does not so much describe the discharge of drive tension, but the return to the mother's womb and the associated state of omnipotence. For Low, it is a principle "beyond" the pleasure principle (Low 1920: 73).

40 On this "unobtrusive" character of the death drives, Freud will later write that these drives are "by their nature mute" (*stumm*) (Freud 1920g: 63; 1923b: 46). Their primal characteristic is to silently work towards reduction of tension and towards stability, and to initiate the displacement and withdrawal of libido. Even before 1920, in the Schreber case, Freud refers to the withdrawal of the libido as a "silent" (*stumm*) process in comparison to the spectacular and noisy *Weltuntergangserlebnis* and delusions (Freud 1911c: 71).

41 In *Group Psychology*, Freud writes "psychic differentiations" and the "discovery of objects" (through binding) increase psychic "instability". The individual then seeks to return to the "former condition of absence of stimulation". According to

Freud, this equals "avoidance of objects" and a return to an initial state of autoerotism and narcissism (Freud 1921c: 130).

42 We can think here of what has been said about panic. Panic cannot be defined solely in terms of the weakening of the bonds between individuals in groups. Panic starts when individuals in a group start to be solicitous on their own account, when they seek to preserve themselves rather than putting their lives in the service of a greater whole. It is characterized by forceful energy, concretely, amounts of senseless anxiety. It is here that we find a phenomenon in which displaceable energy, supporting the libidinal binding between individuals, finds another expression when amounts of drive energy flow into another direction.

43 This explains why Freud will later write that the death drive (like the life drives) employs "displaceable and neutral energy" to dissolve unities (compare Freud 1923b: 44–45).

44 In this context, Freud also associates the life drives, and more specifically the sexual drives, with repetition. He writes that "the sphere of embryonic developmental processes is no doubt extremely rich in such phenomena of repetition" (Freud 1920g: 56). Every coalescence of germ cells produces a next generation, repeating the processes of binding into bodies. And yet, the life drives are neither characterized by blind and endless repetitions for the sake of repetition, nor are they aiming to restore or repeat the same. They never aim to reproduce a previous specific form; in fact, they always produce new unique forms (individuals).

45 In a negative analogy to this capacity, the death drives proceed with chemical process of decomposition (*Abgleichung chemischer Spannungen*) (Freud 1920g: 55).

46 The idea that organic life can be defined in terms of matter that resists entropy, in other words, the idea that seeks to maintain itself against tendencies towards death, can (among others) be found Erwin Schrödinger's 1944 *What Is Life*? (Schrödinger 2020: 67ff). According to Schrödinger, inorganic matter tends towards entropy, whereas organic matter accumulates energy in order to use this for growth and the creation of larger unities. In Freud, both tendencies can be found in organic life; this is expressed in the theory of life drives and death drives.

47 This is analogous to a train of thought in *Three Essays* (1905). Here Freud states that the "finding of an object" (*Objektfindung*) is nothing but a "re-finding of it" (*Wiederfindung*) (Freud 1905d: 222). This seems to suggest that all objects are substitute objects for an original lost object. Lacan, among others, subscribes to such an interpretation in which negativity (object loss) is the motive force in psychic life (Leader 2021: 9). However, this is not what Freud argues. Freud reasons that it is only in puberty, and hence in retrospect, that the first object providing satisfaction (the breast, the mother) acquires any meaning. What one seeks to "re-find" through object relations is the pleasure experienced in non-objectal autoerotic activities. Seen from this perspective, the sexual drive is an energetic drive that pushes life forward towards new constellations in which pleasure (that is, excitation) can be realized (Van Haute & Westerink 2021: 22–23).

48 The term "vital difference" (*Vitaldifferenz*) was coined by the German psychophysicist Richard Avenarius in his *Kritik der reinen Erfahrung* (1888). It describes the imbalance (increase/decrease) in physiological processes caused by stimuli that act upon a system or part of a system (May 2024: 155).

49 In "Analysis Terminable and Interminable", Freud goes a step further: "Only by the concurrent or mutually opposing action of the two primal instincts – Eros and the death-instinct –, never by one or the other alone, can we explain the rich multiplicity of the phenomena of life" (Freud 1937c: 243). The mention of the death drive in the passage of 1937 indicates that the complexity and variety of organic life forms result not only from the unifying processes generated by the

life drives but also include the dissolving and destructive forces of the death drives. This idea follows from Freud's views of the interactions between, and "taming" and fusion of, drives. This is what explains the variety of characteristics of organic life forms. As examples Freud refers to elementary characteristics such as eating (incorporation and destruction of an object) and reproductive activities (aggression as inherent in sexual union) (Freud 1920g: 54; 1940a: 149).

50 In order to account for the element of domination and subjection, Freud had introduced the concept of the drive for mastery (*Bemächtigungstrieb*) in *Three Essays*. In fact, Freud reasoned that the drive for mastery would only be sexualized through a process of anastomosis (Freud 1905d: 193 n.). This remark was deleted from the 1915 version of *Three Essays* and replaced by the suggestion that the drive for mastery belonged to the sphere of sexuality from the outset (Van Haute & Westerink 2021: 52, 66). This change can be understood in the context of Freud's debate with Alfred Adler. Adler had enthusiastically developed the notion of the drive for mastery into a "third drive" alongside the sexual drives and the self-preservative drives. In response to this suggestion of an aggressive drive, Freud had argued, in his case study of Little Hans, that the need for mastery should be seen as the manifestation of sexual drives "becoming aggressive" as a result of the sadistic component of the libido (Freud 1909a: 141).

51 The idea of the sadistic drive being aimed at injuring or destroying an object is new. That is to say, in *Three Essays* and in "Instincts and Their Vicissitudes" Freud had argued that the aim in sadism is to subjugate an object, to exercise power, to humiliate and master an object, and to inflict pain (Freud 1905d: 157; 1915c: 127–128). What is added in *Beyond the Pleasure Principle* is the aspect of destruction and annihilation. It is likely that this shift in the definition of the aim is made under the influence of the study of melancholia. It is in melancholia that Freud finds self-reproaches that can ultimately lead to annihilation (suicide) of the individual (Freud 1917e: 252).

52 This will be further developed by Melanie Klein in her elaborations of the paranoid-schizoid position in which the primitive ego, in fear of its annihilation, "projects" the death drive into the outside world which then give rise to aggressive phantasies of bad objects (to first one of which is the mother's breast) (e.g., Klein 1933: 250–251; 1946: 4–5). In more recent literature Jonathan Lear has interpreted the death drive as a drive towards self-destruction that needs deflection towards external objects to avoid this self-destruction. Aggression is here a defence against self-destructive tendencies (Lear 2005: 160–162).

53 Because Freud in his clinical example only provides evidence for the intermixture of drives, Lacan and also Laplanche and Pontalis could propose that all drives producing change and excitation (the life drives) are also characterized by a conservative tendency (the death drive). The conservative drives are not distinct from non-conservative drives, but inherent attributes or features of all drives (Laplanche & Pontalis 1973: 102; Lacan 1998: 257). In these interpretations, Freud's idea that all drives are conservative is applied to the 1920 distinction between life drives and death drives.

54 Freud had always regarded masochism a secondary phenomenon. This is still the case in "A Child Is Being Beaten", which was written during the period in which Freud was working on the first version of *Beyond the Pleasure Principle*. It is only in 1920 that he reverses the sequence of sadism and masochism.

55 André Green has elaborated on this aspect, arguing that the death drive originates from and manifests itself in object relations as a tendency towards unbinding, and more specifically, as a tendency towards the withdrawal of libidinal investment in objects and the return to a narcissistic position of self-sufficiency

(“*disobjectalisation*”). For Green, the destructiveness of the death drive is thus not to be found in aggression turned outwards and inwards, but in a narcissistic denial (negative narcissism) of the object (Green 1999: 86, 105).

56 Freud had recognized this clearly in his study of melancholic self-reproaches, and would further elaborate this in his discussions of the superego systematically torturing its object, the ego. In this context, Freud moreover puts forward the idea, based on clinical observations, that the death drive is indeed a drive (force): the cruelty of the superego does not correspond with the severity of treatment or upbringing at the hands of others – the cruelty of the superego is “independent” of the severity of treatment by others. If the amount of aggressiveness does not stem from external sources, it must have internal energetic sources (Freud 1923b: 28–29, 51ff; 1930a: 130).

57 This is repeated in later writings such as *New Introductory Lectures*: Only when the destructive drives are directed outwards do they acquire the characteristics of aggressiveness (*damit den Charakter der Aggression erwirbt*) (Freud 1933a: 105). This view of aggressiveness is confirmed in other texts such as *Civilization and Its Discontents* and *Why War?*, in which Freud argues that the death drive turns into a destructive drive when directed at external objects (Freud 1930a: 122; 1933b: 211).

58 Freud’s elaborations on the experience of pleasure in pain are crucial for what Lacan conceptualizes as jouissance. From Freud’s ideas on the fusion of drives in erotogenic masochism, Lacan takes that, beyond the homeostatic pleasure principle, there is an “insisting” desire towards excessive excitation which equals pain and self-destruction. The concept of jouissance refers to the body experiencing excessive and intense unpleasurable excitation that knows no halt or limit. For Lacan, this means that the death drive cannot be defined in terms of a drive towards annihilation of tension (pleasure principle, Nirvana principle), but has to be taken as a (self-)destructive drive (Lacan 1992: 211–212). Beyond the pleasure principle one finds the death drive insisting on *jouissance* – not as a separate drive, but as a characteristic of all drives that “push forward unrestrained” (Lacan 1998: 257).

59 Since Freud distinguishes between processes of unbinding and dissolving, on the one hand, and aggressiveness, on the other, we can say that the notion of “fragmentation” can be used in both contexts but with distinct meanings: fragmentation as silent decomposition of unities; fragmentation as violent self-destruction. On this issue, see also Penot (2016).

60 In passing, Freud mentions another clinical example that can be seen as an immediate manifestation of defused destructive drive impulses: epilepsy (Freud 1923b: 41). He does not discuss this phenomenon any further, but in his 1928 text on Dostoevsky, he returns to the “old morbus sacer” characterized by repeated sudden severe attacks, muscular contractions, loss of consciousness, and deathlike states (Freud 1928b: 179–180, 182). The symptoms of epilepsy appear similar to those of the war neuroses. Freud confirms this implicitly in mentioning fright and the attempts at discharge of large quantities of excitation as possible psychic causes. And yet, in the Dostoevsky text, he does not mention epilepsy – or the traumatic neuroses – as possible manifestation of the death drive; instead, he regards it mainly as a symptom of an oedipal sense of guilt, hence, as sadistic self-punishment for death-wishes against a hated father (Freud 1928b: 183).

61 According to Freud, a variant of such disintegration of narcissistic structures can be witnessed in multiple personality as a severe disruption (*Aufsplitterung* – fragmentation) of the ego (Freud 1923b: 30–31).

62 The conceptualization of the death drive in terms of a destructive drive can also be situated in a context of intense debates with followers on the relation between aggression and libido, and on pre-oedipal and oedipal formations of the super-ego (conscience) and the sense of guilt. In writings from the 1920s and 1930s, Freud vehemently defends the primacy of sexuality, while oedipalizing his theory (Westerink 2009; also May 2023). What preoccupies him in those texts in which he develops the death drive, are processes of desexualization and resexualization associated with the fusion and defusion of life and death drives, the self-destructiveness that manifests itself in the super-ego as the heir of both the narcissistic ego-ideal and the first identifications and object choices, and the struggle between life and death drives on a cultural level (aggression and guilt).

63 Commenting on *Beyond the Pleasure Principle* in a letter dated the 14th of January 1921, Eitingon notes that he finds the text disturbing, but agrees with Freud's "intuition of equating the death drives and ego drives" (Freud & Eitingon 2004: 229). Indeed, Freud moots this idea in the first part of Chapter 6 but then rejects it in favour of the notion of Eros as including the self-preservative drives (Freud 1920g: 53).

64 See also the following remark from a footnote added in 1921: "Our speculations have transformed this opposition [the opposition between libidinal ego and object drives, HW] into one between the life instincts (Eros) and the death instincts" (Freud 1920g: 61 n.).

65 The tendency towards a new opposition between the life drives associated with sexuality, on the one hand, and the death drives as destructive drives, on the other, in later writings leads to the conception of sadism as an intermixture of these two tendencies (Freud 1930a: 107). Sadism is then a perversion in which the sexual aim conflates with the aim of destruction. This is problematic in as far as it reflects a tendency to separate sexuality from aggression as such. Freud's affirmation of Empedocles' distinction between love (*φιλία*) and struggle (*νείκος*) is an illustration of this tendency (Freud 1937c: 246).

66 Deleuze has voiced a similar critique of Freud's persistence in a dualistic drive model, arguing that giving priority to "displaceable energy" would have allowed Freud to give priority to Eros as the source of vital differences and affirmation of life through the creation of new forms (Deleuze 2004: 137; also Somers-Hall 2017: 309–310). Instead, Deleuze and Guattari argue, Freud opted for a dualism in which the death drives seek to destroy the life drives, Eros (Deleuze & Guattari 1997: 331).

67 Ferenczi's conceptualization of trauma as discontinuity and "confusion of tongues" between child and adult implies both a return to Freud's seduction theory and a critique of the concept of death drives. Laplanche can be said to take this position as starting point for his theory of general seduction (Van Haute & Geyskens 2004).

68 Freud notices this also in his obituary of Ferenczi. In his writings from the 1920s Ferenczi "lays stress on the conservative nature of the instincts, which seek to re-establish every state of things that has been abandoned owing to an external interference" (Freud 1933c: 228).

69 In his 1926 "Das Problem der Unlustbejahung", Ferenczi argues that the death drive is not a self-destructive drive but may "accept a partial destruction of the ego" in order to secure and build "a more resilient ego" (Ferenczi 1926: 209). On trauma, fragmentation and the death drive in Ferenczi, see Soreanu (2017; 2023) and Staberg (2023).

70 On Ferenczi's return to the seduction theory, Freud writes in a letter to Anna Freud, dated 3 September 1932: "He has regressed completely to aetiological views, which I held thirty-five years ago and have abandoned, that the regular

cause of neurosis is crude sexual dreams in childhood; he uses almost the same words as I did back then" (Freud & Freud 2013: 386) Another major point of critique concerns Ferenczi's radical ideas on psychoanalytic treatment (Freud 1933c: 229). Ferenczi's late views on psychotherapy result from his theoretical perspective on the death drives as self-preservative restoration of encounters with tender care and love (compensating for inevitable traumas). On these issues, see also Van Haute and Geyskens (2004: 86–101).

71 The ultimate autoerotic pleasurable activity of "the lips kissing themselves" can then be rephrased as "the lips taking each other as object" to reproduce pleasurable sensations (Freud 1905d: 182; Van Haute & Westerink 2021: 22).

72 From his 1917 *Introductory Lectures* we know that Freud had read at least parts of Wilhelm Bölsche's *Das Liebesleben in der Natur* (1898–1903) (Freud 1916–1917a: 354). In this best-selling book, Bölsche argues that cells can be seen as individual organisms with a "body and soul" and an "ego" living together in a "state". The fusions and interactions between cells Bölsche associates with increase of excitation and sexual pleasure. In short, cells have an erotic "love-life" (Bölsche 1898; see also Willner 2024b).

73 The reference to cancer cells was introduced in the 1921 edition of the text – that is, before Freud was diagnosed with cancer in 1923.

74 This line of thought is continued in *The Ego and the Id*: "some degree of communication exists between [miteinander kommunizieren] the component instincts, that an instinct deriving from one particular erotogenic source can make over [abgeben kann] its intensity to reinforce another component instinct originating from another source" (Freud 1923b: 44). Since the life drives are "more plastic, more readily diverted and displaced" than the destructive drives, these drives have the ability to level out intensities, redistribute tensions, obviate blockages, stimulate and inhibit amounts of excitation. We should not be surprised to find references in this context to Fechner's principle of constancy describing the rhythmic intervals of rising and declining levels of drive energy within margins (Freud 1923b: 44–45, 47).

75 These ideas reflect trains of thought from *Group Psychology*. Freud mentions the limits of narcissism when it comes to sexual overvaluation (being in love) and idealization as processes in which "the object has, so to speak, consumed [aufgezehrt] the ego" (Freud 1921c: 113). In group contexts, narcissistic persons are tolerated only for as long as there is mutual advantage gained from collaboration (Freud 1921c: 102–103). Cells are seen to behave like human beings (and other multicellular organisms living in collectives) – and vice versa. And just as soldiers sacrifice their lives to save the life of others and safeguard the fatherland, cells can sacrifice their lives for the well-being of other cells and organs, and thus serve the greater good of prolongation of the life of the unit.

76 See also Grosz (2004; 2011).

77 And he adds: "In the sphere of sexual life we are brought up against peculiar, and, indeed, insoluble difficulties as soon as we try to draw a sharp line to distinguish mere variations within the range of what is physiological from pathological symptoms" (Freud 1905d: 160–161). On this issue, see also Van Haute and Westerink (2021). What Freud suggests here is that the only true pathological sexual activity would be the one in which the activity is reduced to nothing but a purified reproductive act.

78 Another example could be derived from mourning as a phenomenon placed between the poles of, on the one hand, a libido that can easily give up previous objects and move towards other objects and, on the other, a melancholic tendency in which the attachment to the lost object is continued.

79 In *The Ego and the Id*, Freud argues that the defusion of the life drives and the death drive is at the heart of a number of severe psychopathological phenomena such as persecutory paranoia and melancholia (Freud 1923b: 41ff). Normal and healthy life, in contrast, "would be a conflict and compromise between these two trends", that is, between the death drive that seeks to reduce tension and create stability, and the life drives that bring about assimilations of heterogeneous elements, thus complicating life (Freud 1923b: 41, 42ff).

80 Ferenczi's statement reflects his own reading of *Beyond the Pleasure Principle* and his inquiries into the possibilities and limits of applying the libido and trauma theory to ontogenetic and phylogenetic developments. In Thalassa and other writings, he is interested in the processes of condensation, displacement and cathexis of quantities of drive energy in physiological processes, and the "mutual relations of organs" – their interactions, cooperations, disintegrations and individualities. He shows great interest in the theory of the drives as a theory of distribution of libidinal energy in and between cells and organs, their urge to seek autoerotic pleasure, and their "unconscious" motives for transformations (Ferenczi 1924: 81–95). He is intrigued by the potential of the new drive theory to the plasticity of organs and tissues. This plasticity, he argues, cannot only be understood from a functional and expedient notion of use in processes of adaptation, but needs to be considered from an interplay of Eros and death drives, which produces new organic forms. When he remarks that Freud's theory of the life drives comes close to Bergson's *Évolution créatrice*, he is voicing his own initial intuitions on the creativity and productivity of the drives that arise in response to trauma.

81 Notably in section 61 of his *Critique of Judgement*, Kant had argued that mechanistic theories allow for explanations of contingent causations and productions of a variety of life forms, but need to be supplemented with a notion of purpose, that is, a teleological principle of design as a regulative principle or law in nature (Kant 1790).

82 Like Loeb (see Chapter 3), Driesch experimented with sea urchins and concluded that the guidance of cells towards their final form could not be reduced to chemical processes. These experiments led him to put forward the thesis of *Entelechie* (Posteraro 2022: 192–193).

83 With the notion of Entelechie as condition for development in phylogeny and ontogeny, Driesch distanced himself from Roux's developmental mechanics and from Darwinian or (neo-)Lamarckian theories that appealed to circumstantial influences (chances of reproduction and survival; specific needs and use-productions or spontaneous reactive formations to external stimuli) to explain organic variations.

84 On Bergson's *Creative Evolution*, see also Ansell-Pearson (1999; 2016), Bennett (2010: 76–81), Grosz (2011: 26–56) and Posteraro (2022).

85 The main difference between Driesch and Bergson is that for the latter the élan vital is a tendency in life, i.e., the whole of the movement of organic creation, not a principle that safeguards individual development (Bergson 1907: 103; Posteraro 2022: 195).

86 To explain the mechanism of recapitulation in ontogeny Haeckel refers to physico-chemical processes in each individual life form (Gould 1977: 78–79). In *Creative Evolution*, Bergson distances himself explicitly from the orthogenetic theories of Theodor Eimer and his ideas on individual development as organized and directed by physico-chemical processes (Bergson 1907: 86; also Bowler 2003: 247–250).

87 For these reasons, Bergson dismisses notions of hierarchy and fixed developmental stages.

88 It cannot come as a surprise that thinkers influenced by Bergson such as Gilbert Simondon or Deleuze underscore the importance of the concept of the life drives in their reflections on Freud's drive theory. In rethinking the Freudian conceptuality, they prioritize Eros as a creative force that acts from within organic substances. For Simondon, this means taking the starting point in the living being's capacity for self-creation and form-taking (Simondon 2020:184). In *Différence et repetition*, Deleuze reasons along similar lines when arguing that Freud's thought on the compulsion to repeat and to return to a previous state eclipses a more promising train of thought in the new drive theory. It is the life drives that insist on a productive repetition that cannot be defined in terms of the reappearance or confirmation of the same in reaction and opposition to modifying life-threatening forces. Deleuze adds that Freud, on various occasions, had paved the way for such notion of productive repetition, citing the case of Dora – Dora's love for her father expressed repeatedly in a variety of different libidinal investments (Deleuze 2004: 19).

89 Bergson's critique also extends to other positions, such as organicist and orthogenetic theories.

90 Henry Somers-Hall in his reading of Deleuze's critique of Freud in *Différence et répétition* writes that Freud's theory of life and death drives is in clear opposition to Bergson's view of life understood as an affirmative struggling against the entropic nature of matter. This opposition is based on the idea that Freud prioritizes the death drives as an entropic principle for life ("life aims at death"; the drives seek to return to the inanimate). However, with the introduction of the concept of the life drives, the death drives become reactive forces that work against the affirmative and creative tendencies that, in my view, are prioritized in the new drive theory. If one interprets the theory of life and death drives as correction to the idea that "life aims at death", one need no longer assume an opposition between Bergson and Freud (compare Somers-Hall 2017: 310).

91 Freud relates this characteristic of libidinal energy to the thermodynamic notion of entropy, and the gradual decline of psychical and physical plasticity in the course of a lifespan.

92 Freud writes:

> The tenacity [*Zähigkeit*] with which the libido adheres to particular trends and objects – what may be described as the 'adhesiveness' [*Klebrigkeit*] of the libido – makes its appearance as an independent factor, varying from individual to individual, whose determinants are quite unknown to us, but whose significance for the aetiology of the neuroses we shall certainly no longer underestimate.
>
> (1916–1917a: 348)

Freud goes on to suggest that such adhesiveness may be an acquired characteristic enforced upon human beings in prehistoric times. We can think here of Freud's speculations in "Overview of the Transference Neuroses" on the acquisition of character traits in the course of history and sequence of traumatic situations.

93 This allows for another argument on the question as to why Freud introduces sadism and masochism into a text in which various types of neuroses had informed metapsychological speculations. These perversions indicate a tendency towards destruction that opposes the aim of the life drives and must therefore be assigned to other drives. But they also attest to fixation and adhesiveness. It is the same fixated pleasurable sexual (autoerotic) activity that sustains both sadism and masochism. In sadism, one seeks to repeat in relation to an object an earlier fixated autoerotic (erotogenic) pleasurable sensation (Van Haute & Westerink 2021: 16, 97).

94 Freud gives credit to Jung for introducing the concept of "psychical inertia" (*psychische Trägheit*), but also criticizes Jung for limiting the concept to neurotic inhibitions (Freud 1915f: 272; 1918b: 115). In "On the History of the Psychoanalytic Movement", Freud had criticized Jung for substituting the theory of the sexual and self-preservative drives with the idea that the decisive factor in the aetiology of the neuroses consists of a conflict between a "life-task" and "psychical inertia" (Freud 1914d: 68–69). It is precisely this idea that Freud integrates into his new drive theory. On the concept of psychical inertia, see Macdonald (2024).

95 In this context, Freud also refers to phylogeny and acquired characteristics in the form of developmental paths, reaction formations and tendencies – as constitutional factors in psychic resistance.

96 Ferenczi also associates the death drives with exhaustion, albeit not in relation to the vitality of the life drives, but as the gradual abreaction of trauma, that is, of imposed external catastrophes (Ferenczi 1924: 66). In an interesting article from 1930, Antoon Westerman Holstijn interprets the death drives as entropic forces (versus the negentropic life drives) that manifest themselves in exhaustion, rigidity (*Erstarrungsprodukte*), coagulations, and inhibitions and machine-like automatisms, due to the formation of physical and psychical structures (*Strukturbildung*, versus *Plastizität*) (Westerman Holstijn 1930).

97 Gilbert Simondon, among others, has drawn attention to psychic life as the "slowing down" of processes of individuation. The psychical appears when vital forces such as affections and sensations pose problems for the living being and thus provoke interventions (in the form of perceptive-active functions) that aim to slow down and stabilize the living being (Simondon 2020: 177–178). Lyotard has also underscored the tendency towards "slowing down", stabilization and sedimentation in Freudian drive theory as "weakening of intensities" – and intensities as accumulations of energy produced by the life drives (Lyotard 2022: 37–38).

98 Similar suggestions on the concept of the death drives can be found in Moyaert (2013; 2014: 76–86).

99 Hock has argued in this direction when he writes that the death drives must be defined from an economic perspective as the "surplus" energy that cannot used by the life drives and that can be defined in terms of "waste product" and as drives that "abstain from formative processes" and in fact work contrary to these processes in a way analogous to the waste products in metabolic processes that eventually lead to the death of an organism (Hock 2000: 206–217).

100 Of course, this statement and the references to pleasurable sexual excitation in rhythmically repeated "rises and falls in the quantity of stimulus" in the 1924 text are hardly surprising when one calls to mind *Three Essays* (1905). Here Freud had reasoned that what determines the sexual character of the drive is precisely the excitation of erogenous zones, and more specifically, the rhythmic oral activity of sensual sucking. Here, too, he had given the word Lust (pleasure) the full meaning of both need and gratification, i.e., the contribution of sexual tension and the attainment of satisfaction. Remarks on the double meaning of Lust can be found in two footnotes in *Three Essays* (Freud 1905d: 135, 212; also Van Haute & Westerink 2021).

101 Philosophical critiques of Freud's drive dualism can, amongst others, be found in Deleuze (e.g., 2004: 137) and Lyotard (2022: 34, 41ff). Lyotard stresses the indiscernibility of the effects of life and death drives, and writes that the death drives can be seen as forces "slowing down" and "weakening" the "intensities" (quantities of libidinal energy) produced by the life drives.

Bibliography

Alfandary, Isabelle (2019). “Irréductible pulsion de mort?”, in eds. M. David-Ménard & B. Santos, *Pulsion de mort: Destruction et créations*. Paris: Éditions Hermann, pp. 29–44.

Alfandary, Isabelle (2021). *Science et fiction chez Freud. Quelle épistémologie pour la psychanalyse?*. Paris: Ithaque.

Allen, Amy (2021). *Critique on the Couch: Why Critical Theory Needs Psychoanalysis*. New York: Columbia University Press.

Ansell-Pearson, Keith (1999). *Germinal Life: The Difference and Repetition of Deleuze*. London: Routledge.

Ansell-Pearson, Keith (2016). “On Bergson's Reformation of Philosophy”, *Journal of French and Francophone Philosophy* 24 (2), pp. 84–105.

Assoun, Paul-Laurent (1976). *Freud, la philosophie et les philosophes*. Paris: PUF.

Assoun, Paul-Laurent (1981). *Introduction à l'épistémologie freudienne*. Paris: Payot.

Avenarius, Richard (1888). *Kritik der reinen Erfahrung*. Leipzig: Reisland.

Balibar, Étienne (2022). “Dying One's Own Death: Freud with Rilke”, *Angelaki* 27 (1), pp. 128–139.

Benjamin, Walter (1991). “Über einige Motive bei Baudelaire”, in *Gesammelte Schriften*, vol. I-2. Frankfurt: Suhrkamp, pp. 603–653.

Bennett, Jane (2010). *Vibrant Matter: A Political Ecology of Things*. Durham, NC: Duke University Press.

Bergo, Bettina (2025). *The Missed Conversation: Husserl, Freud, and Cognitive Sciences*. Oxford: Oxford University Press.

Bergson, Henri (1907). *Creative Evolution*, trans. A. Mitchell. New York: Dover, 1998.

Bernet, Rudolf (2020). *Force, Drive, Desire: A Philosophy of Psychoanalysis*. Evanston, IL: Northwestern University Press.

Binet, Alfred (1910). *The Psychic Life of Micro-Organisms*. Chicago: The Open Court Publishing Company (originally published in French in 1894).

Bölsche, Wilhelm (1898). *Das Liebesleben in der Natur. Eine Entwicklungsgeschichte der Liebe*. Leipzig: Eugen Diederichs.

Borch-Jacobsen, Mikkel (1988). *The Freudian Subject*, trans. C. Porter. Stanford, CA: Stanford University Press.

Bowler, Peter (1983). *The Eclipse of Darwinism*. Baltimore, MD: Johns Hopkins University Press.

Bowler, Peter (2003). *Evolution: The History of an Idea*. Berkeley, CA: University of California Press.

Brassier, Ray (2007). *Nihil Unbound: Enlightenment and Extinction*. London: Palgrave Macmillan.

Breuer, Joseph & Freud, Sigmund (1895d). "Studies on Hysteria", in ed. J. Strachey, The *Standard Edition of the Complete Psychological Works of Sigmund Freud*, vol. 2. London: Hogarth, 1953–1974.

Burkholz, Roland (1995). *Reflexe der Darwinismus-Debatte in der Theorie Freuds*. Stuttgart: Frommann-holzboog.

Butler, Judith (2020). *The Force of Nonviolence: An Ethico-Political Bind*. London: Verso.

Butzer, Ralph J. & Burkholz, Roland (1991). "Urvater der Eiszeit: Biologisch-evolutionäres und psycholamarckistisches Denken bei Freud", *Luzifer-Amor. Zeitschrift zur Geschichte der Psychoanalyse* 4 (8), pp. 24–49.

Caruth, Cathy (1996). *Unclaimed Experience: Trauma, Narrative, and History*. Baltimore, MD: Johns Hopkins University Press.

Churchill, Frederick B. (2015). *August Weismann: Development, Heredity, and Evolution*. Cambridge, MA: Harvard University Press.

Claus, Carl (1872). *Grundzüge der Zoologie*. Marburg: N. G. Elwert'sche Verlag.

Darwin, Charles (1859). *On the Origin of Species*, ed. G. Beer. Oxford: Oxford University Press, 2008.

Darwin, Charles (1871). *The Descent of Man and the Selection in Relation to Sex*, 2 vols, introduction by J. Tyler Bonner & R.M. May. Princeton, NJ: Princeton University Press, 1981.

Davidson, Arnold (2001). *The Emergence of Sexuality: Historical Epistemology and the Formation of Concepts*. Cambridge, MA: Harvard University Press.

Davies, J. Keith & Fichtner, Gerhard (2006). *Freud's Library: A Comprehensive Catalogue*. London: Freud Museum.

Deleuze, Gilles (1990). *The Logic of Sense*, ed. C.V. Boundas, trans. M. Lester. New York: Columbia University Press.

Deleuze, Gilles (1991). *Masochism: Coldness & Cruelty*, trans. J. McNeil. New York: Zone Books.

Deleuze, Gilles (2004). *Difference and Repetition*, trans. P. Patton. London: Continuum.

Deleuze, Gilles (2006). *Nietzsche and Philosophy*, trans. H. Tomlinson. London: Continuum.

Deleuze, Gilles (2018). *Bergsonism*. New York: Zone Books.

Deleuze, Gilles & Guattari, Félix (1997). *Anti-Oedipus: Capitalism and Schizophrenia*, trans. R. Hurley, M. Seem & H. Lane. London: Penguin.

Deleuze, Gilles & Guattari, Félix (2021). *A Thousand Plateaus*, trans. B. Massumi. London: Bloomsbury.

Derrida, Jacques (1978). *Writing and Difference*, trans. A. Bass. Chicago: University of Chicago Press.

Derrida, Jacques (1987). *The Postcard: From Socrates to Freud and Beyond*, trans. A. Bass. Chicago: University of Chicago Press.

Derrida, Jacques (2020). *Life Death*, trans. P.-A. Brault & M. Naas. Chicago: University of Chicago Press.

De Vleminck, Jens (2013). *De schaduw van Kaïn: Freuds klinische antropologie van de agressiviteit*. Leuven: Leuven University Press.

Doflein, Franz (1919). *Das Problem des Todes und der Unsterblichkeit*. Jena: Fischer.

Driesch, Hans (1905). *Der Vitalismus als Geschichte und als Lehre*. Leipzig: Verlag Johann Ambrosius Barth.

Du Bois-Reymond, Émil (1891). *Über die Grenzen des Naturerkennens: Die sieben Welträtsel*. Leipzig: Veit Verlag.

Exner, Sigmund (1894). *Entwurf zu einer physiologischen Erklärung von psychischen Erscheinungen*. Leipzig: Deuticke.

Fechner, Gustav (1873). *Einige Ideen zur Schöpfungs- und Entwicklungsgeschichte der Organismen*. Leipzig: Breitkopf und Härtel Verlag.

Fenichel, Otto (1935). "Zur Kritik des Todestriebes", in *Aufsätze*, vol. I, ed. K. Laermann. Frankfurt: Ullstein, 1985, pp. 361–371.

Ferenczi, Sándor (1913). "Entwicklungsstufen des Wirklichkeitssinnes", in *Schriften zur Psychoanalyse*, vol. 1, ed. M. Balint. Frankfurt: Fischer Verlag, 1982, pp. 148–163.

Ferenczi, Sándor (1915). "Die wissenschaftliche Bedeutung von Freuds Drei Abhandlungen zur Sexualtheorie", in *Schriften zur Psychoanalyse*, vol. 1, ed. M. Balint. Frankfurt: Fischer Verlag, 1982, pp. 206–209.

Ferenczi, Sándor (1919a). "Die Psychoanalyse der Kriegsneurosen", in S. Ferenczi, K. Abraham & E. Simmel, *Zur Psychoanalyse der Kriegsneurosen*. Vienna: Internationaler Psychoanalytischer Verlag, pp. 9–30.

Ferenczi, Sándor (1919b). "Hysterische Materialisationsphänomene", in *Schriften zur Psychoanalyse*, vol. 2, ed. M. Balint. Frankfurt: Fischer Verlag, 1982, pp. 11–24.

Ferenczi, Sándor (1922). "Die Psyche ein Hemmungsorgan", in *Schriften zur Psychoanalyse*, vol. 2, ed. M. Balint. Frankfurt: Fischer Verlag, 1982, pp. 118–121.

Ferenczi, Sándor (1924). *Thalassa: A Theory of Genitality*. New York: The Psychoanalytic Quarterly Inc, 1989.

Ferenczi, Sándor (1926). "Das Problem der Unlustbejahung", in *Schriften zur Psychoanalyse*, vol. 2, ed. M. Balint. Frankfurt: Fischer Verlag, 1982, pp. 200–211.

Ferenczi, Sándor (1929). "Das unwillkommene Kind und sein Todestrieb", in *Schriften zur Psychoanalyse*, vol. 2, ed. M. Balint. Frankfurt: Fischer Verlag, 1982, pp. 251–256.

Ferenczi, Sándor (1933). "Sprachverwirrung zwischen den Erwachsenen und dem Kind", in *Schriften zur Psychoanalyse*, vol. 2, ed. M. Balint. Frankfurt: Fischer Verlag, 1982, pp. 303–313.

Ferenczi, Sándor (1995). *The Clinical Diary*, ed. J. Dupont, trans. M. Balint & N.Z. Jackson. Cambridge, MA: Harvard University Press.

Ffytche, Matt (2022). *Sigmund Freud*. London: Reaktion.

Fischer-Homberger, Esther (1975). *Die traumatische Neurose. Vom somatischen zum sozialen Leiden*. Giessen: Psychosozial-Verlag.

Fletcher, John (2013). *Freud and the Scene of Trauma*. New York: Fordham University Press.

Fong, Benjamin (2016). *Death and Mastery: Psychoanalytic Drive Theory and the Subject of Late Capitalism*. New York: Columbia University Press.

Freud, Sigmund (1893c). "Some Points for a Comparative Study of Organic and Hysterical Motor Paralyses", in *The Standard Edition of the Complete Psychological Works of Sigmund Freud (SE)*, vol. 1, ed. J. Strachey. London: Hogarth, 1953–1974.

Freud, Sigmund (1895b). "On the Grounds for Detaching a Particular Syndrome from Neurasthenia under the Description 'Anxiety Neurosis'", in *SE*, vol. 3.

Freud, Sigmund (1896c). "The Aetiology of Hysteria", in *SE*, vol. 3.

Freud, Sigmund (1897b). "Abstracts of the Scientific Writings of Dr. Sigm. Freud", in *SE*, vol. 3.

Freud, Sigmund (1900a). "The Interpretation of Dreams", in *SE*, vols. 4–5.
Freud, Sigmund (1905d). "Three Essays on the Theory of Sexuality", in *SE*, vol. 7.
Freud, Sigmund (1905e). "Fragment of an Analysis of a Case of Hysteria", *in SE*, vol. 7.
Freud, Sigmund (1906a). "My Views on the Part Played by Sexuality in the Aetiology of the Neuroses", in *SE*, vol. 7.
Freud, Sigmund (1908c). "On the Sexual Theories of Children", in *SE*, vol. 9.
Freud, Sigmund (1909a). "Some General Remarks on Hysterical Attacks", in *SE*, vol. 9.
Freud, Sigmund (1909b). "Analysis of a Phobia in a Five-Year-Old Boy", in *SE*, vol. 10.
Freud, Sigmund (1909d). "Notes upon a Case of Obsessional Neurosis", in *SE*, vol. 10.
Freud, Sigmund (1910i). "Psychogenic Visual Disturbance According to Psychoanalytical Conceptions", in *SE*, vol. 11.
Freud, Sigmund (1911b). "Formulations on the Two Principles of Mental Functioning", in *SE*, vol. 12.
Freud, Sigmund (1911c). "Psychoanalytic Notes on an Autobiographical Account of a Case of Paranoia (Dementia Paranoides)", in *SE*, vol. 12.
Freud, Sigmund (1912–1913a). "Totem and Taboo", in *SE*, vol. 13.
Freud, Sigmund (1913d). "Dreams in Folklore", in *SE*, vol. 12.
Freud, Sigmund (1913j). "The Claims of Psychoanalysis to Scientific Interest", in *SE*, vol. 13.
Freud, Sigmund (1914b). "The Moses of Michelangelo", in *SE*, vol. 13.
Freud, Sigmund (1914c). "On Narcissism: An Introduction", in *SE*, vol. 12.
Freud, Sigmund (1914d). 'On the History of the Psycho-Analytic Movement", in *SE*, vol. 14.
Freud, Sigmund (1914g). "Remembering, Repeating and Working-Through", in *SE*, vol. 12.
Freud, Sigmund (1915b). 'Thoughts for the Times on War and Death", in *SE*, vol. 14.
Freud, Sigmund (1915c). "Instincts and their Vicissitudes", in *SE*, vol. 14.
Freud, Sigmund (1915d). "Repression", in *SE*, vol. 14.
Freud, Sigmund (1915e). "The Unconscious", in *SE*, vol. 14.
Freud, Sigmund (1915f). "A Case of Paranoia Running Counter to the Psychoanalytic Theory of the Disease", in *SE*, vol. 14.
Freud, Sigmund (1916a). "On Transience", in *SE*, vol. 14.
Freud, Sigmund (1916–1917a). "Introductory Lectures on Psycho-Analysis", in *SE*, vols. 15–16.
Freud, Sigmund (1917a). "A Difficulty in Psycho-Analysis", in *SE*, vol. 17.
Freud, Sigmund (1917d). "A Metapsychological Supplement to the Theory of Dreams", in *SE*, vol. 14.
Freud, Sigmund (1917e). "Mourning and Melancholia", in *SE*, vol. 14.
Freud, Sigmund (1918b). "From the History of an Infantile Neurosis", in *SE*, vol. 17.
Freud, Sigmund (1919a). "Lines of Advance in Psychoanalytic Therapy", in *SE*, vol. 17.
Freud, Sigmund (1919d). "Introduction to Psychoanalysis and the War Neuroses", in *SE*, vol. 17.
Freud, Sigmund (1919e). "A Child Is Being Beaten", in *SE*, vol. 17.
Freud, Sigmund (1919h). "The Uncanny", in *SE*, vol. 17.
Freud, Sigmund (1920a). "The Psychogenesis of a Case of Homosexuality in a Woman", in *SE*, vol. 18.
Freud, Sigmund (1920g). "Beyond the Pleasure Principle", in *SE*, vol. 18.
Freud, Sigmund (1921c). "Group Psychology and the Analysis of the Ego", in *SE*, vol. 18.

Freud, Sigmund (1923a). "Two Encyclopedia Articles: Psycho-Analysis and The Libido Theory", in *SE*, vol. 18.
Freud, Sigmund (1923b). "The Ego and the Id", in *SE*, vol. 19.
Freud, Sigmund (1924c). "The Economic Problem of Masochism", in *SE*, vol. 19.
Freud, Sigmund (1924d). "The Dissolution of the Oedipus Complex", in *SE*, vol. 19.
Freud, Sigmund (1924f). "Short Account of Psycho-Analysis", in *SE*, vol. 19.
Freud, Sigmund (1925a). "A Note upon the 'Mystic Writing-Pad'", in *SE*, vol. 19.
Freud, Sigmund (1925d). "An Autobiographical Study", in *SE*, vol. 20.
Freud, Sigmund (1926d). "*Inhibitions, Symptoms, and Anxiety*", in *SE*, vol. 20.
Freud, Sigmund (1926g). "Freud and Ewald Hering (Appendix A to 'The Unconscious')", in *SE*, vol. 14.
Freud, Sigmund (1928b). "Dostoevsky and Parricide", in *SE*, vol. 21.
Freud, Sigmund (1930a). "Civilization and Its Discontents", in *SE*, vol. 21.
Freud, Sigmund (1933a). "New Introductory Lectures on Psycho-Analysis", in *SE*, vol. 22.
Freud, Sigmund (1933b). "Why War?", in *SE*, vol. 22.
Freud, Sigmund (1933c). "Sándor Ferenczi", in *SE*, vol. 22.
Freud, Sigmund (1937c). "Analysis Terminable and Interminable", in *SE*, vol. 23.
Freud, Sigmund (1939a). "Moses and Monotheism", in *SE*, vol. 23.
Freud, Sigmund (1940a). "An Outline of Psycho-Analysis", in *SE*, vol. 23.
Freud, Sigmund (1940d). "On the Theory of Hysterical Attacks", in *SE*, vol. 1.
Freud, Sigmund (1950c). "Project for a Scientific Psychology", in *SE*, vol. 1, 1895.
Freud, Sigmund (1955c). "Memorandum on the Electrical Treatment", in *SE*, vol. 17.
Freud, Sigmund (1969–1975). *Studienausgabe*, vols 1–10, eds. I. Grubrich-Simitis, A. Mitscherlich, A. Richards and J. Strachey. Frankfurt: Fischer.
Freud, Sigmund (1985a). *A Phylogenetic Fantasy: Overview of the Transference Neuroses*, ed. I. Grubrich-Simitis. Cambridge, MA: The Belknap Press of Harvard University Press.
Freud, Sigmund (1985c). *The Complete Letters of Sigmund Freud to Wilhelm Fliess 1887–1904*, ed. J.M. Masson. Cambridge, MA: The Belknap Press of Harvard University Press.
Freud, Sigmund (2013). "Jenseits des Lustprinzips: Kritische Edition", *Luzifer-Amor. Zeitschrift zur Geschichte der Psychoanalyse* 26 (51), pp. 10–91.
Freud, Sigmund (2016). *Three Essays on the Theory of Sexuality*, ed. and introduction by Ph. Van Haute & H. Westerink, trans. U. Kistner. London: Verso.
Freud, Sigmund (2024). "Beyond the Pleasure Principle", in eds H. Westerink, J. Willner & Ph. Van Haute, *Towards the Limits of Freudian Thinking: Critical Edition and Readings of Beyond the Pleasure Principle*. Leuven: Leuven University Press, pp. 29–80.
Freud, Sigmund & Abraham, Karl (2002). *The Complete Correspondence 1907–1925*, ed. E. Falzeder. New York: Routledge.
Freud, Sigmund & Andreas-Salomé, Lou (1972). *Letters*, ed. E. Pfeiffer. New York: Harcourt Brace Jovanovich.
Freud, Sigmund & Eitingon, Max (2004). *Briefwechsel 1906–1939*, vol. 1, ed. M. Schröter. Tübingen: Edition Diskord.
Freud, Sigmund & Ferenczi, Sándor (1996a). *The Correspondence* , vol. 2: *1914–1919*, eds. E. Falzeder, E. Brabant & P. Giampieri-Deutsch. Cambridge, MA: The Belknap Press of Harvard University Press.

Freud, Sigmund & Ferenczi, Sándor (1996b). *The Correspondence*, vol. 3: *1920–1933*, eds. E. Falzeder, E. Brabant & P. Giampieri-Deutsch. Cambridge, MA: The Belknap Press of Harvard University Press.

Freud, Sigmund & Freud, Anna (2013). *Correspondence, 1904–1938*, trans. N. Somers. Cambridge: Polity.

Freud, Sigmund & Jones, Ernest (1993). *The Complete Correspondence, 1908–1939*, ed. R.A. Paskauskas. Cambridge, MA: The Belknap Press of Harvard University Press.

Freud, Sigmund & Pfister, Oskar (1963). *Psychoanalysis and Faith: The Letters of Sigmund Freud and Oskar Pfister*, eds. E.L. Freud & H. Meng. New York: Basic Books.

Fulgencio, Leopoldo (2005). "Freud's Metapsychological Speculations", *International Journal of Psychoanalysis* 86, pp. 99–123.

Geyskens, Tomas (2005). *Our Original Scenes: Freud's Theory of Sexuality*. Leuven: Leuven University Press.

Gilbert, Scott F. & Sarkar, Sahotra (2000). "Embracing Complexity: Organicism for the 21st Century", *Developmental Dynamics* 219 (1), pp. 1–9.

Gödde, Günther (1999). *Traditionslinien des "Unbewussten": Schopenhauer – Nietzsche – Freud*. Tübingen: Edition Diskord.

Godley, James A. (2018). "Inheritance in Psychoanalysis", in eds. J. Goldbach & J.A. Godley, *Inheritance in Psychoanalysis*. Albany, NY: SUNY, pp. 255–273.

Gould, Stephen Jay (1977). *Ontogeny and Phylogeny*. Cambridge, MA: The Belknap Press of Harvard University Press.

Green, André (1999). *The Work of the Negative*, trans. A. Weller. London: Free Association Books.

Grosz, Elizabeth (2004). *The Nick of Time: Politics, Evolution, and the Untimely*. Durham, NC: Duke University Press.

Grosz, Elizabeth (2011). *Becoming Undone: Darwinian Reflections on Life, Politics, and Art*. Durham, NC: Duke University Press.

Grubrich-Simitis, Ilse (1985). "Metapsychology and Metabiology", in S. Freud, *A Phylogenetic Fantasy: Overview of the Transference Neuroses*, ed. I. Grubrich-Simitis. Cambridge, MA: The Belknap Press of Harvard University Press, pp. 73–107.

Grubrich-Simitis, Ilse (1993). *Back to Freud's Texts: Making Silent Documents Speak*, trans. Ph. Slotkin. New Haven, CT: Yale University Press.

Grubrich-Simitis, Ilse (2007). "Trauma oder Trieb – Trieb oder Trauma: Wiederbetrachtet", *Psyche. Zeitschrift für Psychoanalyse und ihre Anwendungen* 61 (7), pp. 637–656.

Haeckel, Ernst (1866). *Generelle Morphologie der Organismen: Allgemeine Grundzüge der organischen Formen-Wissenschaft, mechanisch begründet durch die von Charles Darwin reformirte Descendenz-Theorie*. 2 vols. Berlin: Georg Reimer Verlag.

Haraway, Donna J. (1976). *Crystals, Fabrics, and Fields: Metaphors of Organicism in Twentieth-Century Developmental Biology*. New Haven, CT: Yale University Press.

Harrington, Ralph (2010). "The Railway Accident: Trains, Trauma and Technological Crises in Nineteenth-Century Britain", in eds. M. Micale & P. Lerner, *Traumatic Pasts: History, Psychiatry and the Trauma in the Modern Age, 1870–1930*. Cambridge: Cambridge University Press, pp. 31–56.

Hartmann, Max (1906). *Tod und Fortpflanzung*. Munich: Ernst Reinhardt.

Helmholtz, Hermannvon (1847). *Über die Erhaltung der Kraft*. Leipzig: Verlag W. Engelmann.

Hering, Ewald (1870). "On Memory", in S. Butler, *Unconscious Memory.* London: A. C. Fifield, 1910, pp. 63–86.

Hering, Ewald (1878). *Zur Lehre vom Lichtsinn.* Vienna: Carl Gerold's Sohn.

Hock, Udo (2000). *Das Unbewußte Denken. Wiederholung und Todestrieb.* Frankfurt: Fischer.

Hock, Udo & Scarfone, Dominique (2024). "An Introduction to Revisiting Freud's 'Remembering, Repeating, and Working-Through'", in eds. U. Hock & D. Scarfone, *On Freud's "Remembering, Repeating, and Working-Through".* New York: Routledge, pp. 1–13.

Holt, Robert R. (1962). "A Critical Examination of Freud's Concept of Bound versus Free Cathexis", in *Freud Reappraised: A Fresh Look at Psychoanalytic Theory.* New York: Guildford Press, pp. 71–113.

Holt, Robert R. (1967). "Beyond Vitalism and Mechanism: Freud's Concept of Psychic Energy", in *Freud Reappraised: A Fresh Look at Psychoanalytic Theory.* New York: Guildford Press, pp. 141–168.

Hume, David (1777). *A Treatise of Human Nature*, eds. D.F. Norton and M.J. Norton. Oxford: Oxford University Press, 2011.

Ingala, Emma (2020). "Freud's Trope of the 'Beyond': On Conditions, Critique, and Violence", *Psychoanalysis, Culture & Society* 25, pp. 576–593.

Janet, Pierre (1919). *Les médications psychologiques*, vol. II: *Les économies psychologiques.* Paris: Félix Alcan.

Johnston, Adrian (2005). *Time Driven: Metapsychology and the Splitting of the Drive.* Evanston, IL: Northwestern University Press.

Jones, Ernest (1919). "Die Kriegsneurosen und die Freudsche Theorie", in S. Ferenczi, K. Abraham & E. Simmel, *Zur Psychoanalyse der Kriegsneurosen.* Vienna: Internationaler Psychoanalytischer Verlag, pp. 61–82.

Jones, Ernest (1957). *The Life and Work of Sigmund Freud*, vol. 3: *The Last Phase, 1919–1939.* New York: Basic Books.

Jung, Carl Gustav (1912). *Wandlungen und Symbole der Libido. Beiträge zur Entwicklungsgeschichte des Denkens.* Munich: DTV, 1991.

Kant, Immanuel (1987). *Critique of Judgement*, trans. and introduction by W.S. Pruhar. Indianapolis, IN: Hacket Publishing (originally published in 1790).

Kant, Immanuel (2004). *Metaphysical Foundations of Natural Science.* Cambridge: Cambridge University Press (originally published in 1786).

Kant, Immanuel (2007). *Critique of Pure Reason*, introduction by H. Caygill, trans. N. Kemp Smith. London: Palgrave Macmillan (originally published in 1788).

Kisner, Manja & Noller, Jörg (eds.) (2021). *The Concept of Drive in Classical German Philosophy: Between Biology, Anthropology, and Metaphysics.* Cham: Palgrave Macmillan.

Kistner, Ulrike (2024). "Traumatic Neuroses and Psychoneuroses in (and) Beyond the Pleasure Principle", in eds. H. Westerink, J. Willner & Ph. Van Haute, *Towards the Limits of Freudian Thinking: Critical Edition and Readings of Beyond the Pleasure Principle.* Leuven: Leuven University Press, pp. 197–224.

Kitcher, Patricia (1992). *Freud's Dream: A Complete Interdisciplinary Science of Mind.* Cambridge, MA: MIT Press.

Kleeberg, Bernhard (2005). *Theophysis. Ernst Haeckel's Philosophie des Naturganzen.* Cologne: Böhlau.

Klein, Melanie (1933). "The Early Development of Conscience in the Child", in *Love, Guilt and Reparation and Other Works, 1921–1945*, ed. H. Segal. London: Vintage, pp. 248–257.

Klein, Melanie (1946). "Notes on Some Schizoid Mechanisms", in *Envy and Gratitude and Other Works, 1946–1963*, ed. H. Segal. London: Vintage, pp. 1–24.

Lacan, Jacques (1988). *The Seminar of Jacques Lacan, Book I: Freud's Papers on Technique 1953–1954*, ed. J.-A. Miller, trans. J. Forrester. Cambridge: Cambridge University Press.

Lacan, Jacques (1991). *The Ego in Freud's Theory and in the Technique of Psychoanalysis 1954–1955. Seminar Book II*, ed. J.-A. Miller, trans. S. Tomaselli. New York: Norton.

Lacan, Jacques (1992). *The Ethics of Psychoanalysis: Seminar Book VII*, trans. D. Porter. New York: Routledge.

Lacan, Jacques (1998). *The Four Fundamental Concepts of Psycho-Analysis*, ed. J.-A. Miller, trans. A. Sheridan, introduction by D. Macey. London: Vintage.

Lacan, Jacques (2004). *Anxiety: Seminar Book X*, ed. J.-A. Miller. Cambridge: Polity.

Lacan, Jacques (2006). *Écrits*, trans. B. Fink. New York: Norton.

Lacan, Jacques (2007). *The Other Side of Psychoanalysis: Seminar Book XVII*, trans. R. Grigg. New York: Norton.

Lacan, Jacques (2019). *Desire and Its Interpretation: The Seminar of Jacques Lacan, Book VI*, ed. J.-A. Miller, trans. B. Fink. Cambridge: Polity Press.

Lamarck, Jean-Baptiste (1910). *Zoologische Philosophie*. Leipzig: Alfred Kröner Verlag.

Laplanche, Jean (1980). *La sublimation*. Paris: Presses universitaires de France.

Laplanche, Jacques (1985). *Life and Death in Psychoanalysis*, introduction by J. Mehlman. Baltimore, MD: Johns Hopkins University Press.

Laplanche, Jean (1989). *New Foundations for Psychoanalysis*, trans. D. Macey. Oxford: Basil Blackwell.

Laplanche, Jean (1999). *Essays on Otherness*, ed. J. Fletcher. London: Routledge.

Laplanche, Jean (2015a). *Between Seduction and Inspiration: Man*, introduction by J. Mehlman. New York: The Unconscious in Translation.

Laplanche, Jean (2015b). *The Temptation of Biology: Freud's Theories of Sexuality*, trans. D. Nicholson-Smith. New York: The Unconscious in Translation.

Laplanche, Jean & Pontalis, Jean-Bertrand (1973). *The Language of Psychoanalysis*. New York: Norton.

Leader, Darian (2021). *Jouissance: Sexuality, Suffering and Satisfaction*. London: Polity.

Lear, Jonathan (2000). *Happiness, Death, and the Remainder of Life*. Cambridge, MA: Harvard University Press.

Lear, Jonathan (2005). *Freud*. New York: Routledge.

Lear, Jonathan (2022). *Imagining the End: Mourning and Ethical Life*. Cambridge, MA: Harvard University Press.

Lerner, Paul (2010). "From Traumatic Neurosis to Male Hysteria: The Rise and Fall of Herman Oppenheim, 1889–1919", in eds. M. Micale & P. Lerner, *Traumatic Pasts: History, Psychiatry and the Trauma in the Modern Age, 1870–1930*. Cambridge: Cambridge University Press, pp. 140–170.

Lipps, Theodor (1883). *Grundtatsachen des Seelenlebens*. Bonn: Max Cohen & Sohn.

Lipps, Theodor (1898). *Komik und Humor: Eine psychologisch-ästhetische Untersuchung*. Hamburg: Leopold Voss.

Lipschütz, Alexander (1914). *Warum wir sterben.* Stuttgart: Franckh'sche Verlagshandlung.

Lipschütz, Alexander (1919). *Die Pubertätsdrüse und ihre Wirkungen.* Bern: Bircher.

Loewald, Hans (1980). "On Motivation and Instinct Theory", in *Papers on Psychoanalysis.* New Haven, CT: Yale University Press, pp. 102–137.

Low, Barbara (1920). *Psycho-Analysis: A Brief Account of Freudian Theory.* London: George Allen & Unwin.

Lyotard, Jean-François (2022). *Libidinal Economy,* trans. I.H. Grant. London: Bloomsbury.

Macdonald, Molly (2024). "Psychical Inertia: Origins and Transformations", *Psychoanalysis and History* 26 (1), pp. 29–54.

Mach, Ernst (1886). *Beiträge zur Analyse der Empfindungen.* Jena: Gustav Fischer.

Malabou, Catherine (2012). *The New Wounded: From Neurosis to Brain Damage.* New York: Fordham University Press.

Malabou, Catherine (2022). *Plasticity: The Promise of Explosion.* Edinburgh: Edinburgh University Press.

Marcuse, Herbert (1955). *Eros and Civilization: A Philosophical Inquiry into Freud.* New York: Routledge, 2023.

Margulis, Lynn & Sagan, Dorion (1986). *Origins of Sex: Three Billion Years of Genetic Recombination.* New Haven, CT: Yale University Press.

Martínez Ruiz, Rosaura (2020). "Collective Working-Through of Trauma or Psychoanalysis as a Political Strategy", *Psychoanalysis, Culture and Society* 25 (4), pp. 594–611.

May, Ulrike (2017). "'Lieben heißt Sterbenwollen. Das Steht felsenfest in mir': Der Todestrieb im Briefwechsel zwischen Freud und August Stärcke", *Luzifer-Amor* 30 (59), pp. 89–120.

May, Ulrike (2023). *Der Abschied vom Primat des Sexuellen. Zum Wandel der Psychoanalyse in Berlin und London zwischen 1920 und 1925.* Gießen: Psychosozial-Verlag.

May, Ulrike (2024). "The Third Step in Drive Theory: On the Genesis of Beyond the Pleasure Principle", in eds. H. Westerink, J. Willner & Ph. Van Haute, *Towards the Limits of Freudian Thinking: Critical Edition and Readings of Beyond the Pleasure Principle.* Leuven: Leuven University Press, pp. 81–164.

May, Ulrike (2025). "Sexual Drives, Eros, and Identification – A Re-reading of Freud's *Group Psychology and the Analysis of the Ego*", in eds. D. Finzi & J. Wolff Bernstein, *Thoughts for the Times on Groups and Masses: A Sigmund Freud Museum Symposium.* Leuven: Leuven University Press, pp. 21–32.

Micale, Mark S. (1995). *Approaching Hysteria: Disease and Its Interpretation.* Princeton, NJ: Princeton University Press.

Micale, Mark S. & Lerner, Paul (eds.) (2010). *Traumatic Pasts: History, Psychiatry and Trauma in the Modern Age, 1870–1930.* Cambridge: Cambridge University Press.

Moyaert, Paul (2013). "The Death Drive and the Nucleus of the Ego: An Introduction to Freudian Metaphysics", *The Southern Journal of Philosophy* 51, pp. 94–119.

Moyaert, Paul (2014). *Opboksen tegen het inerte. De doodsdrift bij Freud.* Nijmegen: Vantilt.

Moyaert, Paul (2022). *De doodsdrift revisited: Een breuklijn tussen Freud en Deleuze,* Amsterdam: Boom.

Müller, Johannes (1834). *Handbuch der Physiologie des Menschen.* Koblenz: J. Hölscher.

Nachmansohn, Max (1915). "Freuds Libidotheorie verglichen mit der Eroslehre Platos", *Internationale Zeitschrift für ärztliche Psychoanalyse* 3 (2), pp. 65–83.

Nietzsche, Friedrich (1882). "Die fröhliche Wissenschaft", in *Werke. Kritische Gesamtausgabe*, vol. 3, eds. G. Colli & M. Montinari. Berlin: De Gruyter, 1999, pp. 343–651.

Nietzsche, Friedrich (1887). "Also sprach Zarathustra", in *Werke. Kritische Gesamtausgabe*, vol. 4, eds. G. Colli & M. Montinari. Berlin: De Gruyter, 1999.

Nietzsche, Friedrich (1901). *The Will to Power*, ed. W. Kaufmann. New York: Vintage Books, 1968.

Oppenheim, Hermann (1915). *Der Krieg und die traumatischen Neurosen*. Berlin: Springer.

Ostwald, Wilhelm (1902). *Vorlesungen über Naturphilosophie*. Leipzig: Veit & Comp.

Pauly, August (1905). *Darwinismus und Lamarckismus*. Munich: Ernst Reinhardt Verlagshandlung.

Penot, Bernard (2016). "The So-Called Death Drive, an Indispensable Force for Any Subjective Life", *International Journal of Psychoanalysis* 98, pp. 299–321.

Posteraro, Tano (2022). *Bergson's Philosophy of Biology: Virtuality, Tendency and Time*. Edinburgh: Edinburgh University Press.

Rank, Otto (1924). *The Trauma of Birth*. London: Kegan Paul.

Richards, Robert J. (2008). *The Tragic Sense of Life: Ernst Haeckel and the Struggle for Evolutionary Thought*. Chicago: University of Chicago Press.

Ricoeur, Paul (1970). *Freud and Philosophy: An Essay on Interpretation*, trans. D. Savage. New Haven, CT: Yale University Press.

Ritvo, Lucille B. (1990). *Darwin's Influence on Freud: A Tale of Two Sciences*. New Haven, CT: Yale University Press.

Rose, Jacqueline (2021). *Den eigenen Tod sterben. Denken mit Freud in Zeiten der Pandemie. Sigmund Freud Vorlesung 2020*. Vienna: Turia & Kant.

Roux, Wilhelm (1881). *Der Kampf der Theile im Organismus*. Leipzig: Wilhelm Engelmann.

Schloegel, Judy J. & Schmidgen, Henning (2002). "General Physiology, Experimental Psychology, and Evolutionism: Unicellular Organisms as Objects of Psychophysiological Research, 1877–1918", *Isis* 93 (4), pp. 614–645.

Schopenhauer, Arthur (1854). *Über den Willen in der Natur*. Frankfurt: Joh. Chr. Hermann'sche Buchhandlung.

Schotte, Jacques (1990). *Szondi avec Freud: Sur la voie d'une psychiatrie pulsionelle*. Brussels: Éditions De Boeck.

Schrödinger, Erwin (2020) *What Is Life? The Physical Aspect of the Living Cell*. Cambridge: Cambridge University Press.

Schröter, Michael (2023). *Auf eigenem Weg. Geschichte der Psychoanalyse in Deutschland bis 1945*. Göttingen: Vandenhoeck & Ruprecht.

Schuster, Aaron (2016). *The Trouble with Pleasure: Deleuze and Psychoanalysis*. Cambridge, MA: MIT Press.

Seeck, Andreas (2021). "Bahnfahrt mit Maxwell – Sigmund Freud und der Energieerhaltungssatz der Physik", *Luzifer-Amor* 34 (67). pp. 92–174.

Semon, Richard (1908). *Die Mneme als erhaltendes Prinzip im Wechsel des organischen Geschehens*. Leipzig: Verlag Engelmann.

Silveira, Lea (2013). "Phylogenetic Schema and Transcendental Field: The Problem of the Universal Character of Fantasy in Freud and Lacan". Paper presented at the conference of the International Society of Psychoanalysis and Philosophy, Nijmegen/Gent.

Simanke, Richard Theisen (2020). "Um reino de possibilidades ilimitadas: as referências biológicas de Freud em 'Além do princípio do prazer'", in ed. G. Iannini, *Sigmund Freud: Além do princípio de prazer. Edição crítica bilíngue*. Belo Horizonte: Editora Autêntica, pp. 369–442 (English translation through private correspondence).

Simondon, Gilbert (2020). *Individuation in Light of Notions of Form and Information*, trans. T. Adkins. Minneapolis, MN: University of Minnesota Press.

Somers-Hall, Henry (2017). "Deleuze, Freud and the Three Syntheses", *Deleuze and Guattari Studies* 11 (3), pp. 297–327.

Soreanu, Raluca (2017). "Something Was Lost in Freud's *Beyond the Pleasure Principle*: A Ferenczian Reading", *American Journal of Psychoanalysis* 77 (3), pp. 223–238.

Soreanu, Raluca (2023). "Catastrophe and the Creativity of Fragments: Towards a Phenomenology of the Scene of Trauma", in eds. R. Soreanu, J. Staberg & J. Willner, *Ferenczi Dialogues: On Trauma and Catastrophe*. Leuven: Leuven University Press, pp. 145–192.

Spielrein, Sabina (1912). "Die Destruktion als Ursache der Werdens", in *Sämtliche Schriften*. Freiburg: Traute Hensch Verlag.

Staberg, Jakob (2023). "Instead of Language: Confusion", in eds. R. Soreanu, J. Staberg & J. Willner, *Ferenczi Dialogues: On Trauma and Catastrophe*. Leuven: Leuven University Press, pp. 23–72.

Stärcke, August (1914). "Inleiding", in S. Freud, *De sexueele beschavings-moraal als oorzaak der moderne zenuwzwakte*. Baarn: Hollandia, pp. 2–8.

Steinach, Eugen (1920). *Verjüngung durch experimentelle Neubelebung der alternden Pubertätsdrüse*. Berlin: Julius Springer.

Sulloway, Frank J. (1979). *Freud: Biologist of the Mind*. New York: Basic Books.

Tran The, Jessica, Ansermet, Jean-Philippe, Magistretti, Pierre & Ansermet, François (2020). "From the Principle of Inertia to the Death Drive: The Influence of the Second Law of Thermodynamics on the Freudian Theory of Psychical Apparatus", *Frontiers in Psychology* 11.

Trotter, Wilfred (1916). *Instincts of the Herd in Peace and War*. London: Oxford University Press, 1953.

Van der Kolk, Bessel & Van der Hart, Onno (1995). "The Intrusive Past: The Flexibility of Memory and the Engraving of Trauma", in ed. C. Caruth, *Trauma: Explorations in Memory*. Baltimore, MD: Johns Hopkins University Press.

Vandermeersch, Patrick (1991). *Unresolved Questions in the Freud-Jung Debate on Psychosis, Sexual Identity and Religion*. Leuven: Leuven University Press.

Van de Vijver, Gertrudis, VanSpeybroeck, Linda & Vandevyvere, Windy (2005). "Reflecting on the Complexity of Biological Systems: Kant and Beyond?", *Acta Biotheoretica* 51 (2), pp. 101–140.

Van Haute, Philippe & Geyskens, Tomas (2004). *Confusion of Tongues: The Primacy of Sexuality in Freud, Ferenczi and Laplanche*. New York: Other Press.

Van Haute, Philippe & Geyskens, Tomas (2007). *From Death Instinct to Attachment Theory: The Primacy of the Child in Freud, Klein and Hermann*. New York: Other Press.

Van Haute, Philippe & Geyskens, Tomas (2012). *A Non-Oedipal Psychoanalysis? A Clinical Anthropology of Hysteria in the Works of Freud and Lacan*. Leuven: Leuven University Press.

Van Haute, Philippe & Geyskens, Tomas (2013). "Woede, wellust en weifelzucht: Een freudiaanse symptomatologie van de dwangneurose", in eds. Ph. Van Haute & J.De Vleminck, *Freud als filosoof. Over seksualiteit, psychopathologie en cultuur.* Kalmthout: Pelckmans, pp. 117–129.

Van Haute, Philippe & Westerink, Herman (2021). *From Pleasure to the Object: Reading Freud's Three Essays on the Theory of Sexuality.* London: Routledge.

Von Felszeghy, Bela (1920). "Panik und Pan-Komplex", *Imago* 6 (1), pp. 1–40.

Wagner, Adolf (1909). *Geschichte des Lamarckismus.* Stuttgart: Franckh'sche Verlagshandlung.

Weismann, August (1882). *Über die Dauer des Lebens.* Jena: Gustav Fischer Verlag.

Weismann, August (1884). *Über Leben und Tod. Eine biologische Untersuchung.* Jena: Gustav Fischer Verlag.

Weismann, August (1886). *Die Bedeutung der sexuellen Fortpflanzung für die Selektions-Theorie.* Jena: Gustav Fischer Verlag.

Weismann, August (1892). *Das Keimplasma. Eine Theorie der Vererbung.* Jena: Gustav Fischer Verlag.

Westerink, Herman (2009). *A Dark Trace: Sigmund Freud on the Sense of Guilt.* Leuven: Leuven University Press.

Westerink, Herman (2015). "De problematische plaats van de woede in het denken van Freud over agressiviteit", *Tijdschrift voor Filosofie* 77 (4), pp. 719–746.

Westerink, Herman (2020). "Pathoanalysis of Existence and the Study of Religion: An Unfinished Freudian Project", *Psychoanalytic Quarterly* 89 (3), pp. 583–611.

Westerink, Herman & Van Haute, Philippe (2025). *Seduction, Drive and Repetition: Freud's Metaphysics of Trauma.* Leuven: Leuven University Press.

Westerman Holstijn, Antoon (1930). "Tendenzen des Toten, Todestriebe und Triebe zum Töten", *Imago: Zeitschrift für Anwendung der Psychoanalyse auf die Natur- und Geisteswissenschaft* 16 (3–4), pp. 207–231.

Willner, Jenny (2022). "The Problem of Heredity: Ferenczi's Organology and the Politics of Bioanalysis", *Psychoanalysis and History* 24 (2), pp. 205–218.

Willner, Jenny (2023). "Catastrophe and Genitality: Ferenczi's *Thalassa* and the Politics of Bioanalysis", in eds. R. Soreanu, J. Staberg & J. Willner, *Ferenczi Dialogues: On Trauma and Catastrophe.* Leuven: Leuven University Press, pp. 91–130.

Willner, Jenny (2024a). "Neurotic Evolution: Bioanalysis against Biologism in *Beyond the Pleasure Principle*", in eds. H. Westerink, J. Willner & Ph. Van Haute, *Towards the Limits of Freudian Thinking: Critical Edition and Readings of Beyond the Pleasure Principle.* Leuven: Leuven University Press, pp. 225–256.

Willner, Jenny (2024b). "Unbehagen am Erbe: Psychoanalyse, Biologie und Neurologie bei Freud und Ferenczi", professorial dissertation, Munich (to be published by Wallstein Verlag, Göttingen).

Wilson, Elizabeth A. (2004). *Psychosomatic: Feminism and the Neurological Body.* Durham, NC: Duke University Press.

Wilson, Elizabeth A. (2015). *Gut Feminism.* Durham, NC: Duke University Press.

Žižek, Slavoj (2004). *Organs Without Bodies: On Deleuze and Consequences.* New York: Routledge.

Zupančič, Alenka (2017). *What Is Sex?.* Cambridge, MA: MIT Press.

Index

For Product Safety Concerns and Information please contact our
EU representative GPSR@taylorandfrancis.com Taylor & Francis
Verlag GmbH, Kaufingerstraße 24, 80331 München, Germany